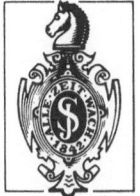

H.A. Bird · Patricia le Gallez
Jacqueline Hill

Combined Care
of the Rheumatic
Patient

Foreword by Verna Wright

With 64 Figures

Springer-Verlag
Berlin Heidelberg New York Tokyo
1985

H. A. Bird, MD, MRCP, Senior Lecturer in Rheumatology, Rheumatism Research Unit, University of Leeds, and Honorary Consultant Rheumatologist, General Infirmary at Leeds and Royal Bath Hospital, Harrogate.

Patricia le Gallez, SRN, Clinical Metrologist, Rheumatism Research Unit, University of Leeds, and Honorary Nursing Sister, Royal Bath Hospital, Harrogate.

Jacqueline Hill, SRN, Clinical Metrologist, Rheumatism Research Unit, University of Leeds, and Honorary Nursing Sister, Royal Bath Hospital, Harrogate.

Library of Congress Cataloging in Publication Data
Bird, H.A. (Howard Anthony), 1945—
Combined Care of the rheumatic patient.
Includes bibliographies and index. 1. Rheumatism—Treatment.
2. Rheumatism—Nursing. 3. Arthritics—Rehabilitation. I. le Gallez, Patricia,
1938—. II. Hill, Jacqueline, 1946—. III. Title. [DNLM: 1. Rheumatism.
2. Rheumatism—nursing. WE 544 B6185c] RC927. B54   1985   616.7'23
84—23618
ISBN-13: 978-3-540-13557-9   e-ISBN-13: 978-1-4471-1365-2
DOI: 10.1007/978-1-4471-1365-2

Product Liability: The publisher can give no guarantee for information about drug dosage and application thereof contained in this book. In every individual case the respective user must check its accuracy by consulting other pharmaceutical literature.

Filmset by Polyglot Pte Ltd, 10 Dundee Road, Singapore 0314.

2128/3916-543210

We dedicate this book to our respective spouses, Anne, Geoffrey and Jeff, who showed outstanding tolerance throughout the writing of this book and to whom we extend our grateful thanks.

Foreword

Gone are the days when the physician could act as God, the orthopaedic surgeon as the Lord God and the nurses as ministering angels. The concept of a team approach with each discipline supplying special yet overlapping skills is accepted in principle, although not always in practice. Physiotherapists and occupational therapists resist integration of their training among the hierarchy; however, on the ground, these remedial therapists often do each other's jobs with remarkable amity. Elsewhere I have discussed whether we need multipurpose professionals or multiprofessional persons (Wright 1982).

At Leeds the close collaboration that exists between rheumatologists and non-medically qualified professionals has resulted in a productive Bioengineering Group for the Study of Human Joints, a Clinical Pharmacology Unit of international renown and a Rehabilitation Unit that consistently produces bricks without straw. One aspect of this combined approach to patient care has been the development of the discipline of clinical nurse metrology (Bird et al. 1980). Skilled nursing sisters have worked in this capacity for a decade in Leeds. Their contribution has not only enhanced the reliability of the results of clinical trials in which they have been engaged, but it has been highly cost effective and greatly appreciated by patients. It has also measurably improved our patient education programme. Moreover, the posts have provided considerable job satisfaction.

This book arises from the expertise gained during these pioneer years. It is not a conventional textbook, but nevertheless contains sound practical advice at many levels. Few books contain a job description for a new breed of paramedical persons, or a template for setting up a similar service elsewhere. Rheumatologists, nurses with experience in caring for rheumatic patients, physiotherapists, occupational therapists, orthopaedic surgeons with a broad view of their specialty, and health planners will gain much from reading these pages. It is to be hoped the book will be read not only in Europe but in the United States, the Antipodes and other countries where combined care by physicians and paramedicals is being developed.

Leeds 1984   Verna Wright, MD, FRCP
                                                Professor of Rheumatology,
                                                University of Leeds

References

Wright V (1982) Multi-purpose therapist or multi-professional team? Occup Ther 1982, 45: 229–230

Bird HA, Galloway D and Wright V (1980) Clinical metrology—a future career grade? Lancet 2: 138–140

Preface

This book has been written in an attempt to bridge a gap. On the one hand there is a variety of advanced textbooks, aimed at medical practitioners and rheumatologists, on the treatment of rheumatic diseases. On the other, there are a few texts covering the same subject but aimed at nurses specialising in rheumatology, physiotherapists and occupational therapists, such as *Rheumatism for Nurses and Remedial Therapists* by Wright and Haslock, an earlier book from this Unit. We hope that our own book will occupy an intermediate position and help to draw together all available expertise in the treatment of rheumatic diseases.

The Rheumatism Research Unit in the University of Leeds has for some time pioneered the use of paramedical workers in the integrated management of patients with chronic rheumatic diseases. In the light of this experience we believe there is an essential need for a more practical (and highly cost effective) level of care in the management of chronic conditions. The concept of 'combined patient care' is perhaps most advanced in the field of anaesthetics, where both recovery room nurses and intensive care unit nurses are trained to a high degree to use complex technological equipment, day and night, in collaboration with physicians.

It is ironic that the concept of total patient care has not been further developed in the treatment of chronic conditions. A general practitioner frequently relies heavily on his district nurse as an early warning or screening system for impending deterioration in the medical state of a patient. It has seemed to us that such combined responsibility in patient care, already applied to the management of diabetes mellitus, can be equally applied to chronic chest disease and many chronic rheumatic diseases.

In the rheumatology clinics at the General Infirmary at Leeds nurses and doctors, each with separate booked lists, consult from adjacent rooms. Only lack of space currently prevents the

allocation of further rooms to occupational therapists and physiotherapists. Patients are booked to see the appropriate specialist
according to their needs. Although this system in part evolved
accidentally in an attempt to extend rheumatology services, in a
financially deprived health service, to those needing them, the
advantages have become obvious. Physicians can devote more
time to using their skills in the art of differential diagnosis and
management of the more complicated patients; 'health professionals' can devote more time to the monitoring of possible
side-effects from toxic drugs such as gold or penicillamine, the
quantitative assessment of a patient's progress in response to new
drugs, and patient education. This system of combined care is
already established in North America and in certain countries,
such as Australia, where the system has proved itself as a method
of stretching limited resources in sparsely populated areas.

One stimulus that prompted the writing of this book was the
need for a more applied nursing text that might further its aims of
advancing 'total care' of the rheumatic patient. A second stimulus
was that the 1983 combined meeting of the professional medical
societies for rheumatology (The Heberden Society, British Association for Rheumatology and Rehabilitation, Royal Society of
Medicine) was the first meeting at which the Rheumatology Forum
of the Royal College of Nurses convened a parallel session with
interchange of delegates—as has long been the practice at meetings of the Pan American Rheumatism Association. Appropriately, this meeting was held in Leeds. Physiotherapists and
occupational therapists also held their own meetings in parallel
with the physicians in Leeds, and it is to be hoped that this
auspicious trend will continue. A third stimulus was provided by
the frequent requests we received from physicians and their
nursing colleagues for help in establishing combined clinics in
hospitals other than the General Infirmary at Leeds.

The book falls into three main sections. The first, comprising
three chapters, commences with a chapter reviewing the common
(and some rarer) rheumatic diseases which are particularly deserv-
ing of multidisciplinary care and will be frequently encountered in
hospital units specialising in rheumatology. Chapter 2 covers
recent advances in investigative techniques of the sort that would
be routine in many hospital rheumatology units, together with
accounts of the ward preparation of patients for such investigations. Chapter 3 reviews recent advances in the treatment of
rheumatic diseases, a rapidly moving and increasingly scientific
field. The second section of the book (Chapters 4–6) commences
with a description of routine rheumatology nursing, which in-
corporates an account of the 'nursing process' recently introduced
in many hospitals in the United Kingdom. There follows a
summary of surgical procedures applicable to rheumatic diseases
and the orthopaedic nursing techniques appropriate to them. This

is followed by a chapter reviewing the role of physiotherapy and occupational therapy in the multidisciplinary approach.

The third section of this book, comprising the last six chapters, then applies the concept of 'combined or total patient care' to this background. We have drawn heavily on our clinical experience both at the General Infirmary at Leeds, with over 8000 outpatient clinic attendances each year, and at the Royal Bath Hospital, Harrogate, which, with 125 beds, is the largest hospital devoted entirely to the inpatient care of the rheumatic diseases in the United Kingdom. Chapter 7 deals unashamedly with patient education. It is placed first in this section in the belief that prevention is better than cure. Nevertheless, rheumatic diseases will still advance in some patients; in such cases physicians are going to be dependent upon their clinical metrologists for an accurate presentation of the progression of disease activity. Chapter 8 describes in detail the wide variety of tests currently performed by clinical metrologists. Chapter 9 deals briefly with the psychological aspects of these chronic disabling diseases. Chapter 10 deals with the evolution of a system of combined patient care in the outpatient clinic and describes how paramedical specialists, initially recruited as clinical metrologists, might aim to be responsible for the total care of their rheumatic patients in a manner akin to the role of the nurse practitioner in the United States. Chapter 11 deals with community care in relation to rheumatic diseases. The final chapter assumes that nurses and other paramedical specialists will wish to conduct their own research in the field of rheumatic diseases and introduces the reader to trial methodology and research techniques.

Although this book has been written by a physician and two nursing sisters, we have drawn extensively on the experience and wisdom of our colleagues. Prof. Verna Wright has shared ideas on administrative and clinical aspects and Dr. Anne Chamberlain on rehabilitation aspects. Physiotherapists and occupational therapists have also been consulted in the hope that at least part of the contents of this book will be of interest to all workers involved in the treatment of rheumatic diseases.

When professional advice has been conflicting (which inevitably occurs in medicine) we have inclined towards description of our own practice and experience. As a result, any errors or omissions are entirely the responsibility of the three authors.

If this book is read by trained nurses who, perhaps after a period of basic nursing on a rheumatology ward, wish to extend their contribution towards the total care of the rheumatic patient, we shall be pleased. If the book is also read by rheumatologists, either established or in training, who, as a result, decide to modify their rheumatology service to allow these specialised paramedical workers to make a greater contribution, we shall be delighted.

Contents

Acknowledgements

We wish to thank all the following people, who have contributed greatly towards the writing of this book: Mrs. Ros Schofield for preparing and typing the manuscript and Miss Patricia Lister and Mrs. Ann Cross for additional typing assistance; Ms. Belinda Moore (artist) for preparing the diagrams; Mr. Michael Jackson and his colleagues at Springer-Verlag for constant support and encouragement; Mrs. Robbie Hopkins SRN and Mrs. Julie McGuire SRN for critical appraisal of sections of the manuscript; Mrs. Evelyn Knaub RN (Greeley), Mrs. Colleen Miller RN, MSN (Denver), Mrs. Pamela Rand-Massey MS, LPT (Pittsburgh), Mrs. Jan Smith-Pigg RN, BSN (Milwaukee) and Mrs. Joan Sutton RN, MSN (Baltimore) for providing insights on patient education, patient care and the work of rheumatology nurse practitioners; Mrs. Joan Hawkes, Miss Mary Jackson and Mrs. Fiona Evard (Physiotherapists), and Miss Joanne Fogden and Miss Sheila Calvert (Occupational Therapists) for supplying us with many ideas.
In addition, Prof. Verna Wright and Dr. Anne Chamberlain have given valuable comment and encouragement throughout, and their help is gratefully acknowledged.

1

The Spectrum of Rheumatic Diseases

Introduction

Rheumatic diseases are extremely common in most populations of the world
and their prevalence is often underestimated. This chapter will present a brief
overview of the spectrum of rheumatic diseases likely to be encountered in
hospital practice in western Europe. Clinical description will of necessity be
brief, since excellent accounts of the common diseases exist elsewhere
(Wright and Haslock 1977; Golding 1979). This chapter will concentrate on
inter-relationships between rheumatic diseases and will also give mention to
some of the rarer conditions that, although rarely seen in general practice
nursing, are likely to be encountered from time to time by nursing rheumatological specialists.

The prevalence of rheumatic conditions in the community is shown in
Fig. 1.1 and is compared to the prevalence of rheumatic conditions amongst
patients attending a specialist rheumatism clinic at Leeds General Infirmary.
It will be noted that in the community undetermined complaints, mainly
non-articular or soft tissue rheumatism, predominate, although disc disorders
and osteoarthrosis are also frequently seen. Rheumatoid arthritis and the
other inflammatory polyarthritides occur only rarely. By contrast, in hospital
practice rheumatoid arthritis looms large, and patients with the rarer conditions are more frequently seen. This spectrum of diseases might well be
different in other parts of the world. In eastern Europe, for example, rheumatic fever, septic arthritis and tuberculosis are much more common than
in western Europe. Although rheumatoid arthritis is the main inflammatory-
polyarthritis in the United Kingdom, in the West Indies and in the western
United States systemic lupus erythematosus (SLE), rarely seen in the
United Kingdom, is sometimes more frequent than rheumatoid arthritis. The
reason for this differential pattern of disease activity in areas with relatively
similar climate is not understood. In many ways the disease spectrum in

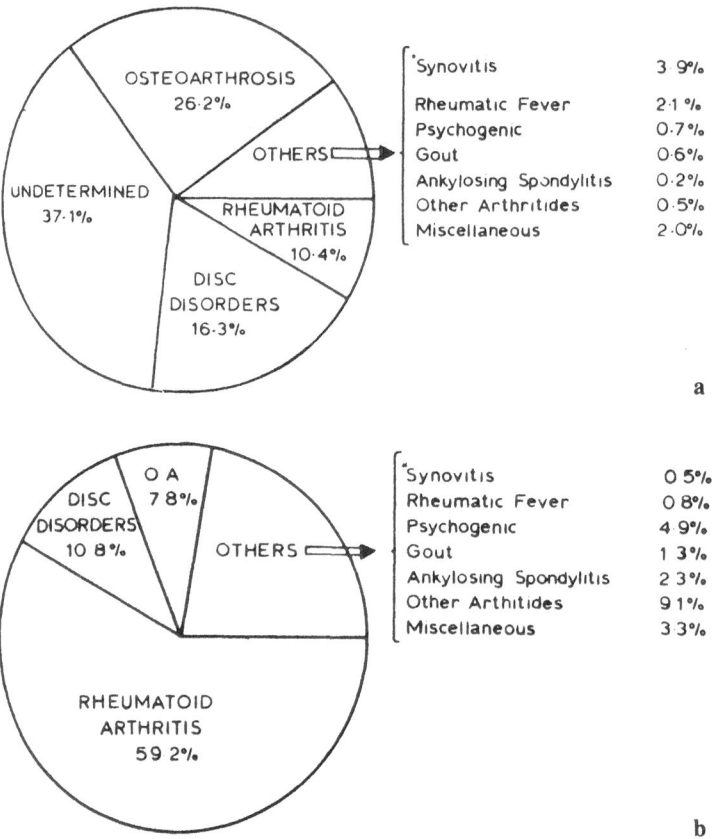

Fig. 1.1a,b. The spectrum of rheumatic diseases. **a** Diagnosis of 1059 patients with rheumatic complaints in the community. **b** Diagnosis of 1061 patients attending a rheumatism clinic at the General Infirmary, Leeds, during a 2-year period. (Wright and Haslock 1977)

eastern Europe resembles that seen in western Europe some 20 or 30 years ago, and it remains a possibility that the prevalence of certain rheumatic diseases ebbs and flows in cycles. Alternatively, improved standards of medical care in western Europe will tend to reduce frank infections allowing alternative conditions to rise to the surface.

In the community, rheumatic diseases account for more days lost from work than accidents, heart disease and infections. The problem of rheumatic disability is even more pronounced in those participating in hard manual labour where the integrity of the musculoskeletal frame is important; as a result, time lost from work because of arthritis and rheumatism is a considerable drain on the economy of a developed country.

This chapter will begin with a discussion of the milder complaints, proceed to the more serious and end up with brief descriptions of some of the rarities.

Non-articular Rheumatism

Although exceedingly common in the community, the causes of musculo-skeletal symptoms that do not cause permanent damage to the joints are ill-understood and underinvestigated. In a sense, everyone experiences non-articular rheumatism when a period of strenuous exercise performed after a period of relative inactivity leaves joints stiff and aching. The condition may be improved by a warm bath and if this fails to relieve symptoms a couple of aspirin tablets are often effective. However, the symptoms are always self limiting and no articular damage is sustained.

One suspects that many of the symptom complexes classified as musculo-skeletal or non-articular rheumatism represent the effects of acute or chronic trauma. It may be that microhaemorrhages occur in muscles or that there is stretching of fibres in ligaments with resultant stimulation of pain-sensitive nerve endings that are common at the site where the ligament is attached to bone. On occasion, a frank tear may occur in a muscle, or the muscular fascia which surrounds and delineates the muscle, or a tendon attached to bone, and this frank damage will take correspondingly longer to heal. If the patient has to continue in active employment using that particular muscle or tendon, healing may be delayed, possibly for several months.

Frank self-perpetuating inflammation may sometimes occur at particular sites where there is redness and swelling of the tendon sheath. Examples of this tenosynovitis often occur in the hands (de Quervain's tenosynovitis of the extensor tendons of the thumb). If a bursa — a synovial sac allowing free play of tendons over a bony or articular surface — becomes inflamed, this is termed a bursitis, and if spontaneous inflammation involves the site where a tendon joins a bone, an epicondylitis may result. Here it is often possible to define the movement that accentuates pain. In tennis elbow, which is a lateral epicondylitis of the elbow, movements that cause tension in the muscles attached to that side will reproduce the pain. A similar situation occurs in golfer's elbow, when the medial epicondyle of the elbow is involved. Similarly, prepatellar bursitis or housemaid's knee is likely to be aggravated by kneeling and is said to be an occupational hazard of both housemaids and clergymen.

The cause for the myalgia that accompanies viral infections, such as influenza, or Coxsackie viral infections, such as Bornholm's disease, is less certain. It is unlikely to be related to trauma and correlates well with the presence of a viraemia. The cause of the non-specific muscle pain that can accompany generalised disorders of connective tissue is also unexplained.

The Painful Shoulder

Assuming that generalised abnormalities such as osteoarthrosis, polymyalgia rheumatica and rheumatoid arthritis have been excluded, a variety of non-articular conditions may cause pain at one or both shoulder joints.

Shoulder pain may also be referred from a pathology in the neck. Rotator cuff disease may result from degeneration of the tendons forming the rotator cuff and this may lead to painful calcifications of the supraspinatus tendon and even rupture of this tendon. Typically patients demonstrate a painful arc. By contrast, 'frozen shoulder' is a blanket term applied to painful stiff shoulders in which all arcs of movement are limited. The cause is not certain, but at operation there may be an adhesive capsulitis of the shoulder. The condition is more common in males over the age of 40, particularly hard manual workers. Subdeltoid bursitis and bicipital tendonitis tend to be less severe. A combination of a painful stiff shoulder with changes in the hand is known as shoulder–hand syndrome and this may follow a variety of disorders of the upper limb including hemiplegia, myocardial infarction and trauma. Finally, general medical conditions such as angina pectoris can cause pain in one or both shoulders.

The Painful Elbow

Tennis elbow and golfer's elbow are likely to be the most common causes of pain in the elbow in the absence of frank arthritis. An olecranon bursitis sometimes occurs, and pain may be referred from the cervical spine. If movements are limited, an intra-articular lesion should be suspected.

Pain in the Hands

An entrapment of the median nerve in the carpal tunnel may cause parasthesiae in the distribution of the median nerve (carpal tunnel syndrome). Sprains, tears and even traumatic dislocations of the joint capsules of the finger joints are relatively common, particularly in hyperextension injury.

Pain in the Hip and Knee

Pain in the hip and/or knee in the presence of normal movements but with reduced movement in the low back suggests referred pain from the lumbar spine, possibly mediated by an entrapment neuropathy. Both these joints are susceptible to strain, and, since the integrity of the joints depends upon the proper functioning of intra-articular structures, cartilage or ligamentous damage inside the joint has to be considered, particularly if joint movements are reduced in the absence of generalised polyarthritis. Internal derangements of the knee are most common and include displaced or torn meniscus and loose cartilage bodies inside the joint (though this may be a variant of the recently recognised crystal deposition disease). Dislocation of the patella may occur if the ligaments are relatively lax.

The Painful Foot

In the absence of frank arthritis, faulty shoes are probably the biggest single cause of foot problems. If the shoes are too tight fitting, as dictated by conventional fashion, the forefoot is compressed and the big toe is deviated into valgus with a resultant bunion on the metatarsal head and ultimately chronic hallux valgus, possibly with secondary osteoarthrosis of this joint. Females are more affected by this than males, and such problems are rarely seen in unshod people. As well as allowing plenty of room for the forefoot the ideal shoe should also clasp the heel firmly from side to side and hold the foot across the tarsus, preferably by lacing. The toes should not be cramped. There should be sufficient space to prevent hallux valgus. The heel should be of modest height and the base of the heel should not be too narrow (Fig. 1.2).

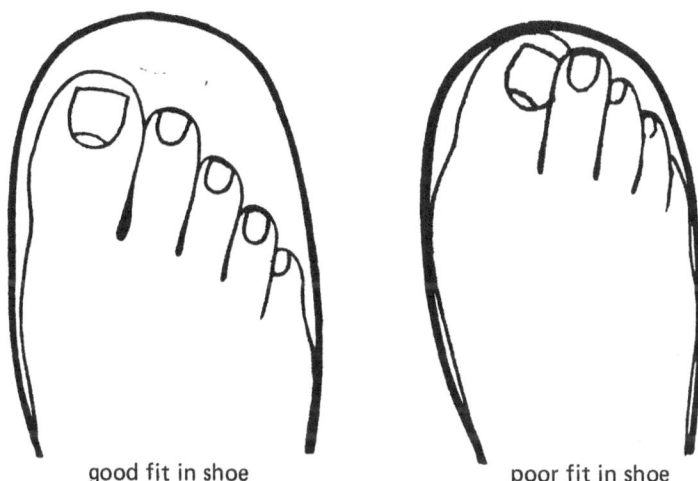

good fit in shoe   poor fit in shoe

Fig. 1.2. The importance of footwear. (After Wright and Haslock 1977)

Forefoot pain may be caused by metatarsalgia (implying flattening of the anterior arch with painful callosities under the heads of the metatarsals in the absence of frank arthritis), march fracture (which is traumatic in origin), osteochondritis or Freiberg's disease, or even the rare plantar digital neuroma.

Midtarsal pain may be caused by flat feet (sometimes secondary to hyperlaxity), inherited pes cavus, or Kohler's disease—osteochondritis of the navicular bone.

Pain in the heel may be due to calcaneal bursitis or plantar fasciitis if inflammatory polyarthropathy is also present.

Hyperlaxity of Joints

Most individuals regard themselves as having a normal range of movement, but a few will be unduly 'stiff' and a few will be unusually 'supple'. Those with supple or hyperlax joints tend to be susceptible to a variety of musculo-skeletal symptoms in the absence of demonstrable arthritis, and the same may apply to relatively stiff-jointed people. Research in this field has been limited by adequate methodology but the advent of machines such as the hyperex-tensometer (see Chap. 8, p. 235) may alter this.

Spinal Disorders

Although spinal pain may be the harbinger of ankylosing spondylitis, the classic inflammatory polyarthropathy of the spine, or of more sinister pathologies such as neoplastic secondary deposits, the majority of patients complaining of a painful neck or a painful back have degenerative spinal disorders. Although the term osteoarthrosis should strictly be reserved for joints with a synovial cavity (the vast majority of joints in the peripheral skeleton), the specialised joints in the spine where the fibrous disc articulates between two vertebral bodies are also susceptible to a comparable degenera-tive change. This can also occur in the apophyseal joints between the arches posteriorly, the only true synovial joints in the vertebral column (Fig. 1.3).

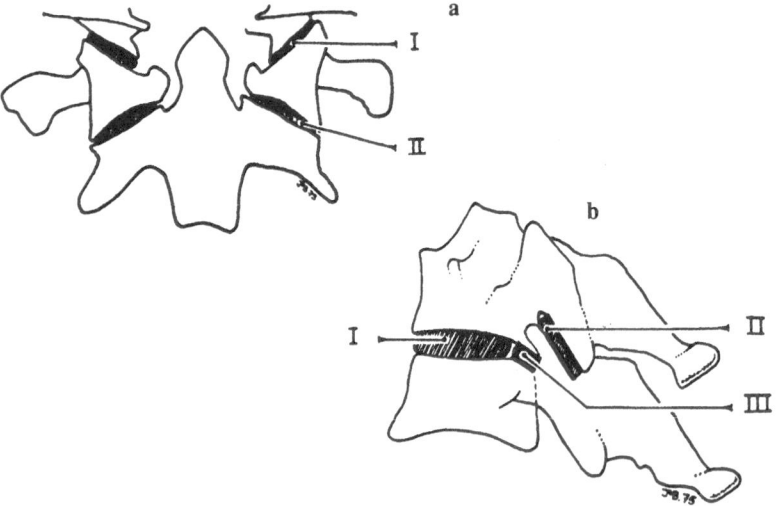

Fig. 1.3a,b. The joints in the vertebral column. **a** Anteroposterior view; **b** lateral view. *I*, fibrous joint between vertebral bodies; *II*, synovial apophyseal joints between the posterior arches of adjacent vertebrae; *III*, the small synovial articulation (of Luschka) between the posterolateral aspects of vertebral bodies (found only in the neck).

Degenerative spinal disease produces a combination of local and referred pain. The disc degenerates throughout the normal life span changing its consistency from a material that resembles hard rubber to a material that resembles crumbling chalk. To some extent this mimics the changes of osteoarthrosis at peripheral joints. With degeneration, the central nucleus may protrude through the annulus in any direction, producing a 'slipped' disc. If the nucleus moves out in a posteriolateral direction, the misshapen disc may produce pressure on the nerve roots, giving referred pain down the arms if this occurs in the neck, or down the legs (sciatica) if this occurs in the lumbar spine, particularly at the level of the fifth lumbar vertebra, where the sciatic nerve is found. A pure posterior protrusion may press on the spinal cord or cauda equina, occasionally necessitating surgical intervention. It is now recognised that individuals who inherit a triangular shaped spinal canal are more susceptible to prolapse of the disc if degeneration in the spine occurs than those who have inherited a round or oval (more capacious) spinal canal. This raises the possibility that with new methods of evaluating spinal canal size, those individuals who will be susceptible to disc disease in later life can be identified and prophylactic advice given at an early stage.

In addition to the frank degeneration at the disc, a variety of congenital anomalies seem to predispose to back pain. Among these are sacralisation of the fifth lumbar vertebra, spina bifida occulta (transitional vertebra) and spondylolysis, which may lead to spondylolisthesis. In this condition, the structural abnormality in the spine (occasionally acquired) causes a slip of one vertebra upon another, and the resultant malalignment probably causes ligamentous strain, which in turn causes pain. A variety of postural faults that may be acquired throughout life are also probably responsible for ligamentous pain and spinal strain. In addition, there may be superimposed lesions of the spinal soft tissues, usually acute and often distinguishable from the history. Finally, some patients almost certainly develop psychogenic back pain, although this diagnosis should be made infrequently; the majority of sufferers (such as the large proportion of nurses who develop back pain once they start lifting heavy patients) undoubtedly have good mechanical reasons for their symptoms.

The importance of correct lifting procedure cannot be overemphasised. The worst way is to bend right forward from the hips with the knees straight and the back in flexion. The best way to lift is to use the legs, bending the knees and standing close to the load so that the back can remain straight and almost erect. The lift is accomplished steadily, and the body should not be twisted once the lift has commenced.

Osteoarthrosis

The condition known as osteoarthrosis used to be considered as a 'wear and tear' arthritis. There are certainly elements of degenerative change in its pathogenesis, but groups of individuals who might be suspected of being at particular risk if its causes were purely mechanical (such as free-fall parachut-ists, athletes and operators of pneumatic drills) do not have an increased incidence of osteoarthrosis. Current teaching suggests that an amalgam of different factors contribute to a final common end point. As more of these factors are recognised it becomes possible to classify more and more examples of osteoarthrosis as being 'secondary'. However, there remains a hard core of patients in whom no obvious predisposing features occur, and these are designated as 'primary' osteoarthrosis.

Primary Osteoarthrosis or Generalised Osteoarthrosis

The terms 'primary osteoarthrosis' or 'generalised osteoarthrosis (GOA)' imply a polyarticular variant of the condition in which no predisposing causes can be identified. The condition tends to occur more commonly in females than males, particularly after the menopause, and is characterised by involvement of the distal interphalangeal joints with Heberden node forma-tion and simultaneous involvement of several other joints, particularly the knees and hips. Involvement at the base of the thumb is common, and a comparable change at the base of the big toe predisposes to hallux valgus. Less frequently, joints such as the shoulder, elbow and ankle are also involved. Although degenerative joint disease in the spine cannot strictly be equated with osteoarthrosis, a large number of such patients seem to have concomitant degeneration in the cervical spine or lumbar spine. The reason why the thoracic spine is spared is uncertain, but this is the part of the vertebral column that exhibits least movement throughout life. Although there is not usually a clear dominant inheritance, a large number of such cases tend to cluster within families, and it seems likely that a combination of acquired, particularly genetic, factors produce the condition. Occasionally the patients have a slightly raised erythrocyte sedimentation rate (ESR) suggesting an inflammatory component, but usually laboratory investigations are within normal limits.

Secondary Osteoarthrosis

The term 'secondary osteoarthrosis' implies that only a small number of joints are involved and that where this occurs there is a clear predisposing cause. Examples of common predisposing factors are shown in Table 1.1. Males or females are affected equally, and normally only a single joint or a small number of joints is involved. This is particularly so when the predisposing cause is localised, as in the orthopaedic causes such as slipped femoral epiphysis, Perthes' disease, a malunited fracture and local aseptic bone necrosis. However, if the predisposing abnormality is more generalised, as in the metabolic disorder or the generalised joint hyperlaxity disorders, the number of joints affected will be larger.

In the case of slipped femoral epiphysis, Perthes' disease and congenital dislocation of the hip, where the abnormality sets up stresses in one (or both)

Table 1.1. Conditions that predispose to osteoarthrosis (Bird and Wright 1982)

Aseptic bone necrosis	Idiopathic
	Thiemann's disease
	Kashin–Beck disease
	Haemoglobinopathies
	Gaucher's disease
Metabolic disorders	Haemochromatosis
	Ochronosis
	Wilson's disease
Joint hyperlaxity	Familial joint hyperlaxity
	Ehlers–Danlos syndrome
	Acromegaly
	Neuropathic joints: Tabes dorsalis
	Syringomyelia
	Diabetes mellitus
	Leprosy
Local articular deformity	Slipped femoral epiphysis
	Perthes' disease
	Malunited fracture
	Meniscectomy (? hyperlaxity)
	Congenital dislocation of the hip (dysplasia)
	Multiple epiphyseal dysplasia
	Mucopolysaccharidoses

hips in childhood, the osteoarthrosis is likely to occur in the affected hip or hips at the age of about 35, although it may occasionally occur before this. Normally the disease remains localised to these sites, but with time secondary changes can occur in other joints. A common pattern is involvement of one hip and subsequent involvement of the contralateral knee, this being simply a function of the mechanical stress in always trying to protect the involved hip. If the neurological supply of the joint is abnormal, extreme mechanical changes occur; it is in this group of patients that the most rapid osteoarthritic changes occur, with severe disorganisation of the joint structure. Individuals with hyperlax joints are probably more prone than most to osteoarthritic changes, possibly through mechanical deformity. In patients with metabolic conditions such as haemochromatosis (abnormal iron metabolism in the body), Wilson's disease (abnormal copper metabolism) or ochronosis (an abnormality of homogentisic acid), the predisposing factor is probably an abnormal chemical composition in the cartilage of the joint that leads to its early breakdown. In such patients the osteoarthrosis is likely to involve many joints, although in ochronosis the spine in particular seems to be attacked.

Radiological Changes in Osteoarthrosis

In the absence of laboratory changes in the blood the diagnosis is usually made radiologically. Fig. 1.4 shows the typical radiological changes of osteoarthrosis. The first pathological change occurs in the cartilage, which becomes fibrillated and ultimately narrowed, although the symptoms may antidate radiological change by several years. The first change is a narrowing of the joint cavity, particularly on weight bearing in the lower limbs, and the

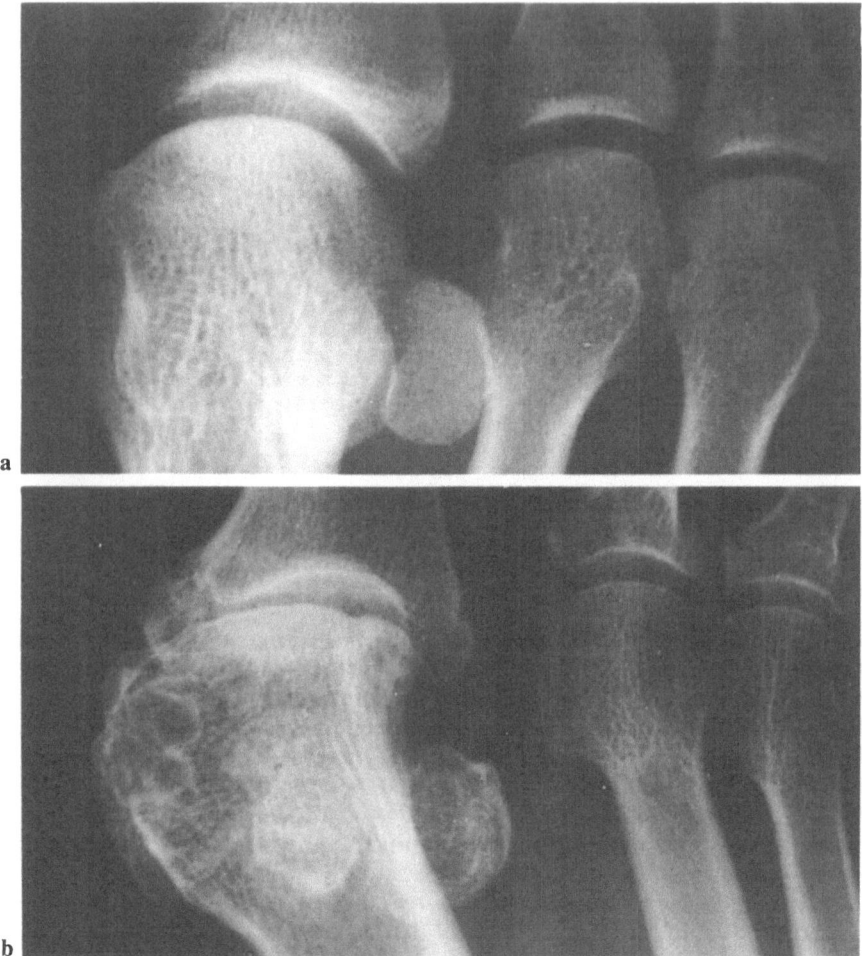

Fig. 1.4a,b. Radiological changes in osteoarthrosis. **a** Normal metatarsophalangeal joints of the feet. **b** In osteoarthrosis changes initially occur at the first metatarsophalangeal joint. The joint space is lost, and increased bone density is seen. Sometimes cyst formation occurs.

radiolucent cartilage becomes narrowed and the bones appear to close together. Subsequently the body responds by attempting to increase the load-bearing surface and osteophyte (new bone) formation and osteosclerosis or increased bone density are very common at osteoarthritic joints and are in complete contradistinction to the rheumatoid radiological changes where osteopenia (reduced density of bone) occurs in the absence of new bone formation. If crystal deposition complicates osteoarthrosis there is likely to be even more calcification in and around the joints.

Crystal Deposition Diseases

The first crystal deposition disease to be recognised was gout. More recently, calcium pyrophosphate deposition disease and hydroxyapatite deposition disease have been identified and are currently the subject of much research.

Gout

Classically, elderly males develop a monoarthritis, usually of the big toe, but sometimes of other joints. The knee joint is the second most common joint to be involved. The pain is intense and acute but of relatively short duration. It follows precipitating events such as an excess of alcohol, a heavy protein meal or trauma such as surgical operation or even an enforced period of bed rest. Certain drugs, particularly thiazide diuretics, may also precipitate an attack.

It is now realised that an acute attack, although triggered, is most likely to occur if superimposed on a hereditary background of hyperuricaemia. Such patients certainly have a high level of urate in the blood either on a hereditary basis or because of underlying metabolic abnormality or disease, but the precise reason why a triggering factor should cause uric acid crystals to initiate an inflammatory reaction in affected joints is not certain. However, this undoubtedly happens, and the diagnosis is confirmed by joint aspiration and visualisation of leucocytes containing uric acid crystals under the polarising microscope. It should be noted that many patients who have gout attacks have uric acid crystals inside the joint, as visualised by the arthroscope, between the acute attacks. Management is with strong anti-inflammatory agents or colchicine for the acute attacks and then with a drug that lowers plasma uric acid (allopurinol or probenecid) for the long-term prophylaxis of the condition.

It should be noted that a certain number of people have idiopathic hyperuricaemia without symptoms and without apparent propensity to gout attacks. It is debatable whether these should be treated; the anxiety is that not treating hyperuricaemia may lead to uric acid calculi and thence to renal failure, although not all physicians accept this. Hyperuricaemia may also be associated with raised blood pressure and abnormalities in lipids.

If gout remains untreated (which, it is hoped, no longer occurs), the patient may be susceptible to a chronic gouty arthritis with tophus formation around joints and bony erosions occurring about affected joints, as seen radiologically.

Pyrophosphate Deposition Disease

The condition characterised by the presence of calcium pyrophosphate crystals inside joints and resultant inflammation has been recognised only within the last 15 years. Chondrocalcinosis, literally calcification within cartilage, is now thought to be a variant of the more ubiquitous pyrophosphate deposition disease. This condition is characterised by acute exacerbations, as in gout, but in general they are not so severe and are confined to different joints, particulary the knees. The disease is more likely to be seen in the elderly, and males and females are involved approximately equally. By contrast, gout is never seen in premenopausal females and thereafter probably does not occur quite so commonly as in males.

Aspiration of joint fluid during an acute attack allows the identification of crystals of calcium pyrophosphate, usually within leucocytes under the polarising microscope. The shape and size of these crystals differs from those of uric acid. Pyrophosphate exhibits a positive birefringence (the position in which the crystals transmit polarised light), whereas uric acid exhibits a negative birefringence. Unlike gout, there appears to be no underlying metabolic abnormality in the blood, although there has been some occasional interest in trying to link the condition with abnormalities of parathyroid metabolism. The condition is also recognised as part of other metabolic disorders such as haemachromatosis and ochronosis.

Most recent interest has centred on the close association between calcium pyrophosphate deposition and osteoarthrosis. There are some who believe that many of the most serious forms of secondary osteoarthrosis merge into calcium pyrophosphate deposition disease with the course of time; others feel that the osteoarthrosis is secondary to the pyrophosphate deposition. Management is with non-steroidal anti-inflammatory agents and analgesics to control attacks; there is no specific drug treatment currently available to prevent pyrophosphate deposition.

Calcium Hydroxyapatite Arthropathy

Even more recently analysis studies of crystals taken from joints have shown the presence of crystals of calcium hydroxyapatite, often in association with calcium pyrophosphate, particularly in joints with severe osteoarthrosis. Calcium hydroxyapatite is a component of normal bone, and discussion centres on whether calcium hydroxyapatite is found in small amounts in normal joints in any case, or whether it is a genuine pathogenetic factor in inflammatory joint disease secondary to crystal deposition.

Degenerative vs Inflammatory Joint Disease

The conditions already described are localised to the joints or musculoskeletal system and can be loosely defined as degenerative or metabolic in aetiology. These arguably less severe conditions contrast with the more severe or autoimmune conditions that are collectively termed 'inflammatory polyarthritis'. The distinguishing features of inflammatory polyarthritis are as follows:

1. Inflammatory polyarthritis tends to be of faster onset and may be more severe than degenerative conditions. It is sometimes characterised by periods of temporary or almost permanent remission, unlikely to be seen in the chronically advancing degenerative conditions.
2. Complex immunological changes can be observed in the blood and tissues of patients with inflammatory polyarthritis, though whether these represent the primary cause of conditions like rheumatoid arthritis or whether they are secondary to acquisition of the disease remains uncertain.
3. Certain haematological and biochemical changes which occur in the blood of patients with inflammatory polyarthritis are not seen in degenerative conditions.
4. Inflammatory polyarthritis involves not only the musculoskeletal system but many other organs throughout the body. In particular, organs involved vary with the different diseases and sometimes provide quite valuable diagnostic clues.

The various forms of inflammatory polyarthritis can be conveniently classified into three main groups:

1. *Seronegative spondarthritides.* The overlapping conditions in this group, summarised in Fig. 1.5, are seronegative for rheumatoid factor. They are certainly less aggressive than seropositive rheumatoid arthritis and the pattern of organ involvement in these conditions differs from that seen in rheumatoid arthritis.
2. *Rheumatoid arthritis*, which is usually seropositive. This denotes the presence of rheumatoid factor, an immunoglobulin complex in the blood of patients, which in turn is associated with severe systemic upset such as the presence of vasculitis, the radiological evidence of erosions

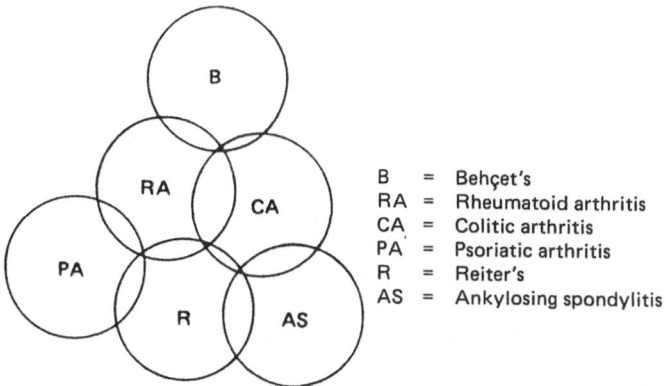

Fig. 1.5. Seronegative spondarthritides. Venn diagram to demonstrate the overlap between these different conditions which share so many common features. (Bird and Wright 1982)

and the rheumatoid nodules which provide a distinguishing pathological feature of this condition. It is likely that over the next few decades, what is conventionally termed 'rheumatoid arthritis' will be subdivided into a collection of different disorders on the basis of serological and clinical features, which in turn may allow us to be more precise in evaluating prognosis in the variants of this condition.

3. *Connective tissue disorders.* The disorders in this group, summarised in the second Venn diagram (Fig. 1.6), are characterised by the presence of abnormal antibodies and organ involvement. In fact, musculoskeletal system involvement is sometimes not very marked in these conditions. Although rheumatoid factor may occasionally be found, most of these conditions are characterised by the presence of other distinctive antibodies, only occasionally seen in rheumatoid arthritis. Nevertheless, there is inevitably some overlap between these different conditions.

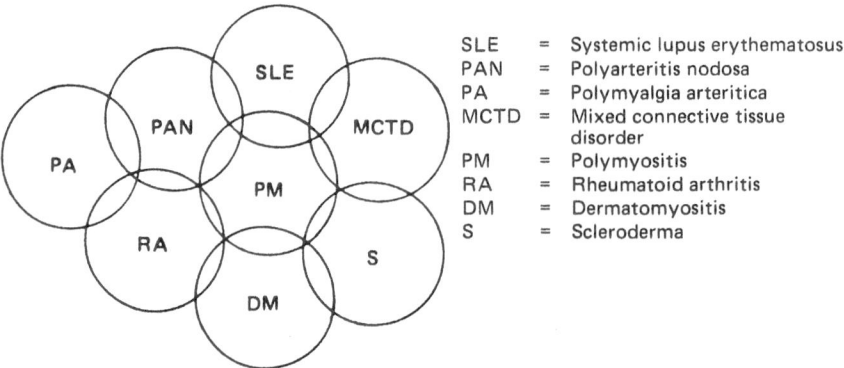

SLE = Systemic lupus erythematosus
PAN = Polyarteritis nodosa
PA   = Polymyalgia arteritica
MCTD = Mixed connective tissue disorder
PM   = Polymyositis
RA   = Rheumatoid arthritis
DM   = Dermatomyositis
S   = Scleroderma

Fig. 1.6. Connective tissue disorders. Venn diagram to illustrate the overlap among this related group of diseases. (Bird and Wright 1982)

It should be noted that rheumatoid arthritis is currently the commonest form of inflammatory polyarthropathy seen in the United Kingdom clinics. Seronegative polyarthritis is seen with about one-fourth or one-fifth of the frequency of rheumatoid disease, and the connective tissue disorders are seen less frequently still.

It must also be acknowledged that the dividing line between degenerative joint disease and inflammatory joint disease is not always quite so distinct as is described here. Some patients with inflammatory rheumatoid arthritis go into a phase of remission when inflammation is barely present and secondary degenerative changes of the osteoarthritic sort may predominate, although the changes revealed by radiographs are always more of a mixture than the pure osteosclerotic changes of osteoarthrosis. In addition, patients with osteoarthrosis sometimes experience inflammatory episodes of disease activity, possibly linked with intermittent crystal deposition, although this is not proven. Such episodes may respond to treatment with anti-inflammatory agents, such as local intra-articular steroid injection. The raised ESR sometimes seen in such conditions is also said to be characteristic of an inflammatory variant of osteoarthrosis, which would rationally be termed 'osteoarthritis'.

Seronegative Spondarthritides

Of the conditions grouped together as seronegative spondarthritides, Reiter's syndrome is the closest to a chronic inflammatory arthritis that has a proven infective aetiology. Psoriatic arthropathy and colitic arthropathy occupy a mid-point in clinical terms, and ankylosing spondylitis shows more distinct clinical differences from the other members of this group. The characteristic feature of these conditions is their association with the B27 antigen, a particular white blood cell group. Although red blood cell groups such as A, B and O do occasionally have minor associations with some diseases such as gastric carcinoma (blood group A) and peptic ulcer (blood group O), in general this has not been of particular diagnostic help in medicine. Extensive mapping of the white blood cell groups has been of value in transplant surgery and it was also natural to consider their appliction to differential diagnosis. Although certain HLA antigens carried on the white cells do bear a relationship to the propensity to contract diseases such as diabetes mellitus and multiple sclerosis, the association is most marked with the B27 tissue antigen and arthritides of the seronegative type. Approximately 95% of all patients with ankylosing spondylitis bear the B27 antigen, although it is seen in only about 10% of a normal United Kingdom population. Approximately 50% of patients with Reiter's syndrome and around 30%–40% of patients with psoriatic arthritis and colitic arthritis, normally those with spinal involvement, also bear this antigen.

Reiter's Disease

There are two variants of Reiter's disease. One is venereally acquired, the initial event being a urethritis which is caused by *Chlamydia*. The other is acquired from food poisoning and starts with diarrhoea, the episode normally being caused by *Shigella*. After appropriate infection, the episode of urethritis or diarrhoea is usually self limiting and rarely lasts for more than 1 week. After a gap of some 10 days, a conjunctivitis occurs, but this again is self limiting, usually after a period of 1–2 weeks, although it may become intermittent in some patients. A few weeks later the arthritis appears, normally being localised to the knees and ankles. This is a disease of young people, males being more commonly involved than females. Sometimes the condition is self limiting, but in about half the patients it progresses to a chronic though relatively mild polyarthritis of the knees, ankles and sometimes of the sacroiliac joints and lumbar spine, with a spondylitic sort of picture.

Psoriatic Arthropathy

Patients with psoriasis are susceptible to polyarthritis. This usually follows skin involvement but may antidate this. There are a variety of clinical presentations, but many patients develop sacroiliitis and spinal involvement (particularly those who have the B27 antigen). Others develop a peripheral arthropathy involving the interphalangeal joints, knees and ankles with sparing of the metatarsophalangeal joints and metacarpophalangeal joints. This is in distinction to rheumatoid arthritis, and it appears that seronegativity is linked to a particular joint distribution. Occasionally a severely mutilating arthritis occurs in the finger joint but it affects only a small proportion of patients suffering from this condition. As a general rule, treatments that help skin lesions and psoriasis do not help the joint involvement.

Colitic Arthritis

Patients suffering from either ulcerative colitis or Crohn's disease are liable to develop a polyarthritis with spondylitis and sacroiliac involvement. The knees and hips are often involved. This tends to be a disease of young people, involving either sex. The peripheral symptoms often seem to resolve with adequate treatment of the ulcerative colitis or Crohn's disease; by contrast the spondylitis, when it occurs (mainly in patients with the B27 antigen), advances more insidiously and independently of the presence of bowel involvement.

Ankylosing Spondylitis

Ankylosing Spondylitis is a disease more frequently seen in males than females, although an increasing number of females who do develop it are now recognised. It is characterised by early morning stiffness in the low back and over the sacroiliac joints occurring normally between the ages of 20 and 30. The disease is insidious in its onset and many patients are misdiagnosed or dismissed as being 'neurotic'. Over a period of several years the disease advances up the spine, causing increased calcification at the lumbar vertebrae and ultimately fusion of the vertebrae to form the classic bamboo spine. The thoracic spine, in particular the costochondral junctions, are involved, causing diminished thoracic excursion and the predominance of diaphragmatic breathing with reduced vital capacity. The disease ultimately involves the cervical spine, where again the final picture is complete fusion. In the early stages patients have difficulty in using a driving mirror.

Visceral complications include an anterior uveitis that responds to local steroid therapy and aortic incompetence caused by inflammatory involvement of the endocardium at the site of the aortic valves. The patients are also susceptible to colitis.

Management has been revolutionised by the introduction of intensive exercise programmes once it was realised that the earlier treatment of complete bed rest accelerated the fusion at the spine. Physiotherapy should be used to correct the dorsal kyphosis that is commonly seen in neglected ankylosing spondylitis, and anti-inflammatory agents may be necessary to relieve pain. At present there is no specific drug therapy to arrest this condition.

Rheumatoid Arthritis

Classically rheumatoid arthritis is a symmetrical small joint polyarthritis involving the hands and the feet. It is more common in females than males and occurs between the ages of 20 and 35 with bilateral pain and stiffness of the metacarpophalangeal joints in the hands and metatarsophalangeal joints in the feet. It is associated with a feeling of tiredness and malaise and is likely to progress to involve the majority of joints in the body. A typical progression would spread both to the wrists and ankles as well as the interphalangeal joints. The elbows, knees and hips and cervical spine would ultimately become involved; however some joints are never affected, for example the sacroiliac joints, which are so commonly affected in seronegative polyarthritis.

In the earlier stages the disease involves the synovium not only lining the joint but also lining the tendon sheaths that pass over the joints. This leads to tendon instability in the hands at an early stage leading to ulnar deviation, swan-neck deformity and boutonnière deformity, although it should be emphasised that these clinical features are not specific for rheumatoid arthritis

Organ involvement is likely to be widespread. Amongst the commonest manifestations are rheumatoid nodules in the myocardium, causing conducting defects on ECG, and pericarditis. In the lungs rheumatoid nodules may mimic neoplastic lesions, and pleural effusions, unilateral or bilateral, may occur. There may be vasculitis, skin lesions best seen as necrotic haemorrhages at the sides of the fingernails on the hands, and it is probably a vasculitic mechanism that causes the sensory neuropathy, motor neuropathy or mononeuritis multiplex occasionally seen. The kidney is spared—in contrast to SLE and connective tissue disorders—unless the disease is of long-standing duration, when amyloid may be deposited in that organ. In the eye, an episcleritis occurs which may even lead to scleromalacia perforans— in contrast to the seronegative polyarthritides, where it is the anterior chamber that is most commonly involved. Sjögren's syndrome, associated with reduced tear formation and reduced salivary flow, may also cause dry eyes and dry mouth.

As the condition advances, secondary mechanical changes occur in the musculoskeletal system. Entrapment neuropathies may be caused by inflammatory synovial tissue at the sites where nerves pass under fascial sheaths. The most important and sinister entrapment neuropathy is where atlantoaxial subluxation occurs as the rheumatoid process eats away the transverse ligament of the atlas vertebra, causing a subluxation that may impinge on the spinal cord, giving paralysis.

The pathological feature is the rheumatoid nodule with characteristic histology that is often found on extensor (possibly pressure-bearing) surfaces such as the back of the elbow. The radiological changes are also characteristic (Fig. 1.7). The earliest changes comprise soft tissue swelling around affected joints and the possible enlargement of the joint cavity. This is because an inflammatory effusion in the cavity distracts the two bones, unlike osteoarthrosis where the two bones move closer together as the cartilage is lost. Subsequently there may be osteopenia around affected joints and the development of bony erosions, initially at the site where the synovium joins the bone, since this is essentially a synovial disease in the early stages. Subsequently as cartilage becomes eroded the joint space will be lost, but this is a relatively late change in rheumatoid arthritis. Ultimately a variety of bony deformities including simple subluxation and even frank disorganisation may occur. If the disease goes into spontaneous remission fewer erosions will be seen and a more stable osteoarthritic-type picture may emerge upon radiological examination. It should be remembered that erosions are evident in the metatarsal heads before they are always apparent at the metacarpophalangeal joints, and this accounts for the frequency with which radiographs of the foot are ordered in patients suspected of having early rheumatoid arthritis.

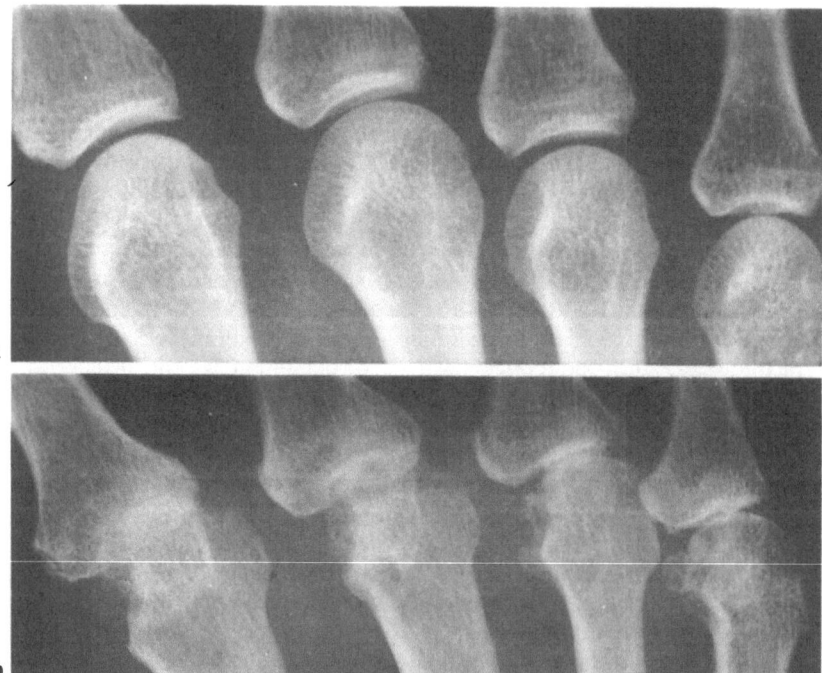

Fig. 1.7 a,b. Radiological changes in rheumatoid arthritis. **a** Normal metacarpophalangeal joints. **b** In rheumatoid arthritis there is initial loss of bone density and subsequently erosions occur. At a later stage there may be subluxation of the joints.

A proportion of patients commence with an episodic sort of arthritis (around 20%). Some of these are described as having palindromic rheumatism. In the remainder the arthritis becomes more persistent, although it should be remembered that ultimately up to 30% of patients have little or no disability and only 10% of patients are completely disabled. It is possible that with modern drug management these figures may be improved upon.

It should be remembered that certain variants of rheumatoid arthritis occur in certain age groups. Although a seropositive rheumatoid arthritis with radiological evidence of erosions can occur in a small number of children, the majority of children who develop chronic inflammatory polyarthritis have a seronegative variant with systemic involvement including lymphadenopathy and skin rashes. In old age, a variant occurs which is characterised by extreme stiffness of the shoulder girdles and, although joint erosions subsequently occur in the hands and feet, the initial presentation mimics polymyalgia rheumatica. There is also a systemic form occurring in middle-aged males that can mimic a lymphoma with gross lymphadenopathy and high swinging fever, sometimes burning out but often leading to a relatively severe rheumatoid joint involvement.

The aetiopathogenesis of rheumatoid arthritis remains unknown but it has recently been linked with particular antigens at the D locus on the sixth chromosome, particularly HLA DW4. This association does not reach the magnitude of some of those seen in the seronegative polyarthritides, but may account, at least in part, for a slight tendency for rheumatoid arthritis to run in families.

Connective Tissue Disorders

Arthralgia or arthritis comprises part of the symptom complex produced by some of the connective tissue disorders; however, they are essentially abnormalities of connective tissue and as such exhibit widespread systemic involvement throughout the body. There are many overlapping features among the different conditions and some of them share some clinical features with rheumatoid arthritis, for example the vasculitis. These conditions are less frequently seen in rheumatic clinics in the United Kingdom but may on occasions be referred for specialist treatment.

Systemic Lupus Erythematosus

SLE is a condition which starts in young females, and is characterised by arthralgia, intermittent Raynaud's phenomenon and photosensitive skin rash, together with a high ESR and specific antibodies. The disease is often benign but in some patients it will run a more malignant course involving the heart (pericarditis and endocarditis), the lungs (pleural effusion and interstitial pneumonitis) and the skin (vasculitis). The two organs most involved, which in turn determine the prognosis, are the kidney and the brain. A glomeru-lonephritis may lead to proteinurea, nephrotic syndrome and moderate hypertension. Central nervous system involvement may be due to epilepsy, psychosis and neurological symptoms mimicking space-occupying lesions.

A positive antinuclear factor provides a useful screening test, but the diagnosis is confirmed by the presence of antibodies to human double-stranded DNA.

Polyarteritis Nodosa

The unusual condition of polyarteritis nodosa, which is usually seen in middle-aged males, is characterised by inflammation of arteries resulting in the formation of painful nodules that have a distinct histological appearance on the arterial wall. The main symptoms are those of vascular insufficiency, claudication and even gangrene. The kidneys may be involved, when the picture is of severe hypertension and only minimal proteinuria.

Polymyositis

Polymyositis is characterised by painful inflammation in the muscles. Muscle enzymes are likely to be abnormal and the patient experiences systemic upset. The diagnosis is confirmed by muscle biopsy, which shows a lymphocytic infiltration throughout the muscles. Treatment is with certain cytotoxic agents. The condition may be associated with malignancy.

Dermatomyositis

In dermatomyositis there is not only inflammation with lymphocytic infiltra-tion of the muscle but a similar lymphocytic infiltration of the overlying skin producing a skin rash and, in some cases, a heliotrope rash around the eyelids. The diagnosis is confirmed on tissue biopsy. The condition is more frequently seen in the elderly but is still very rare. Opinions are divided on whether it is or is not associated with malignancy.

Mixed Connective Tissue Disorder

The syndrome known as mixed connective tissue disorder, recently described from the west coast of the United States, is said to be a distinct entity from other connective tissue disorders, although its symptom complex accumulates different features of many of the disorders already described. Its closest relative is perhaps SLE, although initially it was said to be distinguished from this condition by the presence of a specific antibody, anti-RNA, and the relative infrequency of cerebral and renal involvement. With the passage of time many patients initially thought to have mixed connective tissue disorder are now recognised as having a variant of SLE, and in such patients the renal involvement appears relatively late.

Eosinophilic Fasciitis

In eosinophilic fasciitis eosinophilic infiltration occurs in the subcutaneous tissues producing local pain and tenderness with some tightening of the skin. Treatment may be with cytotoxic agents. The condition has only recently been described. Diagnosis is by histology, and the condition is extremely rare.

Scleroderma

The condition originally described as scleroderma has more recently been divided into three distinct entities. Morphea is a localised variant with a benign prognosis involving the skin, which becomes tethered and contracted, but the condition does not spread. In CREST syndrome (calcinosis, Raynaud's phenomenon, oesophagitis, sclerodactyly and telangiectasiae), there is a relatively benign prognosis but, as described by its name, more parts of the body are involved. Systemic sclerosis represents the most extreme form of the condition in which a widespread fibrosis starting in the skin involves many organs of the body. Typically a female between the ages of 20 and 30 notices a bilateral Raynaud's phenomenon, malaise and tightening of the skin on the fingers and face, such that opening the mouth and smiling becomes difficult. Subsequently fibrosis may extend to involve the majority of organs in the body, producing, for example, a constrictive pericarditis and pulmonary fibrosis. Fibrosis also occurs intermittently throughout the bowel, areas of stenosis being alternated with hypertrophic areas of normal bowel as the bowel musculature attempts to overcome the obstruction. Oesophageal stenosis is also common. There are no specific biochemical features in the blood, but the diagnosis may be made on histology. Treatment is unfortunately unrewarding.

Aetiopathogenesis of Connective Tissue Disorders

The aetiopathogenesis of connective tissue disorders is not known, but it is interesting to speculate that in many ways these disorders represent aberrations (or perhaps physiological excesses) of different parts of the body's protective system. SLE and mixed connective tissue disorder appear to be an aberration of the immune complex wing of the body's defence system. The precise abnormality in animal models appears to be a failure of suppressor T cells (T lymphocytes) which, when present, serve as a brake on the B lymphocytes that produce immune complexes. As a result an excess of B lymphocyte activity occurs with resultant anti-DNA antibodies in the patient's serum. By contrast, polymyositis and dermatomyositis seem more to represent abnormalities of T lymphocyte function, the cellular defence mechanism of the body. Finally, scleroderma appears to be an aberration of fibrosis, the body's natural mechanism of repairing the earlier inflammatory process mediated by B and T lymphocytes.

Polymyalgia Rheumatica and Temporal Arteritis

Polymyalgia rheumatica and temporal arteritis together form an interesting condition which is relatively common and probably underdiagnosed in western Europe and has features in common with both rheumatoid arthritis and the connective tissue disorders. Although polymyalgia rheumatica and temporal arteritis were originally thought to be different conditions, evidence has now accumulated to show that they represent opposite ends of a continuous disease spectrum; indeed, some authorities have suggested the term 'polymyalgia arteritica' to cover both conditions, though this has not found general acceptance.

Polymyalgia Rheumatica

An elderly patient, male or female, complains of a very sudden onset of severe stiffness and, to a lesser extent, pain in the shoulder girdle and sometimes in the pectoral girdle. Such patients are unable to raise their hands to their face to wash in the mornings because of stiffness, but the symptoms often disappear by midday. There may be associated anorexia and depression, and 10%–15% of these patients go on to develop temporal arteritis. There is no diagnostic test, but patients often respond to a single blind therapeutic trial of prednisolone, this drug producing a dramatic relief of symptoms within 1–2 days of starting therapy. The disease is usually self limiting with a mean duration of 2 years (range 6 months to 10 years), and during this time the patients need to be on a small maintenance dose of prednisolone, the dose being increased if patients develop symptoms of temporal arteritis. The ESR is markedly raised in this condition, and the dose of steroids should be adequate to keep the ESR depressed.

Temporal Arteritis

An elderly patient complains of a sudden onset of headache, usually unilateral but sometimes bilateral, over the region of the temporal artery, that is above and behind one of the eyes. This artery supplies the retina and the extraocular muscles, and because of this some patients will notice transient loss of vision, diplopia and even a sudden onset of blindness. About 40% of patients who give a history of temporal arteritis have at some time in the previous 5 years experienced a symptom complex resembling polymyalgia rheumatica. Temporal artery biopsy may show a lymphocytic infiltration of the vessel, most marked at the internal elastic lamina, and the condition is thought to represent an autoimmune reaction to the internal elastic lamina of the arteries. The treatment is with prednisolone in higher doses than that given to patients with polymyalgia rheumatica. Sudden blindness can sometimes be reversed by an intravenous injection of hydrocortisone followed by very high doses of oral prednisolone. The time course for the disease is similar to that of polymyalgia rheumatica. Patients need to be monitored carefully with regular prednisolone until the disease goes into spontaneous remission, although about 10% of patients who are apparently 'cured' of the disease have a further exacerbation during their lifetime.

Septic Arthritis

Infection of a joint with pyogenic bacteria is a rheumatological emergency. The majority of examples are monoarticular; the knee is probably the commonest affected joint in the United Kingdom. If untreated the condition progresses rapidly to joint destruction, and the complications are osteomyelitis, ankylosis of the joint and sinus formation.

The commonest organisms are *Staphylococcus* (almost 50%), *Streptococcus pyogenes*, *Escherichia coli*, *Strep. faecalis*, *Strep pneumococcus* and *Haemophilus influenzae*. *Neisseria gonorrhoeae* may also enter joint cavities, but with this organism (and possibly some of the preceding ones) the evidence slightly favours a brisk inflammatory response to gonococcal antigens circulating throughout the body rather than a proven entry of the organism into the joint cavity.

Any hot swollen joint, disproportionately involved in relation to the other joints, with periarticular oedema and systemic fever, should alert suspicion. Patients with rheumatoid arthritis often develop sepsis in one or more joints, particularly if they are taking steroid therapy, and an isolated joint may show up conspicuously as a high-scoring joint on the Ritchie Articular Index (see Chap. 8, p. 210). Laboratory findings include a neutrophil leucocytosis and often a positive blood culture. Synovial fluid should be aspirated and cultured for organisms, and treatment is urgent with appropriate antibiotics. Provided these are given by satisfactory systemic routes the use of intra-articular antibiotics is rarely required, although daily aspiration of an affected joint may be necessary.

Rarer Arthritic Conditions

Although the majority of arthritic conditions likely to be seen in hospital practice has now been reviewed, a brief description is added of some rarer conditions. A more detailed account of these, if and when required, is available elsewhere (Scott 1978; Kelly et al. 1981).

1. *Psychogenic rheumatism*. Non-disease (normality with symptoms of psychogenic rheumatism) should be diagnosed only with extreme caution, after a full assessment of the patient and exclusion of all likely pathology. Nevertheless, there remains a small group of patients, often habitual hospital attenders, who derive satisfaction from confronting doctors as a sort of challenge. Treatment is often difficult and unrewarding.

2. *Drug-induced arthropathies*. A variety of arthropathies can be induced by drugs. Penicillamine and sulphonamides may exacerbate, and gout may be precipitated by diuretics. A lupus-like syndrome is produced by hydralazine, and fluid retention and sodium depletion and even hypokalaemia can cause painful muscles. High-dose long-term steriod therapy may cause avascular necrosis of the hip, and sulphonamides and penicillin can precipitate polyarteritis nodosa.

3. *Tuberculosis* can involve joints, although this is extremely rare in the United Kingdom. The spine is usually involved, but the hip and knee are also relatively common sites. The arthritis is monoarticular and presents insidiously, often in an Asian immigrant or an individual who has been exposed to tuberculosis.

4. *Pseudohypertrophic osteoarthropathy* presents as digital clubbing and swelling of the distal parts of the limbs (particularly the wrists) caused by periostitis and synovitis. It is associated with malignancy or sometimes chronic pulmonary suppuration, as in bronchiectasis or aortic aneurysm. Irradication of the underlying disease may cure the condition.

5. *Ankylosing vertebral hyperostosis* is a condition of the elderly in which the spine is stiffened with a radiological appearance similar to but distinguishable from ankylosing spondylitis. The condition is benign and does not progress like ankylosing spondylitis.

6. *Avascular necrosis* comprises a group of conditions in which bone infarction is due to interference of blood supply. It commonly involves the hip and is often post traumatic but may be secondary to steroid therapy, existing arthropathies or a variety of rarer conditions.

7. *Behçet's syndrome* is characterised by oral ulceration, genital ulceration and iritis and may be related to seronegative polyarthritis.

8. *Familial Mediterranean fever* causes acute intermittent exacerbations of pain, often in the joint, accompanied by recurrent attacks of fever. It is a condition affecting people of Mediterranean origin, Sephardic Jews or Armenians in the main, and is inherited as an autosomal recessive character.

9. *Haemophilia* can cause attacks of arthritis as the result of haemorrhage into the joints.

10. *Chronic active hepatitis or lupoid hepatitis*, a condition overlapping with systemic lupus erythematosus, can cause a rheumatoid-like arthritis in peripheral joints.

11. *Neuropathic or Charcot's joints*, a variant of premature osteoarthrosis, may be caused by tabes dorsalis (syphilis), diabetes mellitus or syringomyelia.

12. *Paget's disease* is a disorder of unknown aetiology, normally in elderly males, affecting one or many bones, particularly the pelvis, femur, skull, tibia and vertebrae. Radiological changes are quite characteristic; the cause remains unknown but a variety of modern treatments are now available.

13. *Pigmented villonodular synovitis.* This is a rare, benign synovial tumour characterised by synovial proliferation pigmentation with haemosiderin and pannus formation.

14. *Relapsing polychondritis* is a rare condition characterised by inflammation of cartilage in several sites, particularly the pinna of the external ear and the nose.

15. *Rubella or other viral conditions* can cause an arthralgia which may progress to arthritis, particularly in adults who contract these childhood diseases for the first time. It is rare in children. In the case of rubella the wrists and hands are frequently involved. The condition is transient and self limiting but can cause considerable discomfort whilst present.

16. *Sarcoidosis* may produce transient or persistent types of polyarthritis usually involving the knees and ankles and is associated with erythema nodosum.

17. *Multiple epiphysial dysplasia* is a rare hereditary condition, usually inherited as an autosomal dominant. Minimal symptoms may be present in early childhood. However, the significance is that premature osteoarthrosis occurs in a variety of joints in middle life, and radiographs show irregular epiphyses which may become flattened or deformed.

References

Bird HA and Wright V (1982) Applied drug therapy in the rheumatic diseases. Wright, Bristol
Golding DN (1979) Concise management of the common rheumatic disorders. Wright, Bristol
Kelly WN, Harris ED, Ruddy S and Sledge CB (eds) (1981) Textbook of rheumatology. Saunders, Philadelphia
Scott JT (ed) (1978) Copeman's textbook of rheumatic diseases, 5th edn. Churchill Livingstone, Edinburgh
Wright V and Haslock I (1977) Rheumatism for nurses and remedial therapists. Heinemann Medical, London

2

Investigations for Rheumatic Diseases

Introduction

In view of the large number of rheumatic diseases described in Chapter 1, it will come as no surprise that the investigations used in their diagnosis and management are many and varied. This chapter seeks to review those most commonly used and also includes some investigations such as thermography and monoclonal antibody techniques that would be firmly classified as research procedures and are not within the scope of all of the smaller rheumatology units. Where relevant, attention will be directed to important aspects of the nursing care that precedes and follows such investigations. Since the management of rheumatic diseases involves all systems of the body, this aspect will also be reflected in this chapter. For example, a section is included on the investigation of gastrointestinal blood loss, a common problem in patients receiving non-steroidal anti-inflammatory agents.

Routine Haematological Investigations

Routine haematological tests are simple and inexpensive and likely to be performed frequently on many rheumatic patients. The normal range, which is different for males and females and often differs with age, should be obtained from each laboratory since it will differ from centre to centre. As a guideline, the normal values that the laboratories use in Leeds are listed in Appendix A.

Haemoglobin

Haemoglobin, along with other red cell parameters, is normally measured routinely on a Coulter counter which provides a computer print out. The heamoglobin should be interpreted in conjunction with the other red cell findings. Patients with musculoskeletal rheumatism and degenerative arthritis are likely to have a normal haemoglobin unless gastrointestinal blood loss, usually as a result of anti-inflammatory agents, has occurred. If this happens, the resultant anaemia will be microcytic—a low mean corpuscular volume (MCV)—and hypochromic—low mean corpuscular haemoglobin (MCH). A similar anaemia may arise in patients with rheumatoid arthritis who are likely to be treated with similar drugs. In addition, however, the disease, in its own right, may cause a normocytic (normal MCV), normochromic (normal MCH) anaemia. Unlike the iron deficiency type where the marrow produces a large number of small cells in an attempt to compensate for the reduced iron, the anaemia of rheumatoid disease probably results from inappropriate utilisation of iron, the marrow producing smaller numbers of relatively normal cells. A macrocytic anaemia (high MCV) usually develops from B_{12} or folic acid deficiency and in rheumatoid arthritis may occasionally be seen when the condition is treated with sulphasalazine, which causes a folate deficiency anaemia. Patients with polymyalgia rheumatica may also have a normochromic normocytic anaemia, and patients with connecctive tissue disorders who have developed renal failure may occasionally exhibit the normochromic normocytic anaemia of renal disease. In general, patients with active rheumatoid arthritis have a lower haemoglobin than those with rheumatoid arthritis in remission.

White Blood Count

The total white blood count should be reviewed in conjunction with a differential white blood count, showing the proportion of neutrophils and lymphocytes that make up the total numbers of circulating white blood cells. In infectious arthritis, the white blood count is likely to be high, usually because of an increase in polymorphs, although in some viral infections there may be an increase in lymphocytes. The white blood count fluctuates slightly in rheumatoid arthritis, sometimes with a differential increase in lymphocytes, but in our experience is unhelpful in diagnosis or management. However, in Felty's syndrome, where there is a large spleen and sometimes skin rash and oral ulceration in patients with rheumatoid arthritis, there is a leucopenia, almost certainly caused by rapid destruction of cells within the enlarged spleen. The more common cause of leucopenia in rheumatoid arthritis, however, is marrow suppression from toxic drugs such as aurothiomalate or penicillamine, although usually the platelet count drops first and this provides an earlier warning sign.

Platelet Count

One cause of a low platelet count is failure to mix the blood with anticoagulant, since clotting of the blood uses up platelets and there are fewer to be measured by the routine Coulter analysis. If an accurate platelet count is required, the sequestrene anticoagulant tube should be rotated gently for a full minute after the blood sample has been taken. Old specimen tubes which contain outdated anticoagulant will also cause the same problem. In degenerative conditions the platelet count would normally be within normal limits. In active rheumatoid arthritis there is an increased platelet count (thrombocytosis) that drops slowly back to normal as the disease comes under control or goes into remission, and this can be used as a rough test of disease activity. By contrast, in SLE, a distant cousin of rheumatoid arthritis, a low platelet count (thrombocytopenia) is a very characteristic laboratory finding at an early stage of the disease. In addition, drugs used in the treatment of rheumatoid arthritis such as aurothiomalate and D-penicillamine will cause a fall in platelet count. There is a certain laboratory variation, but a platelet count falling steadily over a range of 100×10^9 serves as a warning sign. We try while plotting the platelet count to watch for a fall in the graph, and nurses and secretary are under instruction to draw the attention of the doctor to such a fall or to any platelet count going below 150×10^9.

Erythrocyte Sedimentation Rate

A quantity (1 or 2 ml) of anticoagulated blood is sucked into a capilliary tube and the speed with which the red and white cells settle over a period of 1 hour is observed. Normal values vary with age and sex; although 15 mm/h might be regarded as abnormal for a young person, this might be within normal limits for someone over the age of 60. If inflammation is present in the body the erythrocyte sedimentation rate (ESR) increases. This is in part due to the charges on the red blood cell and also to the inflammatory proteins that are present in the patient's blood. The test is therefore of value in distinguishing inflammatory polyarthritis from the degenerative conditions, providing appropriate allowance is made for the patient's age. Clearly the speed with which the red cells fall will depend in part on their weight. The test is altered by the presence of anaemia, which slightly complicates its use in rheumatoid arthritis (here the plasma viscosity test, described later, is preferred).

The ESR is used as the standard test in many hospitals for evaluating disease activity in rheumatic diseases. Although time consuming for the technician, it requires no sophisticated equipment. It can be used as a monitor of disease activity in seronegative polyarthritis and the connective tissue disorders, and is almost always markedly raised in polymyalgia rheumatica. A very high ESR should prompt the clinician to take a history for polymyalgia and should also alert his suspicion to the possibility of myeloma, a malignant condition of the plasma cells. In the case of the latter, Bence Jones protein, a characteristic protein produced by the cell, may be detected on a 10-ml sample of urine sent to the laboratory; serum electrophoresis on 10 ml of clotted blood may demonstrate the presence of a monoclonal band, produced by the malignant plasma cells.

Routine Biochemical Investigations

As with haematological tests, the normal values vary from laboratory to laboratory and should always be ascertained. Most routine biochemistry is now automated, again with computer print out, and the expense of performing full liver function tests and renal function tests is usually not much greater than performing only a small number.

Biochemical Tests of Renal Function

Electrolytes (sodium, potassium, chloride and bicarbonate or base deficit), together with urea and creatinine are usually measured. The chronic renal failure of connective tissue disorders may produce a high potassium and a low bicarbonate level, and a fast-rising potassium is always a medical emergency; however, on the whole, these investigations have little relevance to rheumatic diseases. Rheumatologists often deal with an age group where the urea and creatinine are likely to be at the upper limit of normal in any case, since renal function deteriorates throughout adult life. The urea may be raised because of dehydration, but creatinine is less likely to be so. The creatinine is the most sensitive simple estimation of renal damage, and a raised level should alert the clinician to the possibility of amyloidosis complicating rheumatoid disease or chronic renal failure from rheumatic disease or other cause. The renal involvement caused by nephrotoxic drugs is more likely to be seen first on routine urine testing.

Liver Function Tests

Bilirubin, SGOT (or SGPT) and alkaline phosphatase estimations are usually made. Sometimes gamma glutamyl transpeptidase, a more sophisticated and specific test of hepatic damage, is given. Total protein, total albumin and total globulin estimates are also provided. In part, these protein estimations reflect hepatic function (particularly albumin, which is made in the liver), although they also reflect factors as diverse as absorption and the inflammation (producing globulins) in the body. Apart from in lupoid hepatitis, which can mimic rheumatoid arthritis, bilirubin and SGOT are likely to be normal. By contrast, alkaline phosphatase is often slightly raised in rheumatoid arthritis, as a function of disease activity. If a raised alkaline phosphatase is noticed, this enzyme may have come either from liver or bone. It is clearly important to determine which, and some laboratories do this by performing tests for alkaline phosphatase isoenzymes, others by determining heat-stable alkaline phosphatase. The resultant laboratory reports will normally indicate whether the raised alkaline phosphatase comes from bone or liver. Gamma glutamyl transpeptidase is sometimes raised in rheumatoid arthritis and may also indicate disease activity, a high value being associated with severe disease and a lower value with disease remission. Some drugs such as azathioprine may cause abnormal liver function tests, and it is possible that salicylates when given for the treatment of systemic lupus erythematosus also cause mild abnormality of liver function.

Biochemical Tests of Bone Metabolism

Laboratories normally provide calcium, phosphate and alkaline phosphatase tests. Calcium is bound to protein and this may need a correction factor if protein levels are abnormal, as often occurs in rheumatoid arthritis. In osteoporosis these values do not change. A slightly raised calcium and a raised alkaline phosphatase level, if of bony origin, should alert the clinician to the possibility of osteomalacia. In Paget's disease there is a markedly raised alkaline phosphatase of bony origin. Radiological confirmation of Paget's disease should be sought, since secondary neoplasms in bone can also cause a raised alkaline phosphatase.

Ward Urine Testing

Urine testing on the ward includes estimation of pH, protein, blood, sugar and ketones. The albumin and blood are of most relevance. Patients with rheumatoid arthritis receiving aurothiomalate or penicillamine check their urine regularly for protein and should report to their physicians if this is seen (although if these drugs, particularly penicillamine, are effective, the physician may be happy to allow a certain amount of proteinuria rather than discontinue the drug). The presence of haematuria in addition to proteinuria in patients receiving either of these drugs is of more sinister prognosis, and if this is seen the drug is normally discontinued. Protein occurring in rheumatic patients who have not received either of these drugs alerts the physician to the possibility of amyloidosis; and renal involvement occurring in connective tissue disorders, particularly SLE, may lead to nephrotic syndrome with resultant proteinuria. More sophisticated tests of renal function (described later) may shortly become more available.

White blood cells should be sought in the urine when infection such as Reiter's disease is suspected; early morning urine specimens are more likely to contain tubercule bacilli than those taken later in the day if this condition is suspected. Glycosuria occurring in the urine of a patient with a rheumatic disease alerts the clinician to the possibility of corticosteriod-induced diabetes mellitus.

Serum Uric Acid

Despite the fact that the serum uric acid level may be raised in patients with gout, there is no alternative for the only reliably diagnostic test, namely the demonstration of uric acid crystals in the affected joint. A certain proportion of the population have a raised uric acid in any case (asymptomatic hyperuricemia), and small doses of aspirin may delay uric acid excretion at the kidney causing a spurious high level. If the patient is taking a uricosuric drug such as probenecid or allopurinol, as used in the treatment of chronic gout, the uric acid will have returned to normal in any case and this is useful in monitoring the effectiveness of this sort of drug treatment in chronic gout. Finally, patients with diseases such as leukaemia and polycythemia will have a raised uric acid level as a result of the increased cell turnover and high production as the white or red cells respectively are broken down.

Immunological Assessment of Rheumatic Disease Activity

Rheumatoid Factor

A circulating rheumatoid factor in the blood (an IgM/IgG complex of two immunoglobulins) occurs in 80% of patients with rheumatoid arthritis. This is more likely to be associated with the radiological evidence of nodules and erosions; nevertheless, if these are seen in the absence of circulating rheumatoid factor it is likely that a 'hidden' rheumatoid factor is present, normally IgG/IgG, which is not detected by conventional tests.

The simplest and cheapest conventional test is the latex fixation test. The serum of blood from patients with rheumatoid factor causes agglutination of latex particles which can be observed on a slide under the microscope. If this is positive, most laboratories proceed to the more sophisticated sheep cell agglutination test (SCAT) in which serum from a patient containing rheumatoid factor, heavy with immunoglobulin complexes, causes the agglutination of sheep red blood cells that have been previously coated with immunoglobulin (IgG). This test is performed at serial dilutions of the patient's serum. If a large amount of rheumatoid factor is present, flocculation of the sheep red cells is likely to be observed with dilutions of the patient's serum as great as 1 in 256. By contrast, if only a small amount of rheumatoid factor is present, flocculation will only occur with relatively undiluted serum, perhaps 1 part in 8, or 1 part in 16. Sometimes patients without rheumatoid factor may also cause this agglutination if not diluted (usually in concentrations of 1 in 4 or 1 in 8); therefore a positive SCAT of 1 in 16 or 1 in 32 is normally sought before making a diagnosis of rheumatoid arthritis. In general, high concentrations of rheumatoid factor are associated with a poorer prognosis.

Since there may be some variation between the batches of sheep cells used, some laboratories perform a duplicate test of 'unsensitised' cells. This is normally positive at a dilution of 1 in 4, but in the unlikely event of the unsensitised cells becoming flocculated at a dilution as great as 1 in 32, a corresponding increase in dilution of the standard (sensitised), SCAT test should be sought before coming to the positive diagnosis of rheumatoid factor.

Diagnosis of SLE

The earlier test, SLE cells, has now been superseded by more modern laboratory techniques. The initial screening test for SLE, which is cheap and easy, is antinuclear factor (ANF). This is occasionally seen in other rheumatic diseases but, if positive, the laboratory proceeds to look at DNA binding in serum from the same patient. The serum is set against double-stranded human DNA material (although this tends to degrade with time to single-stranded human DNA material and sometimes animal material has to be used as a substitute), and the presence of antibodies to this material is estimated by using various dilutions. The result is expressed as a percentage, and figures above a certain percentage for each laboratory will be regarded as being diagnostic for SLE. An alternative test using *Crithidia* is sometimes used in the United States. This flagellated organism has a large amount of DNA and may provide a cheaper alternative test.

Diagnosis of Other Connective Tissue Disorders

Extractible nuclear antigen (ENA) is said to be diagnostic for mixed connective tissue disorder. This test is likely to be performed, if requested, if the ANF is positive. Recent research has suggested that there are a large number of other circulating antibodies in the blood of patients with various connective tissue disorders including patients with severe Raynaud's phenomenon and with scleroderma. The significance, both in terms of diagnosis and prognosis, which may help with management still has to be determined, but there is currently considerable interest in anti-Ro and similar antibodies.

Antibodies to Other Organs

Using tissue sections it is possible to estimate the prevalence of antibodies in the patient's serum to a variety of organs. These include thyroid, adrenal, spleen and lymph nodes, or tissue components such as reticulin. Such antibodies are more likely to be found circulating in the blood of patients with rheumatoid arthritis than in normal individuals, but their significance is not certain. Patients with high levels of antibodies to thyroid tissue, however, should be watched for impending myxoedema.

Immunoglobulins

Estimations can be performed of total IgG, total IgM and total IgE. These are essentially biochemical estimations and relatively crude in relation to function of the immune system. They are likely to be elevated in patients with rheumatoid arthritis, but are not so valuable in determining prognosis as immunoglobulin complexes such as the IgM/IgG rheumatoid factor. However, IgM (which is largely derived from presence of this rheumatoid factor), is likely to be elevated in rheumatoid arthritis and its level may correlate with disease activity. High concentrations of total IgA, an antibody that is connected with the bowel, may be of value in assessing disease activity in ankylosing spondylitis, a condition in which other biochemical and immunological estimations do not appear to be particularly helpful, perhaps because of the chronicity of the condition.

Circulating Immune Complexes

Some patients with classic rheumatoid arthritis and radiological evidence of erosions give negative results to testing for IgM/IgG rheumatoid factor. These patients are thought to have hidden rheumatoid factor (IgG/IgG). Although special laboratory techniques are now available for detecting this, they are not available in all centres. An alternative method is to evaluate total circulating immune complexes present in the patient's serum. This is time consuming and expensive and further work is required to evaluate how closely these complexes correlate with disease activity; however, they may be of use in a difficult differential diagnosis.

Measurement of Complement and Complement Products

The complement system is a complex series of proteins that are concerned in the mediation of inflammation, possibly triggered by immune complex formation. Various complement products can now be measured, C_3 and C_4 being the most readily obtainable. Total haemolytic complement or CH_{50} is also assayed. They are of research interest and in SLE can be used to monitor disease activity; a falling C_3 level taken in conjunction with a rising titre of anti-DNA antibodies sometimes heralds severe renal involvement in this condition.

Monoclonal Antibody Techniques

It is now realised that lymphocytes have many varied functions. The precise function of each lymphocyte may be declared by the type of protein markers that are present on the cell wall, and recently antisera have been developed to detect these. The use of OKT_4 and OKT_8 antisera enables the detection of subpopulations of lymphocytes each as helper T cells and suppressor T cells.

The former probably stimulate B lymphocytes to make more immune complexes; the latter prevent B lymphocytes from making further immune complexes. These can be used to evaluate blood preparations for research purposes and are currently being used to detect the speed with which the different lymphocyte populations occur early in the rheumatoid synovium, when the disease first strikes.

Examination of Synovial Fluid

Synovial fluid is present in very small amounts in normal joints (about 0.5 ml in the knee joint, although this is sticky and hard to aspirate). In inflammatory polyarthritis and even sometimes in osteoarthrosis the volume may be markedly increased so that aspirations of over 100 ml are occasionally made. If the joint is aspirated to dryness the fluid invariably recurs within 24–48 h unless the disease has been brought under control. In degenerative conditions the fluid is likely to be more dense or stickier; in rheumatoid arthritis and other polyarthritides the fluid is more dilute and the speed with which it can be ejected from the syringe and needle after aspiration may provide a clue as to the diagnosis.

Fluid should be observed under the microscope for white cell and differential cell count. A few red cells may be present as a result of a traumatic tap. In pyogenic arthritis there may be over 20 000 neutrophils per cubic millimetre, and tuberculous effusions contain largely lymphocytes. Rheumatoid effusions tend to have a mixture of polymorphs and lymphocytes, although we have not found the actual number or the proportion of different cells of particular value in diagnosis or management, since this is a relatively non-specific finding for rheumatoid disease, seronegative polyarthritis and even occasionally for osteoarthrosis.

Organisms

If white cells are found the fluid should be stained by Gram staining to detect bacteria. It should also be cultured for bacterial growth; special cultures are required if tuberculosis is suspected.

Examination for Crystals

Examination for crystals should be done under a special polarising microscope, and crystals of uric acid or calcium pyrophosphate may be detected. Dirt on the microscope slide or coverslip provides a frequent false positive, and scrupulous attention is required to the cleanliness of the slide. Crystals are more significant if they have been engulfed by white cells.

Further Tests on Synovial Fluid

In the 'mucin clot' test acetic acid is added to the joint fluid, producing a tight mass of precipitated material in osteoarthrosis and a clot which is more stringy in rheumatoid arthritis.

It is perhaps more satisfactory to look for rheumatoid factor in synovial fluid. In the monoarthritis of early rheumatoid disease this may be found in synovial fluid of the single affected joint before it is found in the blood. Tests on immunoglobulins may also be performed on synovial fluid and these, together with the new monoclonal antibody techniques (mentioned later), are likely to supersede the mucin clot test.

Occasionally glucose may be estimated in synovial fluid; it tends to be low in any rapidly metabolising effusion. More sophisticated tests such as for the estimation of histidine and sulphydryl have also been studied, but in general these tend to mirror the alterations that occur in the blood, and, since blood tests are less traumatic to the patient, they are preferred.

Biochemical Assessment of Rheumatic Disease Activity

Although rheumatoid arthritis is essentially an immunological condition, laboratory variation and difficulty with immunological techniques have meant that, in general, biochemical estimations of disease activity are cheaper and more reproducible than immunological assessments. The following tests are of interest in correlating disease activity in rheumatoid arthritis with improvement produced by drugs. Some of them may be of use in certain connective tissue disorders and they are generally of use in seronegative spondarthritides—with the possible exception of ankylosing spondylitis, where biochemical and immunological assessment is much more difficult.

Plasma Viscosity

The plasma viscosity test mimics ESR evaluation but studies the movement of plasma in a horizontal rather than a vertical plane. It eliminates the variation caused by the anaemia of rheumatoid arthritis. High values are found in untreated rheumatoid arthritis and no values are found in remission.

C-Reactive Protein

C-reactive protein is an acute inflammatory protein produced by the liver in response to insult or acute injury. As such it rises in rheumatoid arthritis and falls to normality after the disease comes under control. Changes in C-reactive protein occur faster than in the other biochemical assessments mentioned and, interestingly, it is usually normal in SLE, only rising in the presence of infection.

Other Acute Phase Reactants

A variety of similar proteins behave rather like C-reactive protein and some of these are of particular interest in rheumatoid disease. Fibrinogen, hapto-globin and caeruloplasmin all behave as acute phase reactants, having high values in untreated rheumatoid disease and low values as the disease comes under control. Of particular interest are certain protein fragments that coalesce together to form amyloid. Whether the presence of these in the blood at an early stage in rheumatoid arthritis is a reliable predictor of patients who will subsequently go on to develop renal impairment, as the result of amyloidosis, is the subject of much current research.

Total Serum Sulphydryl

Protein groups containing sulphur atoms have raised levels in the blood in patients with rheumatoid arthritis, although these may also be raised as a result of some of the drugs that are given in this condition, e.g. D-penicillamine. Their assay is not always consistent from laboratory to laboratory.

Serum Histidine

Of the various amino acids found in the body, serum histidine has a particular and uniquely low level in the blood of patients with rheumatoid arthritis. It returns to a normal level as the disease comes under control, and this can be used as an index of response to appropriate drug therapy.

Detection of Infection

As already mentioned, the differential white blood count will give valuable information on the suspected presence of infection. However, this needs to be complemented with various other laboratory investigations.

Antistreptolysin O Titre

The antibody to the product of streptococci, antistreptolysin O (ASO) titre is raised temporarily in patients with rheumatic fever. A streptococcal sore throat is followed by rheumatic fever in less than 2% of patients. However, a raised ASO titre does not necessarily prove the presence of rheumatic fever, which in any case is an extremely rare condition in western Europe at present. Serial ASO titres are required and, even if positive, do not confirm rheumatic fever, since these are likely to have been the result of a simple streptococcal sore throat.

Viral Antibody Assay

Biology laboratories are now able to provide a variety of antibody assays for common viral illnesses. For example, a Paul–Bunnell test is likely to be requested if glandular fever is suspected. The viral illness most relevant to rheumatology is probably rubella. The assay technique requires the provision of paired clotted blood samples, usually 2 weeks apart. In addition, the virologist will need to know the time relation of these samples to the onset of the symptoms before giving an opinion. Such antibody assay techniques are more reliable than the differential white blood count in detecting viruses in the blood of patients.

Blood Culture

In suspected bacterial infections, in contrast to suspected viral infections, blood culture may enable the organism to be detected after a period of growth in an appropriate culture medium. Strict aseptic technique should be used in the collection of these blood specimens (not so essential in the collection of serum viral antibodies).

Gonococcal Complement Fixation Test

If gonococcal arthritis is suspected, the gonococcal complement fixation test (GCFT) is used. Unfortunately, the results are fairly inaccurate, with frequent false positive findings. Blood culture for gonococci or joint aspiration for gonococci is also notoriously unreliable, since the organisms are delicate and are not easily identified outside the body.

Brucella Agglutinins

If brucellosis is suspected, *Brucella* agglutinins may be sought, and this investigative technique is preferable to attempting to grow the organism.

Radiology

Differential Diagnosis

A full description of differential diagnosis is beyond the scope of this chapter. The joints selected for radiological examination are likely to be those giving the symptoms, though in early rheumatoid arthritis the feet and hands, particularly the former, yield the best results. Examples of changes that occur at peripheral joints, already mentioned in Chapter 1, are shown in more detail here. Figure 2.1 shows typical peripheral joint involvement in early and late osteoarthrosis, Fig. 2.2 in early and late rheumatoid arthritis and Fig. 2.3 in gout. Bone sclerosis, osteophytosis and new bone formation is characteristic of osteoarthrosis. Erosions occur both in rheumatoid arthritis and in late

1   2

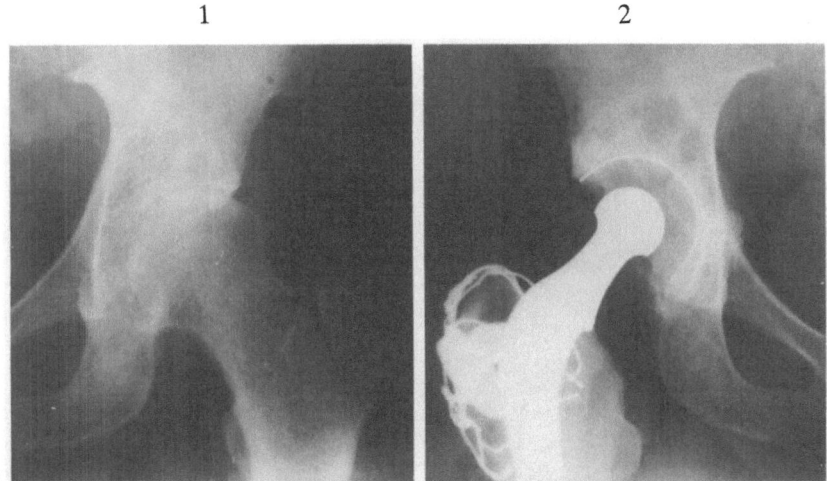

Fig. 2.1a–c. Osteoarthrosis. **a** At the right hip (**1**) there is early osteoarthrosis with loss of joint space and increased bone density around the hip joint. The disease in the left hip (**2**) was more severe and a total hip arthroplasty has been performed.

1   2

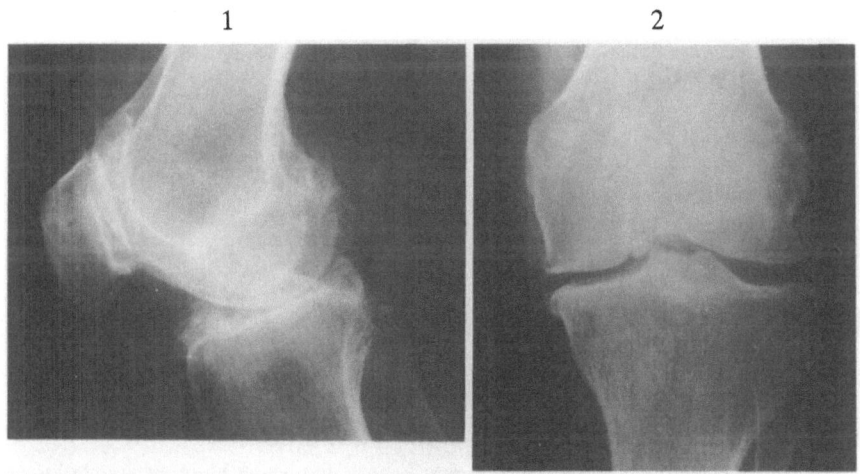

Fig. 2.1b. Lateral (**1**) and anteroposterior (**2**) views of the same knee. There is loss of joint space, particularly in the medial compartment, and osteophyte formation. There is also increased bone density, and the lateral view shows extensive bony proliferation.

1   2

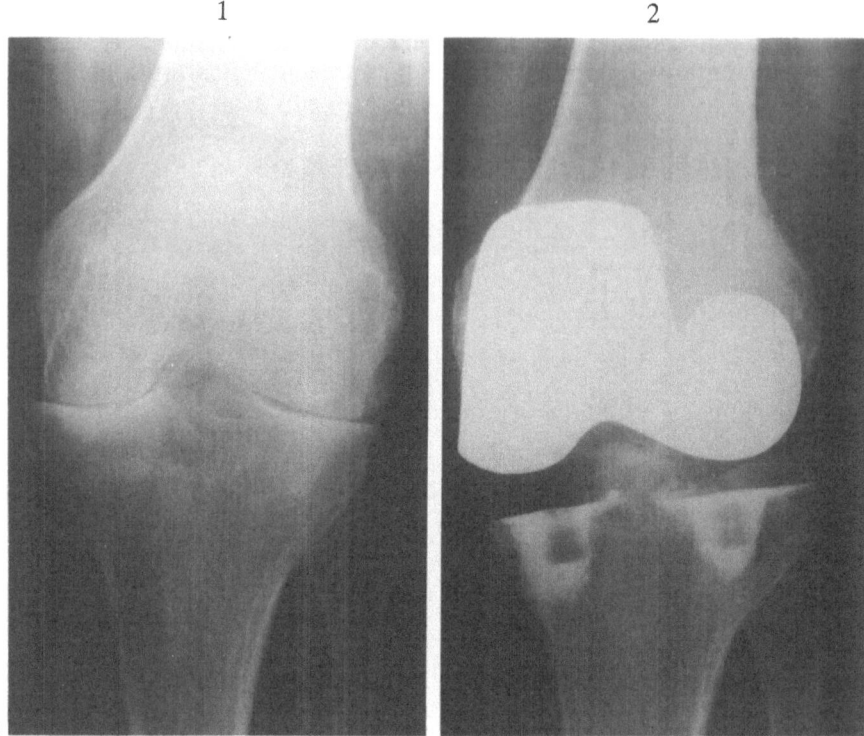

c

Fig. 2.1c. Osteoarthrosis of the knee: before (**1**) and after (**2**) knee joint replacement.

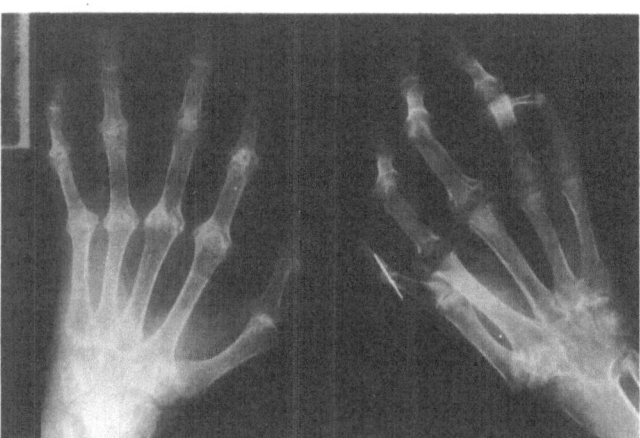

Fig. 2.2. Rheumatoid arthritis. There is severe joint destruction at all metacarpophalangeal joints and proximal interphalangeal joints. Subluxation has occurred at some joints and a pin has been inserted to stabilise the thumb of the right hand. There are Silastic implants at the metacarpophalangeal joints of the right hand.

gout but their size and position differs between the two diseases. Figure 2.4 demonstrates changes of degenerative joint disease in the lumbar spine with a reduction of space between adjacent vertebrae and new bone formation. By contrast, Fig. 2.5 shows the rather different variety of new bone formation that occurs in ankylosing spondylitis with bridging between adjacent vertebrae, the joint space between them being better maintained.

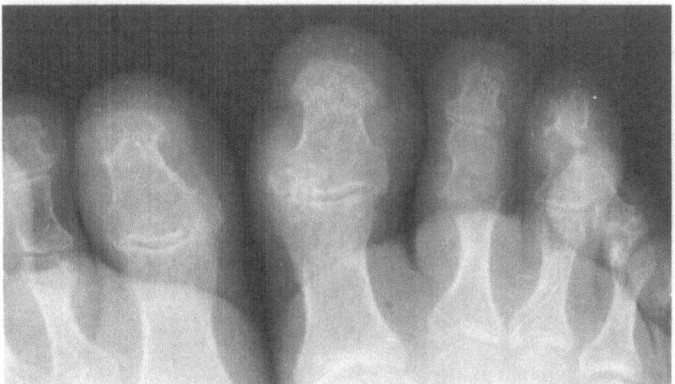

Fig. 2.3. Gout. Large punched-out erosions are present, particularly in the metatarsophalangeal joint of the second toe on the right foot and at the interphalangeal joint of the third toe on the right foot.

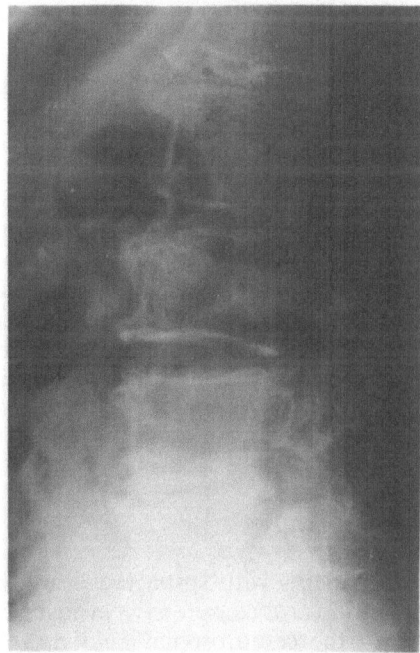

Fig. 2.4. Degenerative joint disease in the lumber spine. There is loss of joint space at the intervertebral discs and osteophyte formation with some bony sclerosis on the vertebral bodies.

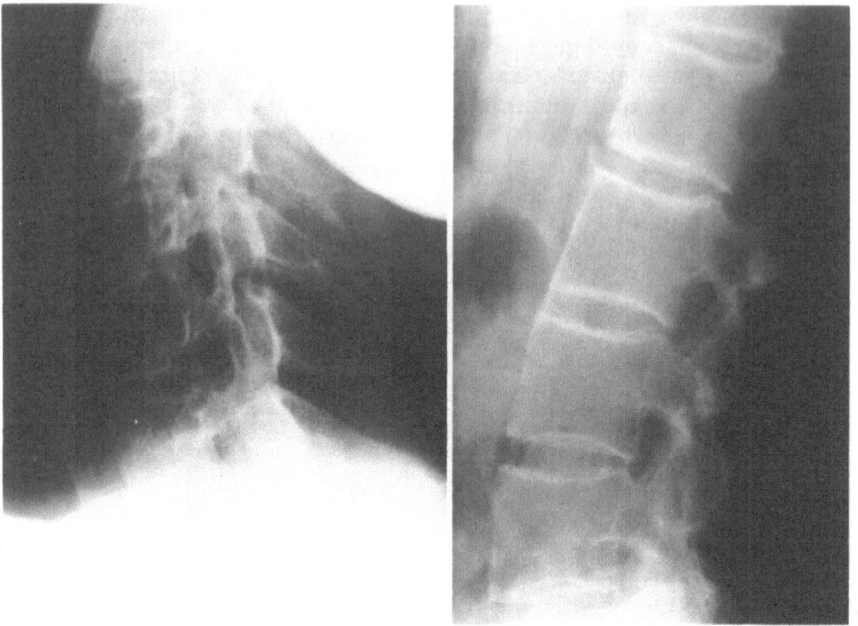

Fig. 2.5a,b. Ankylosing spondylitis. **a** Radiograph of neck. The vertebrae show a squared-off appearance and bony bridges between adjacent vertebrae. **b** Radiograph of lumbar spine. There is bony bridging between adjacent vertebrae, leading to the formation of a 'bamboo spine'.

Use of Radiology in Determining Joint Architecture

If surgical intervention is to be considered, the surgeon is likely to want an appropriate radiograph of the joint in question and possibly of related joints. A new hip replacement, for example, may throw undue strain on the other hip and both knees, and the integrity of these other joints will need to be considered prior to embarking upon surgery. If synovectomy is to be considered it may be of use to have knowledge of joint architecture. This may be best achieved by comparing straight radiographs (which show the bony contour and the soft tissue) with air insufflation studies, where air is injected into the joint cavity and the soft tissue is better delineated, and even with arthrography, where a radiopaque dye is injected into the joint cavity and the resultant synovial contour demonstrated.

Myelography

In patients with suspected disc lesions, particularly if these are leading to neurological compression syndrome, myelography or the introduction of dye into the cerebrospinal fluid may be indicated. Strict aseptic technique is required and the skin of the patient, particularly the lumber spine, should be cleaned appropriately before the investigation. The patient should be rested in a prone position, probably for 24 h, on return to the ward. Since patients occasionally develop an allergic reaction, routine pulse and blood pressure estimation should be performed, at hourly intervals initially.

EMI Scans

The main contribution of the EMI scanner to diagnostic radiology in rheumatic diseases has been the revelation that the spinal canal of different individuals varies from a circular or oval shape to a triangular shape. Patients with a triangular spinal canal are more likely to suffer from prolapsed intervertebral disc, since the shape of the canal allows for more easy nerve entrapment if the disc is out of place.

Microfocal Radiography

Although originally introduced to study trabecular bone structure, the technique of microfocal radiography may be of increasing value in the detection of early rheumatoid disease and crystal deposition disease. At present the equipment required costs something in excess of £50,000 and the technique is only available at one or two centres in the United Kingdom. It would clearly be of value to have 'magnified' radiographs of the joints in the early detection of rheumatoid erosions. Although conventional X-ray films can be enlarged using standard photographic techniques, it is nevertheless impossible to improve upon the quality of the original image. If this failed to demonstrate the erosion in the first place, successive magnification will also fail to reveal it. In microfocal radiography special X-ray apparatus is used to give a picture with higher definition, which in turn is blown up in a photographic sense (Fig. 2.6). This allows for the earlier detection of erosions and may be of value in the early detection of crystal deposition disease. The method is at present only available for the study of small joints, and one possible slight disadvantage is that the period during which the patient is required to keep still is longer than with conventional radiological techniques.

Bone Biopsy

This procedure complements information obtained from radiological examination of bone structure and from blood chemistry on the metabolic state of the bone. It is likely to give more detail, although it is an invasive procedure that is painful for the patient and so can only be attempted, on ethical grounds, in patients where there is a genuine need.

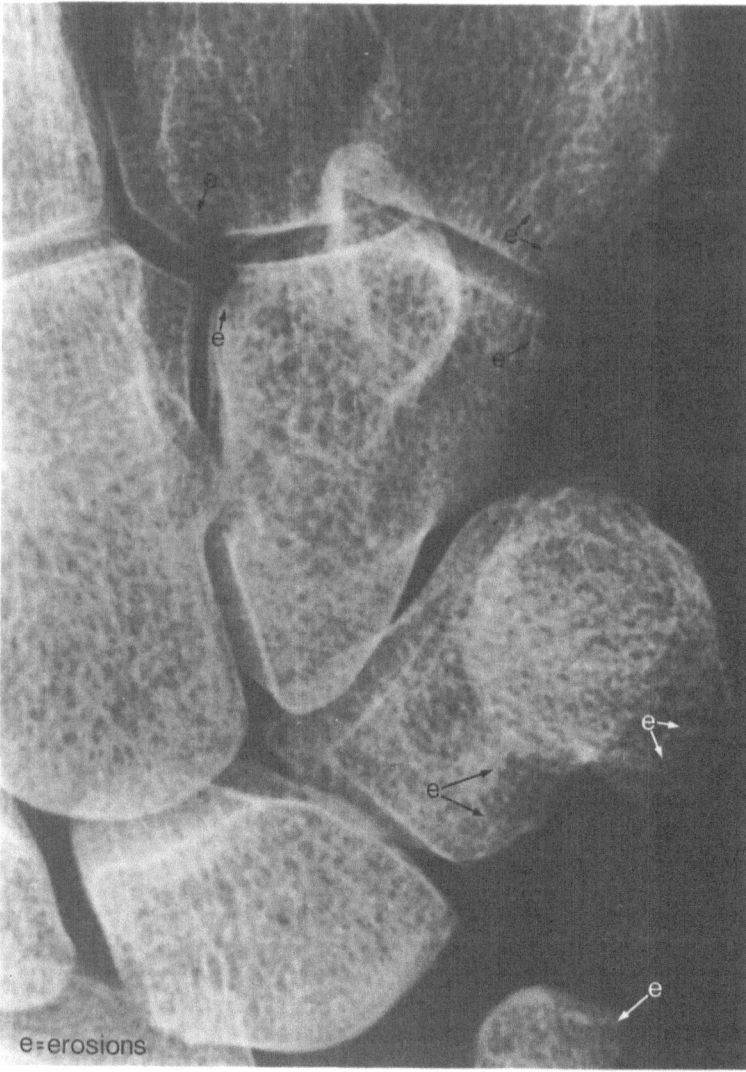

Fig. 2.6. Microradiograph of wrist in patient with early rheumatoid arthritis, demonstrating erosions. (Courtesy of Dr. J.C. Buckland-Wright, Guy's Hospital, London)

The biopsy is normally taken from the iliac bone and can be done in a sterile operating theatre or on a side ward under sterile conditions. Most patients require an injection of pethidine, possibly with intramuscular diazepam half an hour before the procedure. The patient lies on his/her side on a firm immobile bed while the operator scrubs up. An area of skin over the iliac bone is cleaned and the skin, subcutaneous muscle and bony periosteum below is infiltrated with copious amounts of 2% lignocaine. A 1-cm incision is made in the skin with a sterile scalpel blade, and a pair of blunt forceps is entered into the wound and used to dissect apart the muscle bellies until the periosteum is reached. The sterile bone biopsy instrument is then inserted. This comprises two concentric hollow tubes, each about 15 cm long. The outer one is an 'anchor', and the inner one the 'cutter'. Through their centre can be inserted a solid rod which is used to eject the bone biopsy. The outermost concentric tube is anchored onto the periosteum by pressing in the two sharp foot processes. The inner concentric tube, which has a sharp cutting edge, is then used to bore down through the bone, requiring considerable brute force on the part of the operator. Ideally it passes right through the bone, taking a full thickness of core about the size of a cigarette butt. The central tube, with the bone biopsy inside, is then withdrawn and the biopsy ejected using the third central rod into formalin/saline solution. This is forwarded to the laboratory for decalcification and histology. Once haemostasis is achieved by direct pressure, the wound is closed with sutures to the skin and the patient is nursed in bed with a firm pressure bandage to the area of the incision to prevent muscle haemorrhage for the next 8 h. Postoperative pain is common, and patients are likely to need one or two further injections of pethidine to control this.

Quantified histology allows an estimation of the proportion of osteoid in the bone fragment. (Full-thickness biopsy specimens where the biopsy device has passed through the full thickness of the iliac bone are preferable to half-thickness specimens where the biopsy stops short at the bone marrow cavity.) This allows the presence of osteomalacia and/or osteoporosis to be measured.

Investigation of Muscle Disorders

If polymyositis is suspected, there may be a raised level of creatinine phosphokinase or aldolase, both enzymes that are detectable in the laboratory and are present in raised amounts in the blood when inflammatory muscle disease is present. Such patients are also likely to have a raised ESR and raised levels of acute phase proteins.

Electromyography

If muscle disease is suspected, electromyography should be performed. The skin over the muscle is cleaned and appropriate electrodes are connected. During activity the muscle gives off an electrical discharge which can be detected on the oscilloscope and recorded on a moving paper roll (electromyogram) or alternatively the electrical signal can be transformed into sound. The primary disorders of muscle produce specific electrical abnormalities (Fig. 2.7).

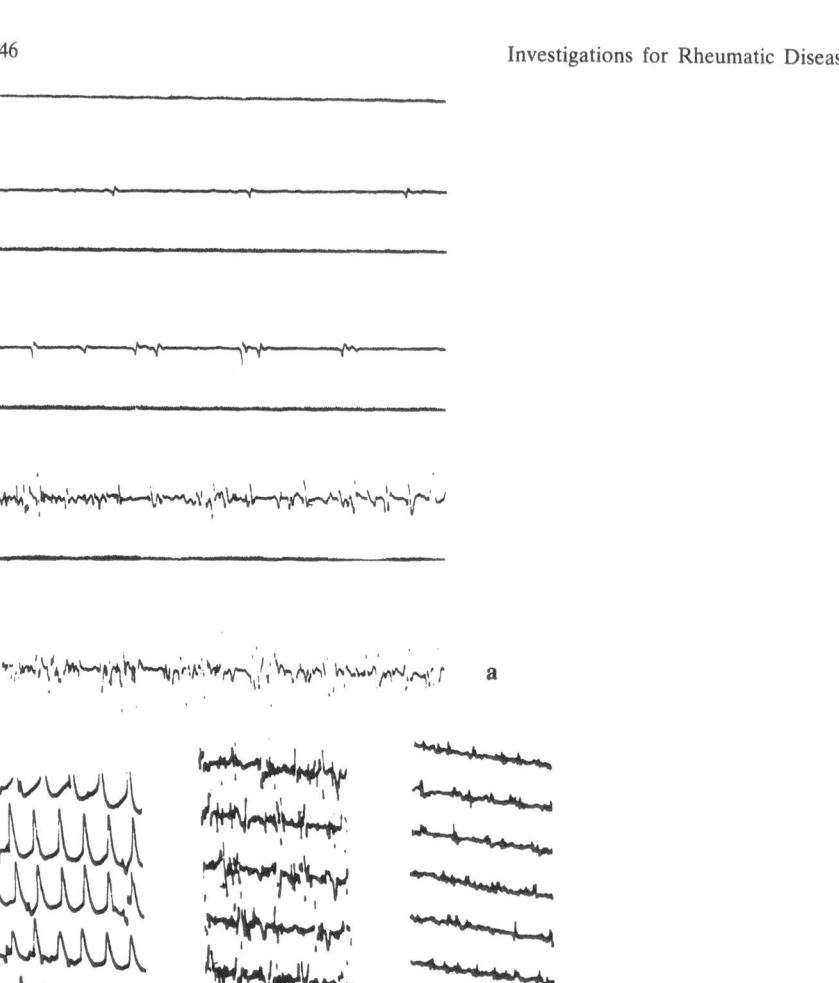

MYOTONIA   NEUROPATHY   MYOPATHY

Fig. 2.7a,b. Normal and abnormal electromyograms (EMGs). **a** Normal EMGs. These vary from minimal contraction (*top*) to strong contraction (*bottom*). **b** Abnormal EMGs.

Muscle Biopsy

If electromyography fails to clarify the diagnosis, muscle biopsy can be performed. This is normally done in a surgical theatre under sterile conditions, since a relatively large amount of muscle may be required, particularly if motor end plate studies are to be performed. The muscle in the upper arm or upper leg is normally used, and an adequate incision is made to allow part of the muscle to be dissected. The muscle is likely to require suturing to provide adequate haemostasis, and the skin should also be sutured. Routine histology can be performed if the diagnosis of polymyositis is suspected; however, if clarification between rheumatoid myopathy and neuropathic myopathy is sought, more sophisticated histological techniques, including motor end point biopsy, are required.

Nerve Conduction Studies

If an entrapment neuropathy is suspected as a cause of symptoms, nerve conduction studies should clarify the diagnosis. Appropriate electrodes are placed proximal and distal to the suspected entrapment on the particular nerve. Clearly a good knowledge of anatomy is required. The nerve is then stimulated and the time required for nervous impulses to reach the distal recording electrode is calculated. This enables the presence or absence of a lesion slow in conduction to be localised. Figure 2.8 shows the sites at which electrodes are placed on the arm over the underlying nerves. The nerve is then stimulated and the passage of the impulse along the nerve is recorded at three separate sites, S_1, S_2 and S_3. Traces taken simultaneously from these three sites show the time interval that elapses (T_1, T_2, T_3 respectively) as the

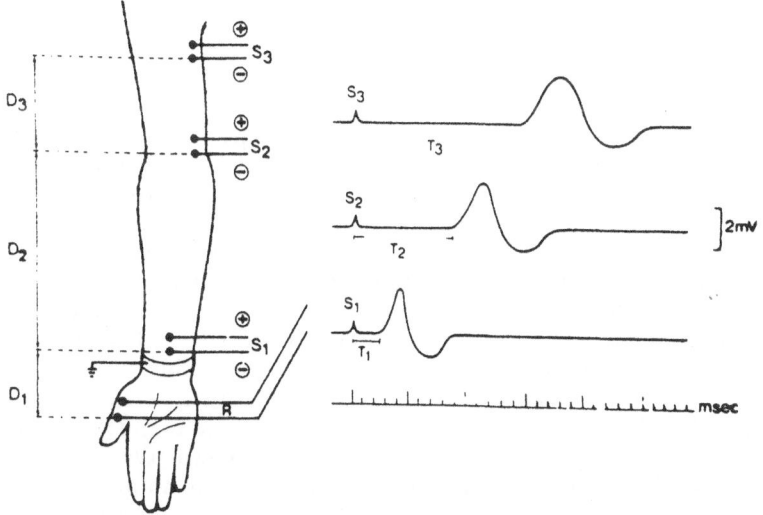

Fig. 2.8. Techniques of measuring nerve conduction studies. [Bradley WG (1974) Disorders of peripheral nerves. Blackwell Scientific, Oxford]

current passes along the arm. A delay in the impulse reaching one of these sites would suggest impaired conduction; comparison of the traces between the sites allow the place at which this is occurring to be identified. Practical examples of the use of conduction studies are in the diagnosis of carpal tunnel syndrome, where the median nerve is compressed under the flexor retinaculum of the wrist in a large number of patients with early rheumatoid arthritis, or in the presurgical assessment of elbow joint arthroplasty, where it is important to determine the extent to which the synovitis at the elbow joint is causing inadequate function in the median, ulnar and radial nerves, all of which pass in close proximity to the diseased elbow.

Tissue Biopsy

Biopsy of a nodule may be indicated if the diagnosis of rheumatoid arthritis is in doubt. Biopsy of skin or muscle may be necessary for the diagnosis of dermatomyositis and polymyositis respectively. Biopsy of skin lesions may be necessary to clarify diagnosis, as in the case of rheumatoid vasculitis, although the findings here are relatively non-specific. Occasionally biopsy of the lymph nodes may be necessary in the early stages of rheumatoid disease in order to exclude lymphoma, since the systemic variant of rheumatoid disease with gross lymphadenopathy can mimic this condition.

Arthroscopy

Arthroscopy is a surgical procedure to visualise the interior of a joint, to take photographs if required and to biopsy under direct vision. The knee joint is the most common joint to be examined by arthroscopy, but machines are available for arthroscopy of the shoulder, wrist and joints of comparable size.

Arthroscopy of the knee is probably best performed in a sterile operating theatre; if rheumatologists perform this technique themselves they are likely to borrow an operating theatre from their orthopaedic colleagues. The procedure can be performed under local anaesthetic. However, if this technique is used, flexion of the knee joint is relatively painful; therefore for full visualisation of articulating surfaces, as may be necessary if a meniscus lesion is suspected, general anaesthetic may be preferable. When the procedure is performed under local anaesthetic the patient is likely to be given a premedication of pethidine and/or diazepam 1 h before. The patient should be sent to the operating theatre in a theatre gown. On arrival in theatre the knee is washed and appropriate sterile drapes applied. Up to 20 ml of 2% lignocaine are injected into the joint cavity, and two needle tracts from the skin to the joint cavity are also anaesthetised. Into one of these a polythene intravenous cannula is inserted and this is connected to

1 litre of sterile dextrose saline solution. The joint is distended with the solution and the volume of fluid that runs in gives some idea of the capacity of the joint, which in turn may be relevant to diagnosis. Osteoarthrosis tends to produce a joint of small capacity; seronegative polyarthritis and rheumatoid arthritis tend to produce a joint of large capacity. With the knee joint fully distended a small skin incision is made, normally on the opposite side to the knee, and the arthroscope is inserted along the second anaesthetised needle track. Once in the joint the sharp trochar is removed and the blunt trochar placed inside the arthroscopic cannula for further manipulation within the joint. When the cannula is well within the joint the telescope is inserted and connected to the light source. The operator scrutinises the inside of the joint, then takes photographs using a special camera attachment and finally, using biopsy forceps, takes segments of synovium as required. Those for conventional histology are placed into formalin/saline; those for crystalline studies are placed in absolute alcohol. The anaesthesia provided by this technique lasts about 40 min, and it is unusual for the procedure to last any longer. After further joint irrigation, running the fluid in through the intravenous cannula and out through the wide-bore arthroscopic cannula (which may in itself have a therapeutic value), the irrigation is stopped and the joint compressed to eliminate all surplus fluid. At this point a single suture is used to close the skin wound. Figure 2.9 shows the component parts of the arthroscope.

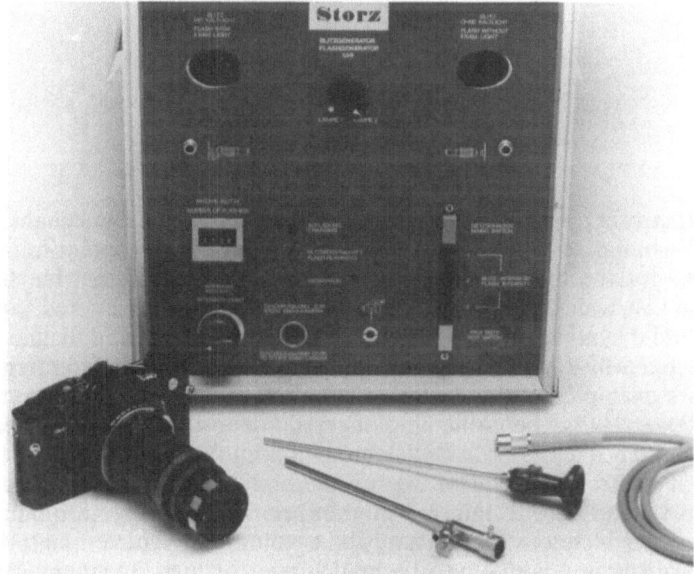

a

Fig. 2.9a, b. Arthroscope. **a** The component parts are assembled and connected to a light source.

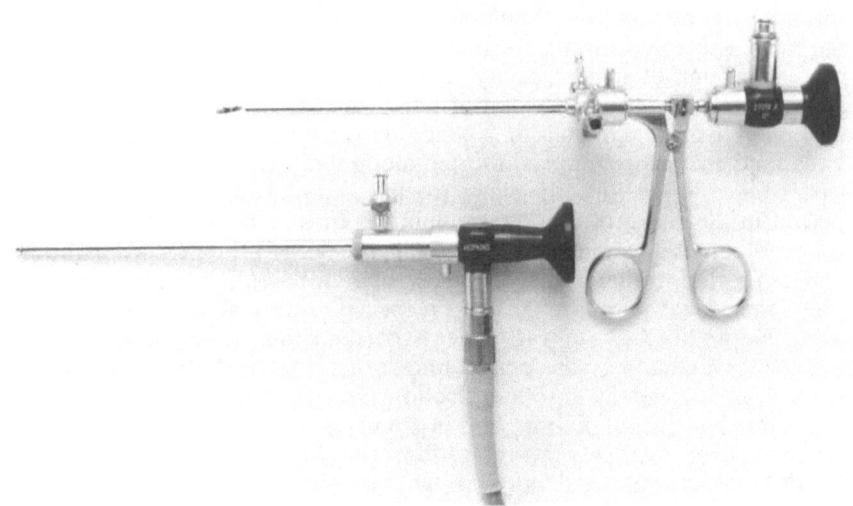

b

Fig. 2.9b. The telescope in place in the cannula. The cannula *above* contains a narrower telescope and biopsy forceps so that biopsies can be taken under direct vision. (Courtesy of Storz)

Although arthroscopy may be of value in diagnosing local mechanical lesions, many rheumatologists feel it has been slightly disappointing. It certainly allows for the biopsy of the synovium under direct vision, but the number of ways in which the synovium responds to disease is limited, and consequently blind synovial biopsy studies do not really clarify the diagnosis when this has been in doubt. Nevertheless, certain broad patterns emerge; Fig. 2.10 shows examples of osteoarthrosis, rheumatoid arthritis and crystal deposition disease. It may be in the field of crystal deposition disease, where crystals that would not necessarily be detected on joint fluid aspiration can be visualised, that arthroscopy will prove most useful in the next few years. There has also been recent interest in monoclonal antibody techniques applied to synovial histology. Regrettably, the volume of synovial material obtained on arthroscopy is likely to be inadequate for these techniques on most occasions, and surgical open biopsy as at synovectomy may well be preferable.

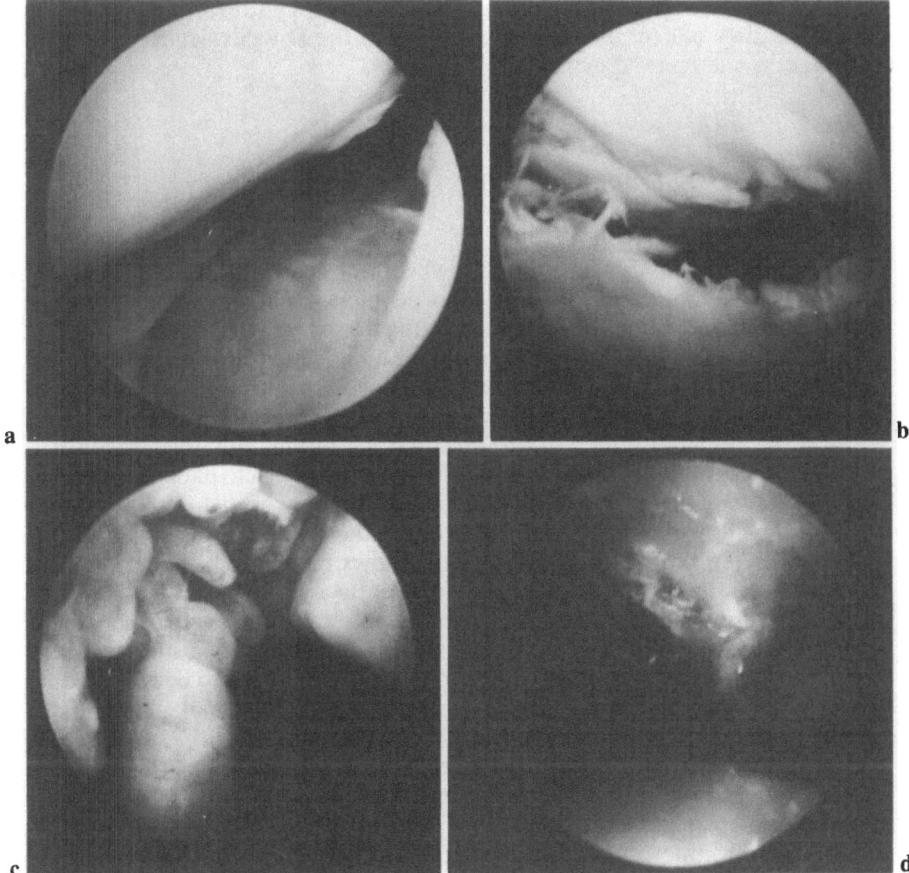

Fig. 2.10 a–d. Arthroscopic appearances. **a** The articulating surfaces are almost normal, with only a minor degree of degenerative change. **b** In advanced osteoarthrosis the articulating surfaces are roughened with fibrillation and loss of the cartilage. **c** In rheumatoid or other inflammatory arthritis there is proliferation of the normally smooth synovium into thick villus formation. **d** In crystal deposition disease, crystals (in this case calcium pyrophosphate) are deposited in the synovium.

Study of White Cell Blood Groups in Rheumatic Diseases

The study of HLA typing is sometimes of use in the management of rheumatic patients, but it has been deliberately left until late in this chapter since in our view it is no substitute for careful clinical diagnosis. Blood samples must be forwarded to the laboratory promptly for HLA studies, which are costly and time consuming. At present tissue typing at the B locus, of use in ankylosing spondylitis, is available in most centres; however, only a limited number of centres offer tissue typing at the D locus, which may be of some use in rheumatoid arthritis.

Evaluation of Faecal Blood Loss

Patients are frequently encountered who are receiving anti-inflammatory agents for rheumatic diseases and who develop a microcytic hypochromic anaemia which is proved beyond reasonable doubt by subsequent studies on iron binding capacity or ferritin to be the iron deficiency anaemia rather than the anaemia of rheumatoid disease. This anaemia is invariably caused by anti-inflammatory agents; however, in an elderly age group one can never exclude the possibility of a gastrointestinal neoplasm. For this reason it is probably preferable to investigate the majority of such patients, and we currently favour the early use of endoscopy. Patients are admitted on a day basis and swallow the endoscope while under the influence of a small dose of diazepam, often given intravenously. This allows visualisation of the whole of the upper gastrointestinal tract, and frequently evidence of hiatus hernia, gastritis or duodenal or gastric ulcer that would account for the bleeding is found. Our own practice is then to treat this by appropriate measures and re-endoscope later if necessary. Further investigation tends to be reserved for those patients in whom no obvious cause of gastrointestinal blood loss is found on endoscopic examination and who are subsequently submitted to barium enema. It should be remembered that iron deficiency anaemia in rheumatoid arthritis often responds better to intramuscular iron injections than to oral iron therapy.

Of research interest is the technique of labelling red blood cells to determine the faecal blood loss that results from existing and novel anti-inflammatory agents. A blood sample is taken from patients and their blood cells are tagged with 100 μCi of chromium 51. The tagged red blood cells are re-injected into the venous circulation, and for a subsequent period of about 6 weeks any blood loss occurring through the gastrointestinal tract can be detected by counting the radioactivity of stool specimens. In the Leeds Unit we ask patients to provide stool specimens throughout four consecutive 24-h periods in every week. This allows the mean daily faecal blood loss to be calculated and we find that 4 days of stool collection over every week is sufficient to eliminate the day-to-day variation that may occur. During the period of the study patients take the various anti-inflammatory agents under test. It should be remembered that the faecal blood loss resulting from an anti-inflammatory agent continues for several weeks after the drug has been stopped (this is particularly true for the new long-acting drugs of the oxicam series), and the study design should make allowance for this. Stool specimens are collected into cellophane bags, which are deposited in hygenic disposable plastic containers. These are forwarded to the medical physics department for counting in a special counting apparatus.

Use of Radioisotopes in Rheumatology

Radioisotopes may be used diagnostically for the imaging of bone and bony lesions or for joints. Radioisotope visualisation of the sacroiliac joints is sometimes of value in the early diagnosis of ankylosing spondylitis, since changes can be detected earlier by isotope then by X-ray. Similarly, it has been suggested that isotope scans are of value in detecting those suspected joint lesions resulting from rheumatoid arthritis that might advance. Isotopes that localise in bone are also available.

Isotopes are also used in quantity to aid assessment of inflammation. An injection of isotope may be made into the joint and the subsequent loss of isotope measured from the joint by regular counting. Alternatively, isotope may be injected intravenously and the uptake by inflamed joints measured, again by regular counting. The techniques are invariably invasive and subject the patient to a small but definite amount of extra radiation and have therefore found more favour in early differential diagnosis than in quantitive assessment of inflammation. Technetium counting is the method most frequently employed. The isotope has a short half-life and joints are usually counted 20 min after the isotope has been given. Indium and xenon are alternative isotopes, but they have not found universal acceptance for various technical reasons. Figure 2.11 shows a typical scan of the hands in a patient with early rheumatoid arthritis.

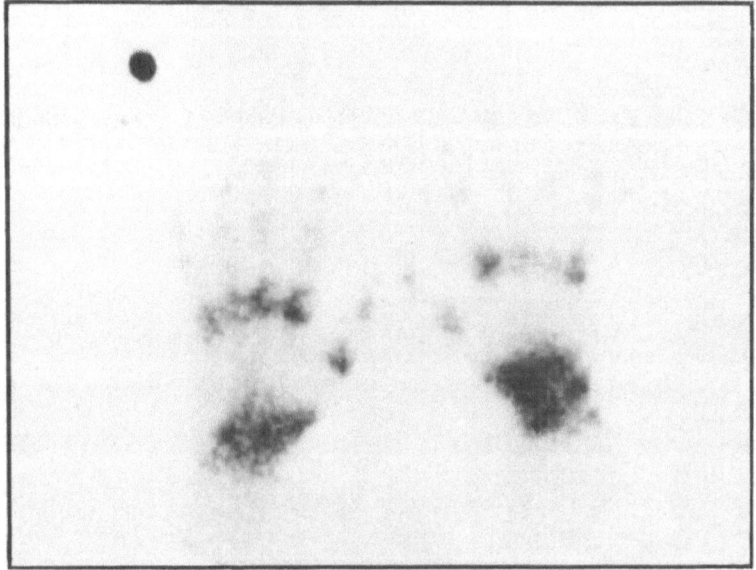

Fig. 2.11. Joint scan of the hands and wrists of a patient with rheumatoid arthritis. The isotope (which appears dark) accumulates in diseased joints. In this case the disease is localised in the metacarpophalangeal joints and the wrists.

Thermography

Infrared thermography provides an alternative method of quantifying in-flammation in joints. The patient is taken to a temperature-controlled room and asked to undress. The joints to be surveyed then equilibrate with the relatively cold room temperature. The patient is asked to stand in front of an infrared heat camera and infrared pictures of the hot joints are taken. Although these thermograms allow visual representation (Fig. 2.12), it is of more use to feed data calculated from the thermograms into a computer, which will provide a single numerical value, the thermographic index. This will

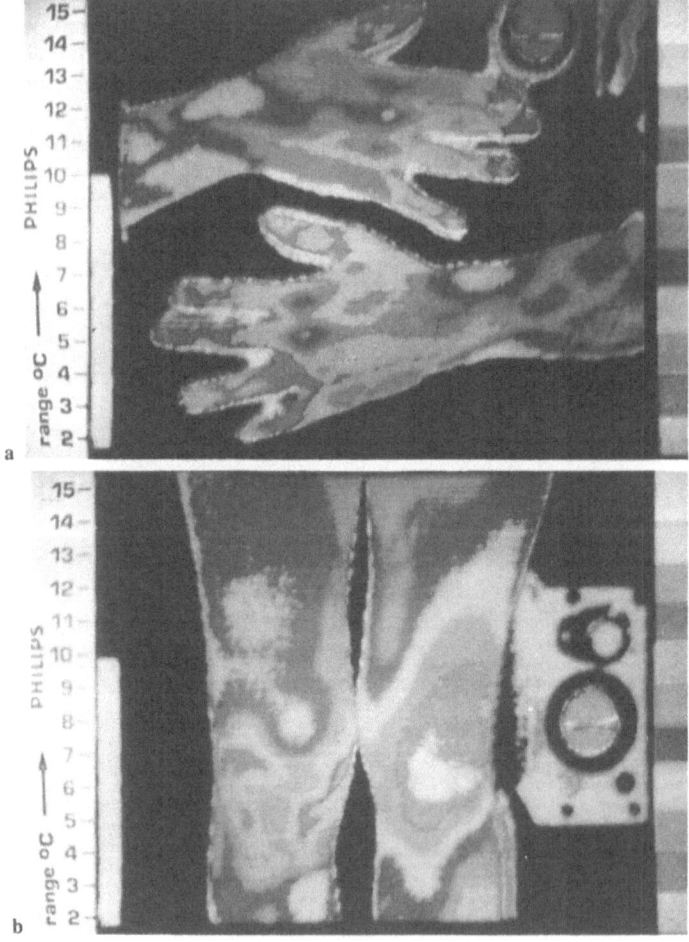

Fig. 2.12. Thermograms of the hands (**a**) and the knees (**b**). The contours of the joints are outlined in different colours from red (hottest areas) to blue (coldest areas).

fall as an administered drug acts to improve the arthritis. Figure 2.13 shows the way in which the thermographic index will change both with conventional non-steroidal anti-inflammatory agents and also, to a lesser extent, with second-line drugs like penicillamine, but not with pure analgesics such as paracetamol. No special preparation is required for this procedure, and serial thermographic indices of the patient's worse joints (hands and knees are normally surveyed) can be entered into the case notes.

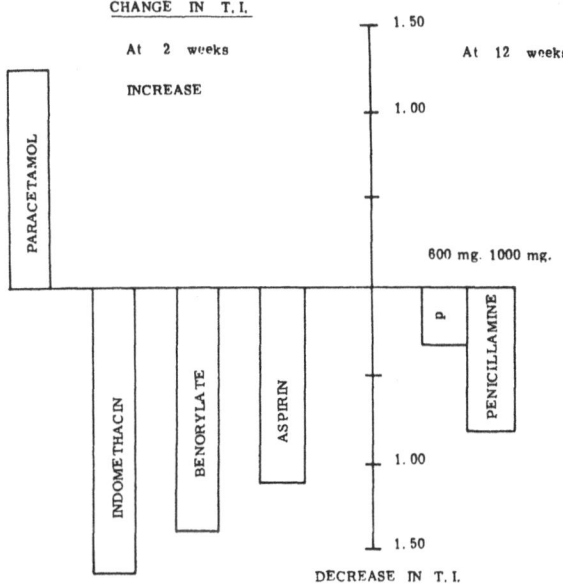

Fig. 2.13. Change in thermographic index (*TI*).

Research Investigation on Urine

Although most rheumatic disease centres will not have the facilities to cope with more than routine dipstick assessment of urine, it should be noted that further sophisticated investigations are available. The *N*-acetyglucosamine (NAG) creatinine ratio is said to be one of the earliest indicators of drug-induced renal damage, and we have used this routinely in our own group in various drug trials, mainly to confirm that drugs are not nephrotoxic. The research assessment of other proteins in the urine such as alpha 1 micro-globulin and beta 2 microglobulin may also be of use in detecting whether certain drugs have a damaging effect on the proximal renal tubule.

3

Treatment of Rheumatic Diseases

Introduction

In spite of the large number of different pathological conditions that can involve the joints, management and treatment are at present less variable. Many conditions such as osteoarthrosis are the end result of a wide variety of initiating factors, and management often has to be based upon relief of symptoms in the absence of a definitive cure. As a result, the spectrum of treatment available is relatively limited.

The rheumatic diseases comprise a large variety of conditions that can involve all age groups of the population. Taking into account childhood arthritis and the relatively young onset of ankylosing spondylitis and rheumatoid arthritis, hospitals devoted to the treatment of rheumatic diseases often attract a relatively young patient compared with acute general hospitals. Consequently, the challenge to the paramedical professions is made more varied and interesting, because of the wide variety of clinical material encountered.

This chapter attempts to discuss some of the treatments available for rheumatic diseases. In the space available we do not attempt to be comprehensive. Furthermore, certain aspects of treatment such as that contributed by the physiotherapist and occupational therapist are dealt with later (see Chap. 6). This chapter deals mainly, though not entirely, with general aspects and drug management of rheumatic conditions. In parts it is speculative as well as authoritative.

Plan of Patient Care

Many rheumatic diseases are chronic disabling conditions. Patients will benefit from a full explanation of their condition and from advice on what they might do to help themselves, to improve their symptoms and how they might best prevent deformity. (Patient education is dealt with in full in Chap. 7.) Patients will also be referred to the physiotherapy and occupational therapy departments at an early stage in their disease (see Chap. 6). Consideration may also be given to patient care in the home environment, with special regard to the social benefits and allowances for which the patient may be eligible (see Chap. 11).

The physician will then turn his attention to the amelioration of symptoms by drugs. Attention will be given in the first instance to general systemic needs. The correction of congestive cardiac failure and of iron deficiency anaemia are examples. The physician will then prescribe drugs that will be specifically active for rheumatic diseases, and a discussion of this occupies the rest of this chapter. Finally, consideration must be given to whether surgery would improve the patient's symptoms and function. (For discussion of the surgical aspects of rheumatic diseases see Chap. 5.)

Analgesics

The majority of patients with rheumatic diseases experience pain sooner or later. Traditionally physicians have concentrated on relieving inflammation, believing that the inflammatory process was the prime cause of these conditions. This may have been slightly misguided; although anti-inflammatory agents relieve inflammation and this in turn may improve pain (most of them act as minor analgesics in their own right in any case), much of the pain in rheumatic conditions arises from mechanical factors. If the joint is eroded, or becomes diseased, the nerve endings may become exposed, and the abrasion of roughened articular surfaces may initiate pain sensation.

Unfortunately, the range of analgesics available in the United Kingdom is not as large as the range of anti-inflammatory agents. Table 3.1 lists the commonest ones that are currently available. Clearly one would wish to avoid the majority of narcotic analgesics listed in this table for the long-term management of rheumatic conditions; however, some of the most popular and successful analgesics do contain small amounts of dextropropoxyphene and codeine, often in combination with other drugs, and there is inevitably a risk of habituation. Nevertheless, it has to be admitted that many of these more potent drugs often work and help the patient when minor drugs such as paracetamol alone have failed to do so. If, after appropriate discussion and having been fully informed by his practitioner, a patient elects to remain on a combination of paracetamol and dextropropoxyphene for the pain relief that it gives him, this decision should be respected. It is of interest that some conventional studies of high-dose paracetamol against comparable doses of paracetamol plus dextropropoxyphene combinations have claimed that the analgesic effect from the paracetamol alone is equal. This would seem to suggest that the addition of a drug with a more potent central nervous system action (e.g. dextropropoxyphene, which one suspects may have mildly

Table 3.1. Classification of analgesics available in the United Kingdom[a]

Peripherally acting drugs	
Drugs with minimal anti-inflammatory action	Paracetamol
	Aspirin (low dose)
	Diflunisal
	Mefenamic acid
	Flufenamic acid
Non-steroidal anti-inflammatory agents	Aspirin group (high dose)
	Pyrazole group
	Indole group
	Propionic acids
Narcotic analgesics	
Methadone group	Methadone
	Dipipanone
	Dextromoramide
	Dextropropoxyphene
Pethidine group	Pethidine
	Fentanyl
	Phenoperidine
	Ethoheptazine
Morphine group—Natural	Papaveretum
	Morphine
	Codeine
—Synthetic	Diamorphine
	Levorphanol
	Phenazocine
	Pentazocine
	Oxycodone
	Dihydrocodeine

[a] Bird HA and Wright V (1982) Applied drug therapy in rheumatic diseases. Wright, Bristol

euphoric properties) may modify pain perception. It remains a possibility that a search for safer analgesics that act via the central nervous system higher centres, possibly without the risk of habituation, may be a more cost-effective exercise for the pharmaceutical industry than the routine trailing of further anti-inflammatory agents.

We have recently constructed a sleep laboratory at Leeds for the evaluation of pain relief in patients with rheumatic diseases. Almost half of all rheumatic patients complain of sleep disturbed by pain, and little research has been done on whether these patients should be given an analgesic (for pain), an anti-inflammatory agent (to relieve stiffness) or a hypnotic (to promote sleep). EEG electrodes are connected to the patient's skull and an EEG machine records the brain potential throughout an 8-h period of sleep. Subsequent analysis enables the sleep records to be scored into epochs, and the proportion of each epoch spent in the various stages of sleep, some deep and some shallow, graded from I to IV, allows direct comparison of different treatments to be made in the same patients. It remains a possibility that psychotropic agents (in combination with analgesics) may exercise more effective analgesic action than the use of non-steroidal anti-inflammatory agents together with analgesics.

Non-steroidal Anti-inflammatory Agents

A selection of these non-steroidal anti-inflammatory drugs (NSAIDs) recently available in the United Kingdom are listed in Table 3.2. It is easiest to arrange these into families since all the drugs are distant relatives either of salicylic acid, indomethacin, phenylbutazone or the propionic acids. Rational management consists of selecting a drug from each of these families in turn and evaluating its performance in the patient in maximum tolerated doses. All these drugs have side-effects, and those produced by phenylbutazone, including the potentially fatal blood dyscrasia, may restrict its use in routine management; however, its successors, although in our opinion not quite so potent, are said not to cause this problem. In the United Kingdom,

Table 3.2. Classification of NSAIDs[a]

Aspirin family (salicylic acids)	
Soluble aspirin	
Effervescent aspirin	
Slow release aspirin or enteric-coated aspirin	
Relatives of aspirin:	Benorylate
	Salsalate
	Choline magnesium salicylate
	Diflunisal
	Aloxiprin
Indomethacin family (indole and indene acetic acids)	
Indomethacin	
Sulindac	
Phenylbutazone family (enolic acids)	
Phenylbutazone	
Oxyphenbutazone	
Azapropazone	
Other acidic drugs	
Anthranilic acids:	Mefenamic acid
	Flufenamic acid
Arylpropionic acids:	Ibuprofen
	Flurbiprofen
	Ketoprofen
	Naproxen
	Fenoprofen
	Indoprofen
	Fenbufen
Arylacetic acids:	Diclofenac
Oxicams:	Piroxicam
	Isoxicam
	Tenoxicam

[a] After Bird HA and Wright V (1982) Applied drug therapy in rheumatic diseases. Wright, Bristol

phenylbutazone has recently been withdrawn from use, except for the treatment of ankylosing spondylitis in specialist centres. Aspirin is likely to cause tinnitus, and indomethacin can cause headaches and fluid retention. Their close relatives are also likely to provoke these side-effects, and it is interesting how patients often seem to respond better to a particular NSAID, there being no 'best buy' for the whole spectrum of rheumatic diseases. Propionic acids sometimes cause skin rash but are arguably the safest of the NSAIDs. Some of the newer propionic acids, for example the oxicams, have the benefit of once daily dosage, although the disadvantage of this is that if side-effects occur it takes correspondingly longer for the drug to work out of the body and their duration may therefore be longer lasting. Oxicams have a long half-life (i.e. the time for the drug to be excreted from the body), which allows for less frequent administration.

All the anti-inflammatory agents cause gastrointestinal side-effects, and this is their main disadvantage. This is because they inhibit formation of protective prostaglandins in the stomach. In general, attempts to alter formulations have not minimised these side-effects. Examples are enteric-coated aspirin tablets (Nu-Seals Aspirin) and slow-release derivatives (such as Indocid-R, which is a slow-release preparation of indomethacin). Some propionic acids have been marketed as 'pro-drugs' (e.g. Fenbufen), the concept being that an inactive metabolite that does not cause gastrointestinal side-effects is taken by mouth and is subsequently converted by the liver into a more active metabolite that spares the patients from nausea and abdominal pain. In general, however, gastrointestinal side-effects are as much a function of systemically circulating metabolites of the drug as of local gastric irritancy when tablets are swallowed, and unfortunately many of these pro-drugs have not achieved the desired effects of sparing patients from gastrointestinal side-effects.

A recent advance has been the mapping out of the metabolism of derivatives of arachidonic acid, called prostaglandins. Most NSAIDs are thought to be inhibitors of prostaglandin synthetase, and this is said to account for their efficacy as anti-inflammatory agents, since prostaglandins are one of the main causes of inflammation. Since prostaglandins have a locally protective effect in the bowel, the propensity of these drugs to cause gastrointestinal side-effects is held to be a direct result of the lower prostaglandin levels produced by them in the gastric mucosa. It is now recognised that there are two main families of prostaglandin metabolites: those derived from PGG_2 (first discovered pathway) and those derived from 5-HPETE. The majority of prostaglandin inhibitors fall into the former group, but a minority (possibly those with longer duration of action and those particularly effective on cellular processes) fall into the latter group. Some recent anti-inflammatory agents have shown specificity for one side of the pathway or the other. Unfortunately, the drugs synthesised so far have seemed particularly liable to produce side-effects, but if safer analogues can be produced it would be of interest to see whether future NSAIDs might have specific actions within prostaglandin metabolism, thus potentially separating the adverse effects of blocking prostaglandin from the beneficial effects. Figure 3.1 shows the main prostaglandin metabolic pathways.

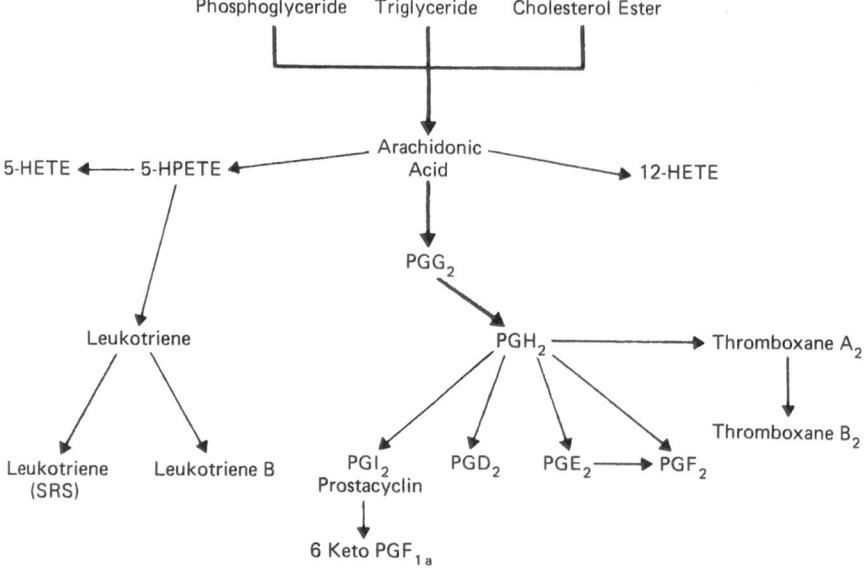

Fig. 3.1. Metabolic pathways of arachidonic acid (prostaglandin metabolism).

Disease-Modifying Agents for Rheumatoid Arthritis

The last 10 years have seen a proliferation of drugs that are claimed to have disease-modifying action in rheumatoid arthritis or second-line activity. Unlike NSAIDs, which simply relieve the symptom and can be used in almost any arthritic condition for this, these drugs are specific (usually) to rheumatoid arthritis and are claimed to actually slow down the rheumatoid disease process. Suggestion has already been made (see p. 36) of the various tests that might separate this property from conventional NSAIDs. It has to be said that final confirmation that a drug 'arrests' the rheumatoid arthritis process (which is as near as rheumatologists can possibly get to a cure) can only come from detailed follow-up of careful radiological studies, possibly over a 10-year period. Microfocal radiography (see p. 43) may bypass this lengthy period of trial, cutting it down to 1–2 years or even less, but nevertheless some rheumatologists still have grave doubts about the ability of these 'disease-modifying agents' to actually modify the disease. There is more unanimous agreement that the quality of life when patients are receiving these drugs is better, even if the actual structural joint damage remains almost unaltered.

The wide variety of drugs that are claimed to have this second-line action is demonstrated in Table 3.3. The conventional drugs are hydroxychloroquine, sodium aurothiomalate and D-penicillamine, together with a group of immunoactive drugs that will be discussed in more detail shortly. To these have been added a collection of compounds, some of them relatives of gold

Table 3.3. Drugs or methods of treatment with proved or possible antirheumatoid activity[a]

Drugs of proved antirheumatoid activity in standard use
  Chloroquine/hydroxychloroquine
  Sodium aurothiomalate
  D-penicillamine
  Sulphasalazine

Drugs of accepted antirheumatoid activity in occasional use
  Gold thioglucose
  Auranofin
  5-Thiopyridoxine
  Pyrithioxine
  Thiopronine
  Dapsone

Drugs with possible antirheumatoid activity
  Zinc sulphate
  Fenclofenac
  Benoxaprofen
  Clozic
  Orgotein

Immunoactive drugs or mechanical methods with proved or suspected[b] antirheumatoid activity

Azathioprine	Thymopoetin[b]
Methotrexate	Antilymphocyte serum[b]
Chlorambucil	Thoracic duct drainage[b]
Cyclophosphamide	Total body irradiation[b]
Thiotepa	Plasmapheresis[b]
Levamisole	Lymphopheresis[b]

---

[a] After Bird HA and Wright V (1982) Applied drug therapy in rheumatic diseases. Wright, Bristol

(such as auranofin), others relatives of penicillamine (pyrithioxine). Others are more novel, such as clozic (since withdrawn) and some are more conventionally classified as non-steroidal anti-inflammatory agents (fenclofenac; also withdrawn in the United Kingdom) that may also have second-line activity in addition to their anti-inflammatory properties. One drug, sulphasalazine, was recently re-introduced for the treatment of rheumatoid arthritis after a gap of some 20 years. It had originally been synthesised for this condition but was borrowed by the gastroenterologists when early trials had suggested that it might not be effective. Recent and more sophisticated work sugggested the early conclusions of rheumatologists might have been incorrect, and the drug has now been shown to be almost as effective as penicillamine in controlled trials.

In general, the use of this group of drugs is limited by their side-effects. Hydroxychloroquine can cause retinal damage; sodium aurothiomalate can cause severe skin reaction, nephrotic syndrome and marrow aplasia, any one of these side-effects being capable of causing death; and D-penicillamine can cause loss of taste, skin rashes, nephrotic syndrome and marrow depression. In general, the side-effects from D-penicillamine, although perhaps slightly more frequently encountered than with gold, are less severe, and this has led many rheumatologists to prefer it; however, many patients feel that the remission they obtained on gold was much more convincing than the re-mission they achieved with penicillamine. The risk of these side-effects has to be balanced against the poorer quality of life if the disease is left untreated and the possible risk that more severe joint damage may accrue if the drug is not given. Our own view is that the value of these drugs more than compensates for the risk of side-effects, although this may reflect the very careful precautions that can be afforded to the patients by the use of clinical metrologists to follow up such patients in special clinics. Patients who default from their series of booked appointments in these clinics place themselves at special risk, and we have found a wide variation in the standard of care amongst our general practitioner colleagues, some being quite assiduous in their scrutiny of patients taking second-line drugs, others preferring to remain completely uninvolved on the basis that they have neither the time nor inclination to take routine blood tests.

The frequency with which precautions should be taken to guard against side-effects is a decision for the physician, who will make it in the light of current progress in clinical pharmacology. The more recent the introduction of the drug, the closer must be the scrutiny for side-effects. Our current policy is to submit patients on hydroxychloroquine to 6-monthly eye assessments once they have been receiving the drug with success for 9 months; patients who have an eye condition that would make such assessment technically difficult should not be started on the drug in the first place (though others would argue that the frequency of retinal toxicity is so slight that this may be an overcautious precaution). Patients on gold and penicillamine have their urine checked with Albustix at weekly intervals while they are receiving the drug and have monthly full blood and platelet counts once they are receiving stable doses. By contrast, drugs such as sulphasalazine cause less serious side-effects. The problem here is that up to 30% of patients develop gas-trointestinal side-effects even with the use of enteric-coated sulphasalazine tablets, so limiting the use of this drug. However, if patients can tolerate it, the only subsequent serious side-effect seems to be a macrocytic anaemia that responds to folic acid and occurs after 6 months of drug therapy in a small number of patients.

The recent plethora of second-line agents for rheumatoid arthritis seems to have two important implications for the future. First, some of the safer drugs such as sulphasalazine may be routinely monitored from general practice rather than from hospital clinics, thus reducing the work load in areas of the country that are deprived of rheumatologists. Second, because the wide variety of drugs available come from a large number of different families, combination therapy may be of particular value. In Hodgkin's disease—a chronic condition characterised by abnormalities of the autoimmune system, which therefore has certain similarities with rheumatoid arthritis—a major therapeutic breakthrough was achieved when anticancer drugs were used in combination rather than alone. The use of gold and penicillamine together in rheumatoid arthritis has hitherto been felt to be inappropriate because both are toxic drugs with a very similar range of side-effects that might have aggregated (although a recent study from Switzerland suggested that this risk may have been exaggerated in the past). Now that drugs are available with similar action but with different spectra of side-effects because they are chemically distinct, polypharmacy may be much safer. We envisage that in the near future more drugs will be given in combination. We also envisage that drugs may be given in series rather than alone. Major breakthroughs in the treatment of ulcerative colitis, for example, came with the realisation that if a remission could be induced by high doses of steroids, this could be maintained by switching to an alternative and safer agent such as sulphasalazine. In Leeds we are currently evaluating the use of pulse methyl prednisolone therapy to initiate a remission in rheumatoid disease followed by the use of a subsequent second-line agent to try and keep symptoms in remission and to enable us to wean patients off the steroids initially used to achieve this remission. Our current studies are evaluating both solu-medrone followed by sulphasalazine and solu-medrone followed by D-penicillamine, as well as repeated solu-medrone alone.

Immunoactive Drugs in Rheumatic Diseases

Although immunoactive drugs have been used in rheumatoid arthritis and connective tissue disorders, particularly SLE and polymyositis, for many years, the precise choice of drugs used varies between countries. Azathioprine is mainly used in the United Kingdom, whereas methotrexate is often preferred in the United States and chlorambucil has most devotees in continental Europe. Cyclophosphamide is regarded as the most potent of the group; however, since its side-effects include alopecia and haemorrhagic cystitis, which can itself lead to cancer, in addition to the skin rashes, hepatotoxicity and risk of marrow aplasia common to all members of the group, there are many who feel that it should not be used routinely in the management of non-life-threatening diseases such as rheumatoid arthritis.

The main problem with all these compounds has been the lack of specificity. It is becoming increasingly clear that the various rheumatic conditions differ in pathogenesis, certain conditions being associated with specific abnormalities of the immune system. The advent of monoclonal antibodies is likely to enable rheumatologists to pinpoint these abnormalities more precisely, and it is hoped that, once this has been achieved, drug therapy can be more specifically matched to the various conditions. This in turn may pave the way for immunomodulating drugs that do not have serious systemic side-effects.

There has been recent interest in drugs that appear to stimulate rather than depress the immune system. Levamisole, a drug originally used for the treatment of worm infections, is one such example, although at present its side-effects seem to outweigh its advantages, even when one uses the modified dosage regimens recently recommended. Thymopoeitin, which is essentially a thymic hormone and may in turn stimulate parts of the immune system, also falls into this category; however, it is not yet commercially available, although it is currently under assessment in a few selected centres.

Mechanical methods of immunomodulation, again restricted to a limited number of research centres, include thoracic duct drainage (the insertion of a surgical cannula into the thoracic duct to remove lymphocytes), total body irradiation (again to destroy surplus lymphocytes) and plasmapheresis and lymphopheresis in which blood from the patient is centrifuged and the different component parts of the blood such as lymphocytes or plasma containing large numbers of immune complexes are removed. Plasmapheresis has recently been the subject of controlled trials in SLE and other rheumatic conditions, with apparently conflicting and not always encouraging results.

Management of Seronegative Spondarthritides

In general, the peripheral presentation of psoriatic arthritis and colitic arthritis responds to some of the second-line agents that are used in rheumatoid arthritis. By contrast, the central spinal involvement of these conditions is less likely to respond, and management more closely resembles that of ankylosing spondylitis, described below.

There has been some discussion that hydroxychloroquine and gold might exacerbate the skin lesions of psoriasis. In our experience this is not necessarily the case and we have occasionally seen dramatic responses in psoriatic arthropathy following the use of gold and azathioprine, though less frequently with penicillamine. Now compounds such as tigason are particularly effective for the skin lesions of psoriasis, and the use of psoralen and ultraviolet therapy (PUVA) is currently under evaluation, but in general the arthropathy does not normally respond to the drugs that are effective in controlling the skin lesions of psoriasis.

Management of Connective Tissue Disorders

Gold and penicillamine are not effective in SLE and related diseases. By contrast, hydroxychloroquine is the only drug that appears to be effective both in rheumatoid disease and SLE, perhaps suggesting completely different mechanisms of action for this particular compound. Management of SLE is with anti-inflammatory agents in the first instance, then possibly with hydroxychloroquine; if the disease advances, the choice is between systemic steroids, cytotoxic drugs such as azathioprine and the perhaps relatively unproven plasmapheresis technique to remove circulating immune complexes.

Management of Ankylosing Spondylitis

At present no drugs are available that arrest the insidious progress of ankylosing spondylitis. This is ironical since the understanding of the aetio-pathogenesis of this condition has advanced recently in comparison to rheumatoid disease. It appears that when the appropriate genetic background—the HLA B27 antigen—and a possible infective stimulus, still to be identified, come together the disease may be triggered. The search for a possible infective agent has been handicapped by the lack of tests that indicate when disease activity is present (ESR provides only limited information). Although IgA currently seems the most likely contender for monitoring serial disease activity (and can even be measured in salivary samples, obviating the need for regular phlebotomy), studies on the use of thymic hormones at times of exacerbation as judged by the presence of clinical uveitis, have not been promising. Our own studies on antirheumatoid drugs have also lacked promise; none of the conventional agents tested have been shown to alter disease progression in ankylosing spondylitis.

Management therefore rests with adequate analgesic and anti-inflammatory control and regular physiotherapy. This is one field where paramedical management is of paramount importance, and several studies have shown that intensive periods of regular physiotherapy, covered by adequate analgesic therapy, have improved the range of movement in involved joints. Clearly this is unlikely to have any effect on the underlying disease pathogenesis, but the symptomatic benefit to the patients is considerable and many patients feel better for regular exercise in formal classes. The exercise classes that have been established in the larger rheumatic disease hospitals in the United Kingdom over the last 10 years bear witness to the advantages of regular exercise. However, some patients are unable to take 2 or 3 weeks off work to come into hospital each year, and for such patients we have recently established regular outpatient evening exercise classes and education sessions at Leeds General Infirmary. It is hoped that more vigorous quantification of improvement should be possible now that remedial exercises have been introduced, and this provides a challenge to the physiotherapy profession. It also remains a possibility that the value of physiotherapy can be enhanced by the concomitant use of adrenocorticotropic hormone (ACTH) injections or even a short, sharp course of systemic steroids, although this also requires critical evaluation before being accepted as fact. The provision of exercise classes for ankylosing spondylitics also enables such patients to meet together in a group and to discuss mutual problems.

Osteoarthrosis and Crystal Deposition Disease

Although a combination of physiotherapy, analgesics, occasional NSAID therapy and particularly replacement surgery usually provides adequate control for this disease, hopes for a drug that might arrest the condition are slim. The first symptoms and radiological confirmation probably occur some considerable time after the basic damage has occurred in the cartilage, which seems to be the first insult. Although it would be theoretically possible to reverse a chemical change in cartilage by chemical means, detection of those individuals who would be at risk and therefore need this intervention would be much more difficult. Some interest has recently centred on a group of people with hyperlax joints who are susceptible to premature osteoarthrosis on a familial basis. These might be particularly suitable subjects for the evaluation of new compounds that might alter the progress of osteoarthrosis, but to date such compounds that have been suggested have not seemed particularly promising. Diphosphonates and superoxide dismutases, for example, have not seemed to be particularly efficacious, although this may be because the correct form in which to deliver a drug that might chemically alter osteoarthrosis is not yet known.

Interest has also focused on the way some variants of osteoarthrosis seem to lead to crystal deposition disease. This is suggested by our own work at Leeds, although not all researchers are in agreement, some feeling that crystal deposition disease occurs before the osteoarthrosis. Assuming that crystal deposition disease is a late consequence, this again may be capable of therapeutic attenuation by drugs that might reduce crystal formation or prevent their seeding. Such therapies would provide relatively strong symptomatic relief at a late stage in the disease rather than prevent the disease from occurring.

Arthritis in Childhood

Many of the drugs that are used for adult rheumatoid arthritis may be tried in childhood arthritis; however, it should be remembered that this is often seronegative and so some of the constraints applicable to adult seronegative spondarthritides seem to occur. Children are also reluctant to have regular injections, and therefore drugs given by the oral route are preferred. Drugs that would alter reproductive cell function such as cytotoxic agents should only be used as a very last resort. Patient education, parent education and patient counselling are particularly important (and rewarding) in this group of patients. Some can be pinpointed as being particularly at risk; children with a positive ANF are more susceptible to anterior uveitis than those with a negative ANF. Such children require careful surveillance.

Patient Compliance

Cooperation from the patient is important in any form of treatment. The return tablet counts and patient education on the taking of drugs will aid compliance; however, studies in which the actual drugs consumed by patients, as measured by the presence of the metabolites of these drugs in their urine, have been compared with the quantity the patients claim to be taking have suggested that even in the best regulated centres as many as 30% of patients are guilty of not following instructions.

One important aspect that is frequently forgotten is the provision of the correct sort of container. Although childproof containers are in vogue, many arthritics find these impossible to open. Blister packs are also found to be particularly difficult to break open by patients with severe arthritis. We have recently completed a comparison of 12 different bottles currently available for the dispensing of common NSAIDs in the United Kingdom (Fig. 3.2). One drug container was outstanding when compared with all the others (Fig. 3.3) and four bottles were judged well above average (Fig. 3.4). The cap and base of the container should be differently shaped, preferably one of them being angulated, so that they can be opened easily. The container should be about 8 cm high. There should be only a short thread on the screw of the cap, and the base and cap should both be of a convenient size for arthritic hands. Glass is unpopular with patients, who generally prefer the safer and less slippery plastic containers.

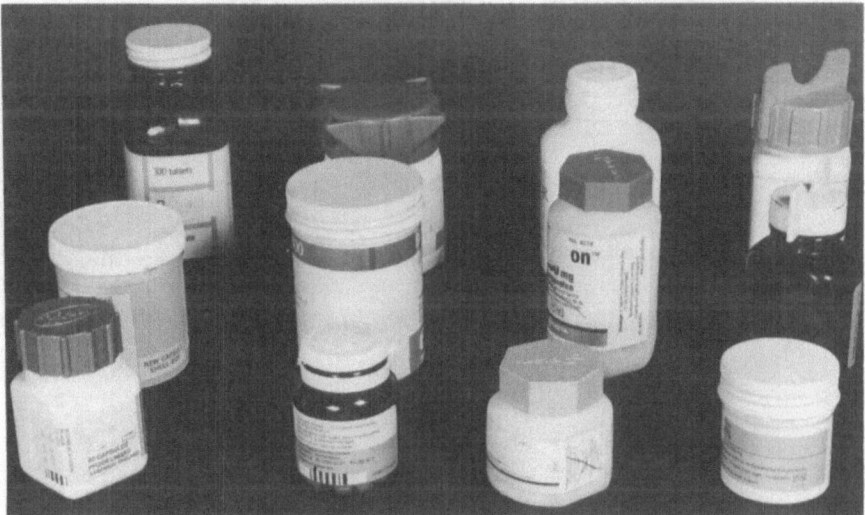

Fig. 3.2. Twelve containers currently used for the dispensing of anti-inflammatory drugs in the United Kingdom. These were the subject of a recent study in Leeds and Harrogate to determine which was the easiest to open by patients with arthritis in the hands.

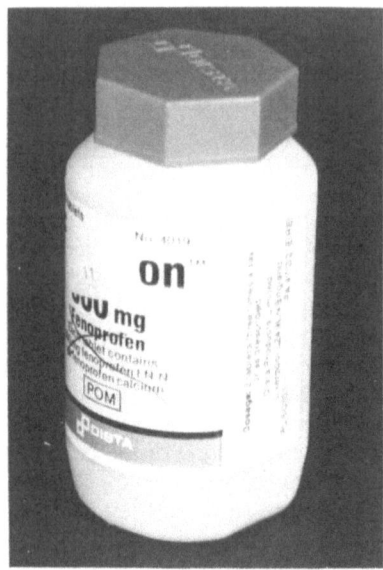

Fig. 3.3. The 'best buy' among the containers
tested.

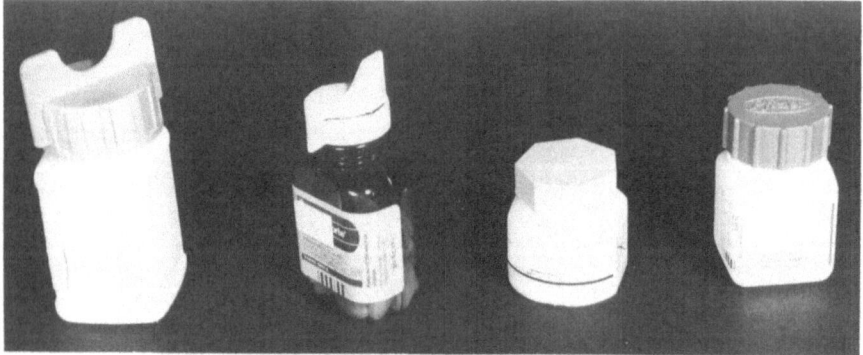

Fig. 3.4 Four containers that were judged as close runners up in the comparative study.

4

The Nursing Process and Rheumatology Nursing

Introduction

Planning of nursing care by use of the nursing process was first introduced into this country by the Department of Nursing in the University of Manchester in 1973.

Over the past 10 years the method has probably caused more consternation, frustration and possibly even resignations than any previous nursing intervention. A large proportion of nurses throughout the country have been consistently vocal in their rejection of the process, on the basis of various aspects which usually revolve around the sheer impracticality of it all. The medical fraternity, who have suddenly become aware of its existence in the more recent past, are in the main suspicious and have criticised it as 'time wasting and an attempt by the nurses to build their own empire', and, most important of all, have asked 'why were [we] not consulted in the first place?' (Joint Consultants' Committee Meeting 1983)

In this chapter a brief outline of the nursing process will be provided, together with case studies to illustrate how it can be applied in rheumatology. For the benefit of non-nursing readers mention will first be made of the more traditional method of nursing—that of 'task allocation'—in order to give a comparison with the nursing process.

Nursing Care by Task Allocation

Under the task allocation system the ward sister has full responsibility for each patient on her ward, and it is she or her deputy who delegates individual patient care to the nurses.

Traditionally, nursing is divided into 'tasks'. Therefore, shortly after arriving on duty, and having listened to the ward report, the nurse will make it her priority to perform as quickly and efficiently as possible as many tasks as the ward sister may care to give her. Throughout the day, as each separate task requires attention, the nurse who is available will be sent to cope with it. During the course of a day she will find herself bathing some patients, dressing the wounds of others, feeding those she has time for, in between escorting patients to and from the operating theatre, the X-ray department or for other forms of diagnostic treatment. Her aim will be to complete her task as soon as possible in order to perform the next task the sister has organised for her.

The nurse will have little time for recognising individual patient problems, or for producing an individual care plan. Evaluation of the care she is giving will evade her as she dashes backwards and forwards from one task to another, attempting to spread herself among the 30 or so patients being cared for in the ward and in the process being able to give only a little of her time to each. The end result is that the nurse becomes 'task orientated' instead of 'patient orientated'.

The patients meanwhile have to contend with the continual staff changes. They must decide for themselves which nurse they can best relate to and hope to catch her eye as she passes on her way to yet another task. Alternatively, they must wait until the ward sister is on duty and free. Very soon after admission they will have realised that if they require information (which is what all patients require) they must ask at the top. A patient's individual needs become swamped by the demands of the other 29 patients all vying for attention from the nurse who happens to be within calling distance.

How different is the philosophy behind the nursing process, which states that every patient must be seen as an individual, with individual problems, and that each patient must be involved in the decisions affecting his or her treatment. In addition, the role played by patients' families must be recognised as an important part of the patients' overall treatment.

It would be impossible to record here in any depth the entire philosophy behind the nursing process. All we can hope to achieve is a brief yet concise outline of the aims of this entirely new approach to nursing. Many books have been written on this subject, and all are well worth reading, though initially they may appear conflicting. Some authors suggest that five stages are required to identify each problem, others postulate four. Some have a concept of the process as a circle, whilst others visualise a spiral. We, however, use five stages as a basis for implementation in rheumatology. Yet each unit must make this decision for themselves. In identifying each stage they may well choose different names, though essentially they will be describing the same thing.

The Nursing Process

The nursing process is a problem-solving approach to nursing. Its methodology is based upon a nursing history which involves discussion with the patient and his relatives and which may incorporate observation and clinical measurements. Following from this discussion an assessment of the individual patient is made which involves identification of patient problems, goals to be achieved and nursing action to be taken. Finally, an overall evaluation is made of the nursing care given.

The five stages are:

1. Nursing history
2. Assessment
3. Planning
4. Implementation
5. Evaluation

Stage 1. Nursing History

Ideally the nursing history will be taken as soon as possible after admission. Sufficient time must be spent over this, otherwise problems will be missed. To aid the nurse and also save time, predetermined questions can be drawn up and assembled onto charts. Well-planned charts will ultimately produce information, for identification of individual patient problems, although it should be remembered that not all patients will have problems. These may be identified by the patient, nurse or relative, though it is usually by a combination of all three. Problems may be physical, emotional or social. With experience, charts may eventually be replaced by a written case history taken either in front of the patient during interview or immediately afterwards. Other documents from which information may be taken to complete the nursing history are the medical notes and the notes of the medical social worker. Observation of the patient is a crucial aspect of the history, and it would be helpful if the nurse involved could accompany the doctor during the medical examination, thus eliminating duplication of notes.

Figure 4.1 is an example of a history chart divided into sections to facilitate the easy recording of personal details, medical history, clinical assessment and medication details.

a

NURSING HISTORY	NAME OF ASSESSOR	DATE	TIME	WARD

CONSULTANT:

NAME:

ADDRESS:

D.O.B.:   AGE:

HOSPITAL NO.:

DATE OF ADMISSION: TIME:

ADMITTED FROM:

RELIGION:

MARITAL STATUS:

NEXT OF KIN:

NAME:

ADDRESS:

TEL. NO.:

HOME: WORK:

G.P.:

DISTRICT NURSE:

HOME HELP:

DAY CENTRE:

VISITORS: YES/NO

IF NO, WHY?:

GENERAL APPEARANCE/MENTAL STATE

SOCIAL HISTORY

OCCUPATION:

CHILDREN: AGES:

OTHER DEPENDANTS:

LIVES ALONE/WITH RELATIVE

HOUSE   FLAT   BUNGALOW

PART 3   SHELTERED

RESIDENTIAL CARE

TOILETS   BEDS

HEATING

PAST MEDICAL HISTORY

OPERATIONS:

PROSTHESIS   YES/NO   (See page 2)

HEALED GASTRIC/DUODENAL ULCERS

CONCOMITENT DISEASE - SPECIFY

PSYCHIATRIC ILLNESS:

VALUABLES HELD:

REASON GIVEN TO PATIENT FOR ADMISSION:

PROVISIONAL DIAGNOSIS:

URINE:

WEIGHT: HEIGHT:

PRESENT MEDICAL HISTORY AND REASON FOR

ADMISSION

ACUTE FLARE

REHABILITATION

DIAGNOSIS

SOCIAL

RA   OA   AS   PMR

C. SPINAL

OTHERS

ANAEMIA   YES/NO   Hb

CHEST   YES/NO

ULCER   YES/NO

GASTRIC   DUODENAL

CLINICAL ASSESSMENTS ON ADMISSION

CONDITION OF:	Joints A.I.	Pain 0,1,2,3	Swollen	Prosthesis Date	I.A.I. Date	MORNING STIFFNESS HOURS MINS
MOUTH GOOD/POOR	Temporomandibular					
DENTURES CROWNS	Cervical spine					
	Sternoclavicular					T
EYES GOOD/POOR	Acromioclavicular					P
GLASSES CONTACT LENSES	Shoulder R L					R
HEARING GOOD/POOR	" R L					
AIDS	Elbow R L					
	" R L					
SPEECH GOOD/DIFFICULTIES	Wrist R L					B/P
	" R L					
APPETITE	M.C.P. R L					FUNCTIONAL GRADE
DIET – NORMAL/SPECIAL	P.I.P. R L					1
SPECIAL DISLIKES	Hips R L					2
SLEEP PATTERN	Knee R L					3
BLADDER	Ankle R L					4
BOWELS	Talocalcaneal R L					5
SMOKES	Midtarsal R L					
ALCOHOL	M.T.P. R L					
CONDITION OF PRESSURE AREAS	Score					

MOBILITY:	GOOD	FAIR	POOR
AIDS:			
WALKING STICK		CALLIPERS	
ZIMMER		CRUTCHES	
SPINAL COLLAR	NIGHT – DAY		
WRIST SPLINTS:			
RESTING WORKING			
SHOES			
OTHERS			

		GRIP STRENGTH			GONIOMETER READING	
		R	L		R	L
1.						
2.						
3.						
TOTAL						
MEAN						

LEG ULCERS   YES   NO

WHERE

PATIENTS ASSESSMENT OF PAIN ON ADMISSION

1   2   3   4   5

b

c

MEDICATION SHEET

PAST MEDICATION	DATE	PRESENT MEDICATION		COMMENCED	MEDICATION ON DISCHARGE	
		DRUG	DOSAGE		DRUG	DOSAGE

PAST MEDICATION

I.M. MYOCRISIN

PENICILLAMINE

HYDROXYCHLOROQUINE

PREDNISOLONE

SULPHASALAZINE

IMMUNOSUPPRESSIVES

HAS PARTICIPATED IN SELF MEDICATION
PROGRAMME   YES/NO

KNOWN ALLERGIES TO DRUGS

N.S.A.I.   YES/NO - PLEASE SPECIFY

    1.

ANALGESICS   2.

    3.

    4.

    5.

OTHERS   KNOWN SIDE EFFECTS TO DRUGS

    YES/NO - PLEASE SPECIFY

       DRUG   S/E

    1.

    2.

    3.

HAS PARTICIPATED IN DRUG TRIALS   4.

    5.

YES/NO   OTHER ALLERGIES - SPECIFY

WHICH?

ADDITIONAL COMMENTS BY ASSESSOR

FOLLOW UP SERVICES ON DISCHARGE

1. O.P.A.

2. DISTRICT NURSE

3. HOME HELP

4. MEALS ON WHEELS

5. TRANSPORT REQUIRED/ORDERED

6. SOCIAL WORKER (MEDICAL)

7. DATE OF DISCHARGE

    WHERE TO:

HAS HAD X-RAYS OF: DATES:

PATIENT EDUCATION CLASSES   YES/NO

Stage 2. Assessment

Assessment is made by interpretation of the nursing history to identify, in order of priority, the actual and potential patient problems. Identification of a problem, however, does not automatically mean that it can be resolved. A patient problem can be defined as 'anything which causes concern to either the patient or nurse' and which can be improved or resolved by specific nursing action.

Stage 3. Planning

A methodical care plan for the individual patient (see Figs. 4.6, 4.8) will contain the following elements:

1. Summary of actual and potential patient problems in order of priority
2. Determination of goals/expected outcome
3. Specific nursing action
4. A review time or date

Planning of nursing action, as with the history and assessment, should be the province of the nurse into whose care the patient has been placed. However, if team nursing is the method employed on the ward, then the team leader will adopt this responsibility.

The ward sister's traditional role will undergo a complete change. She will now delegate tasks which were previously her sole responsibility and at the same time she will diversify her role to include that of coordinator, clinical expert and, most important, teacher. The main benefit of this change will be that she will now have the time to teach and therefore pass on her specialist skills, having delegated much of her previous workload to others.

Stage 4. Implementation

Implementation simply means putting the planning stage into action. The following are essential considerations before adequate intervention can take place:

1. The degree of self-care that a patient can maintain (e.g. the patient may be a child or severely crippled)
2. The various categories of nursing skills which may be applied (e.g. manual skill, psychological skills, counselling, communication and teaching skills)
3. Provision of a suitable environment (e.g. a rheumatic patient will respond and benefit from a slow, cautious, almost leisurely pace)
4. The prearranged organisation of nursing care. This can either be primary nursing, team nursing or patient assignment (see p. 79).

Stage 5. Evaluation

Evaluation is the comparison of goals set with goals attained. This is an *ongoing process*, and obviously goals decided upon during the planning stage will eventually require evaluation. One important point is that all goals must have a time limit. In other words, goals must be accomplished within a time considered reasonable for outcome to be achieved. Above all, goals must be realistic. Should it be found that the goals set have not been achieved, alterations to the treatment plan must be considered. Luker (1979) has devised a simple format of alterations for consideration as follows:

1. Change goal, keep treatment the same
2. Change treatment, keep goal the same
3. Change goal and treatment
4. Change evaluation date and keep treatment and goal the same

Summary

The way is now open for any nurse interested in clinical research to make a contribution which will not only confound the critics but also, and more importantly, improve in every aspect general nursing care.

By keeping detailed and accurate records of planned patient care, the nurse, regardless of status, will have at her disposal for the first time the means to evaluate the care that she has been giving. Much criticism has been aimed at the nursing profession because this element of evaluation is missing from traditional nursing care.

Planning care, as just described, may well involve the nurse in more paperwork than she has previously been acustomed to. However, the end result is the elimination of much unnecessary and repetitive treatment, and ultimately better individual patient care.

To the careful reader it will have become apparent that each of the five stages mentioned overlaps with the neighbouring stages. This is inevitable and merely serves to prove the point that no individual part of nursing care can be looked at in isolation. Everything that nurses do for their patients, no matter how trivial or important, reflects upon the care given as a whole.

Other Methods of Staff Deployment

At this point it is essential to give a description of the three ways in which nursing staff can be organised, apart from the traditional method of task allocation. Obviously the choice of method of staff deployment will be largely dictated by available resources of finance and personnel. Ideally primary nursing is the method of choice; however, it requires a normal staff allocation which includes an adequate proportion of trained nurses. Unfortunately, current staff shortages and the preponderance of untrained personnel do not augur well for establishing primary nursing within the nursing process.

Organisation of nurse deployment can be governed by one of the following concepts:

1. Primary nursing
2. Patient assignment
3. Team nursing

Primary Nursing

Primary nursing (PN) is an entirely new concept on the wards which consists of a trained nurse having total responsibility over a group of patients in a ward. The primary nurse assesses, plans, implements and evaluates the 24-h care of each patient under her jurisdiction until they are discharged or transferred. Working in conjunction with the primary nurse is an associate nurse (who could be a nurse learner), who takes over the care of the patient while the primary nurse is off duty. The primary nurse/patient ratio should be in the region of one to four on day duty (McFarlane and Castledine 1982), depending on the type of care required. This concept could be considered impractical at the present time, because of the constraints of low staffing levels. With foresight and good planning, however, it may well become the model for the future, especially if nurse learners are transferred from the wards and into colleges of further education. The consequence should be a sufficiency of trained nurses to care for all patients (United Kingdom Central Council 1982).

Patient Assignment

The most obvious differences between PN and patient assignment (PA) are that the nurse responsible need not be trained and will not have total charge of the patients and their care from admission to discharge, as will the primary nurse. Instead she will be allocated a small group of patients for whom she will take responsibility for either a single day, a week at a time, or even longer. If she is not yet qualified, the actual assessment and planning of the patient care may remain in the hands of trained staff. However, the assigned nurse will be encouraged, and provided with the opportunity, to take on this responsibility under trained guidance and supervision.

It is essential for the trained delegator, usually the ward sister, to match the ability of the nurse to the individual needs of the patient.

Team Nursing

As the term 'team nursing' implies, the work on each ward is apportioned to teams of nurses comprising all grades and headed either by a staff nurse or by a senior student nurse. Each team (usually two) will have a balanced number of trained staff, learners and auxilliary staff. The ward sister retains overall charge, her role being that of a teacher, counsellor and manager as well as supervisor. The main difference from the traditional role is that she will now delegate more individual patient care to each team on her ward.

Summary

There are some distinct advantages to be found within all three systems as compared with the more traditional method of task allocation.

The nurse will have the opportunity to become totally involved in the care of those patients directly in her charge, and will make herself available for ward rounds and case discussions with all other disciplines. This intense involvement allows for a greater depth of understanding to develop between nurse and patient. The result is better communication, the cornerstone upon which to build a satisfactory relationship that is ultimately beneficial to both.

Within this new framework accountability plays an important role. The nurse must now question 'Why?'. She can no longer assume the cloak of ignorance, merely carrying out orders or treatment by rote. By question and inquiry, by recognising the need for change, she will progress towards research, which is now acknowledged as the natural development in nursing.

Fragmentation—the accepted word to describe the disadvantages of task allocation—will be lessened. Patient care must become the focus of attention upon which, not only the nurse, but indeed all disciplines will unite. Role changing will undoubtedly take place from the top down. The medical staff must learn to accept the new role of the nurse in caring for her patients and must be prepared to relate directly to her (as opposed to the ward sister) for consultation or for giving instructions on a change of treatment. Also, they must appreciate fully the advantages to the patient of being an active participant instead of the more usual submissive, almost detached, onlooker. The ward sister may well experience a complete change of role, and this may be hard to accept, especially for those nurses in whom traditional methods of nursing are ingrained.

Rheumatology Nursing

A patient suffering from one of the many rheumatic diseases requires a unique form of nursing. Unfortunately, this is not readily available on a general ward, and therefore many nurses do not appreciate the special needs of the rheumatoid patient.

It is regrettable that the care of patients suffering from arthritis and rheumatism has, over the years, become synonymous with geriatric nursing. Without wishing to denigrate geriatric care in any way, it is essential that the two specialties are recognised as being separate and entirely independent of each other.

Reasons for Hospitalisation of Rheumatic Patients

Admission may be for any one, or a combination of, the following reasons:

1. Acute flare
2. Rehabilitation
3. Diagnosis
4. Social admission (family holiday etc.)

Acute flare accounts for probably the largest percentage of admissions, followed closely by rehabilitation, with diagnosis and social admissions accounting for only a very small number. It seems sensible, therefore, to consider the essentials of rheumatology nursing care in relation to a patient suffering from an acute flare. Much of what is written will, of course, apply to most rheumatic conditions to a lesser or greater degree. To assist the nurse in preparing her nursing care plan brief mention will be made of the other reasons for admission, with emphasis placed on the differing priorities.

Acute Flare

The patient diagnosed as experiencing an acute flare of rheumatoid arthritis (RA), or certain other conditions, will be suffering extreme misery, coupled with excruciating pain emanating from diseased, swollen and stiffening joints. Movement, however slow or minor, will only serve to exacerbate the patient's agonising condition. In many cases they will exhibit symptoms of deep depression and also despair.

The environment into which this patient is to be admitted is therefore all important. The patient's main concern will be for relief of pain and rest. They will therefore wish to be treated in a tranquil, peaceful atmosphere by professional caring staff conversant with their suffering. At this stage the patient will be assessed by a nurse who will compile the individual care plan in conjunction with the patient. An example of such a plan can be seen in Fig. 4.6a–f.

Rest

Periods of rest are essential to help conserve energy and to allow the patient the opportunity to regenerate, physically and spiritually.

The exact amount of bed rest will vary from patient to patient. Unless complete bed rest is ordered, as it will be in the case of septic arthritis, then intermittent bed rest (i.e. rest alternating between bed and chair) should be considered. Complete bed rest could result in the development of pressure sores, particularly in patients who are receiving steroids, although any rheumatic patient is vulnerable. Because of their individual disabilities, rheumatic patients find alternating position in bed from side to back to side both painful and difficult, especially while trying to keep their limbs in the optimum position. If patients change into day clothes and lie on top of the bed, they can move with some independence from bed to chair as they feel the need. For patients who are more ambulant, definite periods of rest should be set aside each day, and the patient encouraged to take advantage of them.

Pain Control

Night sleep is generally considered essential for the maintenance and promotion of health. Deprivation of sleep means that a patient does not receive its restorative benefits. Pain must therefore be adequately controlled to achieve this result.

Certainly pain relief must receive priority soon after admission, for until pain is brought under control all other forms of treatment fall into abeyance. A patient will not readily comply with any form of treatment, especially of a physical nature, not even a bath, if they are experiencing severe pain. We are not suggesting that drug therapy alone can alleviate pain; rest and the application of heat or cold also play a major role. Figure 4.2 shows an information sheet given to patients at Leeds to explain the principles behind the application of heat and cold.

Admission of a patient suffering severe pain stemming from an acute attack of inflammatory arthritis, does not automatically suggest that the patient's existing drug therapy is non-efficacious. A 'flare' can result from other causes, such as physical trauma (a fall) or from mental or emotional stress (death of a loved one or divorce). A secondary illness such as a chest infection or gastrointestinal upset, or any pre- or postoperative procedure can also predispose a patient to a flare. All of these factors should be taken into consideration when an assessment is being made and drug therapy is under review.

Drug Therapy

Drug therapy plays an extremely important part in the overall treatment of any rheumatic patient. Therefore, once decisions as to drug treatment have

Heat

This helps to decrease pain and stiffness by relaxing you. This in turn results in better mobility, which then makes exercise less painful.

Types of Heat

Moist	Dry
1. Hot shower/bath	1. Electric pad/blanket
2. Wax	2. Hot water bottle
3. Oil	3. Hydrocollator pad
4. Bowl of hot water	

Cold (ice)

This does everything that heat does. It is simply a matter of personal choice.

Types of Cold

1. Ice (crushed) pack
2. Frozen peas (pack)
3. Cold water
4. Freezer pack (normally used in conjunction with an ice box)

Use of both heat and ice

1. Day of a 'flare' (even if only one joint is involved)
2. Prior to exercise
3. First thing in the morning

Additional Information

1. If taking a bath or shower as little as 10 min can be beneficial.
2. When using individual heat appliances, i.e. hot water bottle, apply for 20 min.
3. If using cold appliance, i.e. freezer pack, apply for 10 min initially, then leave for longer if required.
4. Always cover involved joint with a towel before applying heat or cold, otherwise the skin may be burned in both cases.

Fig. 4.2. Patient education sheet, Leeds University: Principles behind the use of heat/cold.

been made, education—preferably in the form of a self-medication pro-gramme—should be considered. If self-medication is considered inappro-priate, for whatever reason, then education of the patient's relatives or friends, as suggested in Chapter 7 (see p. 197) becomes imperative.

If self-medication is not accepted as a normal part of patient care on a particular rheumatology ward, then the timing of the 'medicine round' becomes all important. NSAIDs must be administered with food if gastrointestinal upsets are to be avoided. Ideally, D-penicillamine should be taken 1-h before food for satisfactory absorption to occur. Patients who are receiving oral iron are advised to take the tablets after meals. These are only a few of the drugs dispensed on a rheumatology ward. Rheumatic patients in particular cannot order their pain to suit the medicine round and require access to pain relief when they need it, not when tradition dictates. Self-medication for rheumatic patients must be seen as an advance in patient management and care. Providing patients are nursed in specialist wards—and not among general patients—we feel there is no valid reason for hospital management to refuse to allow self-medication to take place (see Chap. 7, p. 194).

Many patients will be receiving daily a multitude of tablets (polypharmacy), which include analgesics, NSAIDs, second-line action drugs, diuretics, antidepressants, hypnotics, laxatives, 'the pill', etc. Each tablet has been prescribed in good faith by the medical staff and accepted in equally good faith by the patient. It is therefore a shared responsibility of all the medical and nursing staff to ensure that the patient is fully aware of the benefits or otherwise of every tablet recommended and administered by them. To discharge a patient involved in polypharmacy, yet ignorant of the facts about the medication, would be tantamount to negligence.

Other Methods of Pain Control

Drugs are not the only means of controlling pain. Indeed, counselling can do much to relieve anxiety, and, consequently, pain and depression may drift away. Often the unexpected visitor can help to ease tension, thereby reducing the need for more drugs.

Relaxation Therapy. This is an alternative method of pain control, usually used in conjunction with conventional forms of therapy. We appreciate that not every hospital will be in a position to provide these facilities, or indeed will wish to do so. However, a brief description of the method is given here.

A small room should be set aside and decorated to give a soothing atmosphere. It need only be furnished with a firm couch and small side table. On the table should be placed a tape recorder containing a relaxation tape. Windows are not essential and the lighting should be subdued. All patients should be allowed free access to this facility, particularly when depression and despair have intensified. By lying down in such surroundings and listening to, and participating in, the relaxation programme on the tape, most patients benefit by varying degrees. The tape should be available for purchase for home use on discharge.[1]

---

[1] Progressive Relaxation Tapes by Dr. Ian Martin. Supplied by: Graves Medical Audio Visual Library, 220 New London Road, Chelmsford, Essex CN2 9BJ.

Positioning and Splinting

When joints are hot, swollen and inflamed, positioning becomes all important. It is all too easy to place the involved limb in the most comfortable
position to ease the pain and leave it there. Unfortunately, this position is
usually the most damaging and contractures quickly develop. Correct positioning, and, if necessary, splinting, must be initiated immediately. The
patient may lie in the most comfortable position, providing that upper and
lower limbs are kept in the optimum position (Fig. 4.3a, b). As can be seen in
the illustration, the optimum position is where the limb is maintained in the
extended state to allow for normal usage once inflammation has subsided.

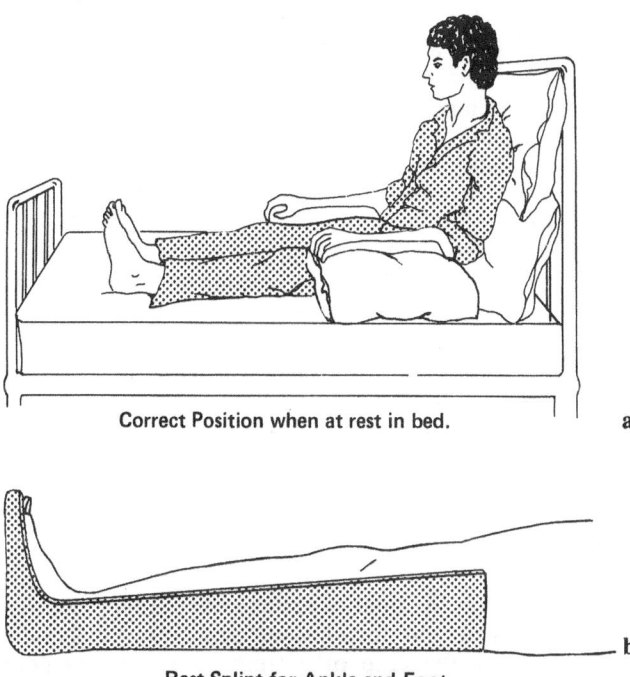

Correct Position when at rest in bed.   a

Rest Splint for Ankle and Foot.   b

Fig. 4.3. Splinting of the hands and legs in the position of optimum function.

Bed cradles may be provided, particularly at night, to help reduce the
weight of bedclothes on the painful lower limbs. Also, provision of a small
soft pillow for placement between the legs can prove most beneficial when
knee and ankle joints are painful. Additional support may be provided by
using pillows along the length of the involved limb. A pillow should *never* be
used to support a knee or elbow in a flexed position. To do so, certainly with
the lower limb, would result in the patient being unable to walk, as flexion
contractures would quickly occur. There may actually be something to be said

in favour of flexion deformity developing at the elbow. If damage to the joint is inevitable then a fixed flexion at the elbow may in fact result in a more useful position than one which is fixed and fully extended.

Patients with early rheumatic disease or those who have little or no deformity, should be instructed to lie in the prone position with the head supported by one pillow and with the feet hanging over the end of the bed. A minimum period of 10 min daily spent lying in this position, whether at home or in hospital, should help to maintain a good hip and knee alignment.

The cervical spine, when involved, can give rise to severe headaches plus restricted head movement. Collars can be provided to help alleviate both conditions. A soft collar is used at night and a firmer, more supportative one during the daytime. Should atlantoaxial subluxation be suspected, great care must be taken when moving the patient. Always ensure that sufficient pillows are at hand to provide support for patients with fixed spinal deformities.

Specialised custom-made splints are the province of the occupational therapy or plaster departments. One of the most commonly prescribed is the serial splint. This is used in an attempt to reduce fixed flexion deformity at the knee or elbow. As the name implies, it is a series of splints, each applied over a period of days or weeks until the optimum extension has been achieved. Once this has occurred, the final splint can then be cut in half lengthways (bivalving) and used as a resting splint in an attempt to prevent further flexion deformity developing. Other joints suitable for custom-made splinting are the metacarpal phalangeal (MCP) and proximal interphalangeal (PIP) joints, particularly as a preventive measure when ulnar deviation seems likely to occur.

Patients wearing splints will require encouragement from the nurse in their use, for splints are not popular with patients. Often they find them painful to wear at the start, heavy and cumbersome, certainly restricting and even ugly. The advantages of wearing them must be reinforced continually.

Lifting and Manoeuvring

Before attempting to move any rheumatic patient the nurse must be certain which joints are involved and to what degree. Slow, calculated movement should be routine; in the case of extreme joint involvement, sufficient members of staff should be on hand to assist in the procedure. LISTEN TO THE PATIENTS. Take their advice, for only they know how bad the pain and stiffness is. Be governed by them as to speed and actual manoeuvrability.

Allow patients as much independence as possible. If at first, because of acute illness, patients are almost totally dependent upon nursing care, then the gradual re-introduction of independence becomes of paramount importance to their rehabilitation.

Most patients have devised ways of manoeuvring. Unless the nurse has a better solution, they should be allowed this individuality. Providing patients are unhurried they can usually succeed on their own with only a minimum of assistance. This is infinitely better than one or two nurses attempting to get a patient either in or out of bed, at speed, causing unnecessary suffering in the process.

If a patient must be lifted, then it is important to avoid placing too much stress upon the involved joints, particularly the knees, hips and shoulders. Special care must be taken while lifting not to cause further damage, not only to the involved joints, but also to the patient's skin. The fragile skin of patients on steroids tears easily and once broken is very difficult to heal (see Care of Leg Ulcers, p. 88). Therefore nurses should take care not to drag the patient's skin against their own skin in the process of lifting. The application of talcum powder to the nurses' arms before proceeding to lift may help to alleviate this problem. Also care should be taken not to knock the patient's limbs against sharp objects. A nurse should never attempt to drag a patient up the bed single handed, but always seek assistance. The cradle method of lifting (Fig. 4.4) can be used, with the patient's arms folded in front. Certainly the Australian lift is a method to be avoided.

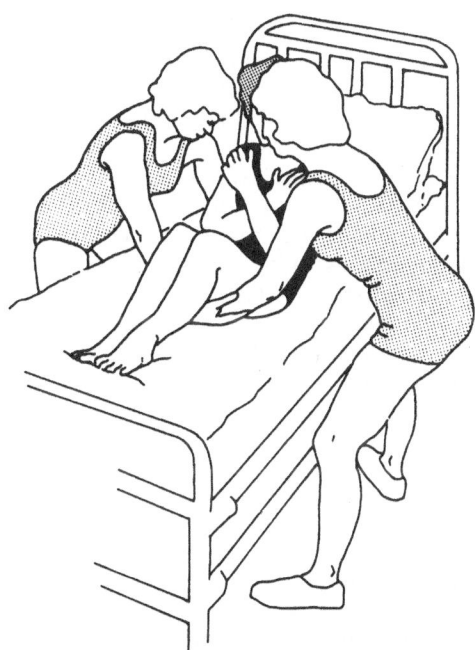

Fig. 4.4. Cradle method of lifting.

Patients should be encouraged to use the toilet facilities whenever possible and can be assisted by the nursing staff when necessary. As an alternative a commode may be used by the very ill and severely disabled. A bedpan is only to be used when the previous suggestions prove impracticable, and is therefore to be considered as a last resort. A patient should never be left unsupported on a bedpan, yet at the same time the need for privacy must be respected. The patient must be provided with the necessary equipment to ensure that personal hygiene can be carried out. Many acutely ill patients will find this task impossible and will require assistance from the nurse.

Care of Leg Ulcers

The main causes of leg ulcers include gravitation, vasculitis and/or steroid therapy. With a gravitational ulcer, the patient may have a poor arterial blood supply, with incompetence of communicating veins in the lower half of the lower leg. The patient may or may not have RA. With a vasculitic ulcer, the patient will undoubtedly have been diagnosed as suffering from inflammatory polyarthritis, particularly the systemic connective tissue disorders. Patients receiving steroid therapy, especially those who have been taking steroids for some years, suffer a reduction in collagen fibre, making the skin more fragile, easily broken and susceptible to bruising. In addition, steroids modify tissue reaction to infection. Consequently, there is a proliferation and spread of bacteria and viruses. The surface area of an ulcer therefore becomes an ideal breeding ground for organisms.

As certain patients are undoubtedly more susceptible to leg ulcer than others, prevention is therefore better than cure. Patient education on how to avoid sustaining an ulcer is invaluable information, and should be a priority.

Ulcers usually follow trauma, and treatment must be started immediately. If the patient is in hospital, the damage may be the result of careless handling of the patient, ill-fitting splints or even damage following collision against sharp objects, for example bed cradles, chairs, trolleys, or even the walking aids of other patients. Damage sustained by a patient at home usually follows a fall or a collision against a sharp object.

A recent survey carried out in Southampton found that 9% of 215 patients diagnosed as suffering from RA had at some time sustained leg ulcers (Thurtle and Cawley 1983).

The method of healing leg ulcers varies from hospital to hospital. As with the treatment of bed sores, each ward sister has her own preference. Description of a less conventional method, that of 'moist wound healing', combined with conventional nursing techniques, is offered here for consideration.

'Wet Method'

1. Elevation of the leg should be achieved as soon as possible, taking into account the stiffness and pain which may well ensue from placing the patient in this fairly static position for prolonged periods.

2. Following elevation, the ulcer must be kept clean and moist. The theory behind moist wound healing is relatively new and postulates that epithelialisation occurs more rapidly under moist conditions than under dehydration. Moisture also slows down the development of eschar (scab) formation and thus helps to protect the epidermal remnant that serves as a source of new epithelial cells. Moist wound healing, however, necessitates an extremely careful technique on the part of the nurse in order to minimise infection, for bacteria will flourish in a moist

wound environment. Therefore, it is essential to take the following precautions:

a) Always adhere closely to the aseptic technique, for infection will delay healing.

b) Debridement of necrotic tissue is essential. Removal will promote healing and deprive bacteria of a rich medium in which to breed. It also allows the cleansing agent to thoroughly penetrate the ulcer. Culture of any ulcer exudate should be sought and appropriate action taken. Because steroids modify skin reaction to bacteria, local antibiotic cream may be more beneficial to patients on steroid therapy than would a systemic antibiotic.

c) Avoid overfrequent wound changes, as these can disrupt epithelial growth by removing new areas each time a dressing is removed. Careful thought must therefore be given as to how often a change of dressing should be made.

d) Lengthy dressing changes result in heat loss as well as exposing the wound to infection and dehydration. These should therefore be avoided.

These steps should help to create the optimum environment for the healing process to take place. Yet success can still elude the diligent nurse, and skin grafting can therefore be considered.

3. Once healing is achieved, a firm elastic bandage from the base of the toes to just below the knee—not forgetting to include the heel—should be applied each morning before the patient gets up. Some rheumatic patients will of course find this a difficult procedure to carry out alone when at home. An 'all in one' elastic stocking could be tried as an alternative, providing a relative is on hand to apply it.

An alternative method said to promote healing is the application of ultraviolet light to the ulcer. This treatment is the province of the physiotherapy department.

'Dry' Method

1. Elevation of the leg should be achieved as soon as possible, with due consideration being given to the stiffness and pain which this may cause to the patient over a prolonged period.

2. The ulcer must be kept both clean and dry. Should sloughing have occurred, the ulcer will require debridement at least twice a day until all necrotic tissue has been removed. Culture of the ulcer exudate should be sought and appropriate action taken. Local antibiotic cream may well be more beneficial than systemic antibiotics if the patient is on steroid therapy.

3. Once the ulcer is clean and dry, it should start to heal. Granulation, however, is difficult to achieve. The whole process can take many weeks and success can still elude the diligent nurse. Skin grafting can be considered as a last resort.

4. As with the wet method, once healing is achieved the daily application of a firm elastic bandage or elastic stocking is essential before the patient gets up.

As mentioned already in relation to the wet method, ultraviolet light may be used by the physiotherapy department to promote healing of the ulcer.

Bathing

Unfortunately, in many British hospitals, bathing facilities do not meet the standard required by rheumatic patients. It would be equally fair to say that bathrooms in many private homes also fall short of these standards. The latter deficiency, however, is slowly being remedied by occupational therapists with the support of local social services.

Meanwhile, some hospital patients and staff have to battle with outdated equipment. This problem is not as trivial as it may sound, as most patients suffering from rheumatoid arthritis experience early morning stiffness. This harmless-sounding complaint can in fact render the patient almost totally immobile. The stiffness which can affect every joint often lasts 2–3 hours; indeed some patients say it lasts even longer. One very simple form of treatment for easing and relieving stiffness is the taking of a bath or shower. By soaking the affected joints for as little as 10 min in hot water, the stiffness decreases and the patient is once more able to resume movement. In other words, the joints become viable, an all-important goal for all patients, especially first thing each morning. The degree of movement gained will vary, and 'normal' may differ for each individual patient.

When at home a patient has no need to jostle for the bathroom, but in a hospital ward three baths may have to cater for the needs of 30 patients. Although not all of them will suffer from early morning stiffness, the majority will. The provision of shower facilities for each ward will help to circumvent or at least alleviate this distressing problem. The showers must be equipped with adapted mixer knobs (for patients will have hand involvement) set low down in the shower cubicle so that the patient sitting on a plastic stool or chair will be independent of staff. Furthermore, as stiffness returns (which is inevitable for many patients as the day progresses), the patient can take advantage of the shower facilities again without having to rely upon staff. This is a marvellous morale booster for any patient. Should hydrotherapy facilities be limited, or non-existent in a hospital, then occasional quick showers will help the patient remain mobile and also enable the patient to exercise more freely.

The availability of showers could also be of enormous benefit to a night nurse when faced with a patient unable to sleep, complaining of pain and possibly depression. The nurse could recommend a warm shower followed by a cup of tea. This might eliminate the need for further analgesia or at least a reduction in dosage might be achieved. Unfortunately, noisy plumbing could be a drawback; therefore, this nocturnal showering may be unrealistic in some hospitals. However, the advice is invaluable for patients at home.

A more obvious use of bathing facilities for any patient is for personal hygiene. For rheumatic patients, however, involvement of the upper extremities may well result in their inability to wash themselves. Female patients who are menstruating have added problems; therefore, daily bathing or showering is to be recommended. Taking a shower is quicker and much less tiring for the patient than taking a bath, and showers are cheaper in use than the conventional bath.

Elderly patients, however, may not take kindly to showers, considering them to be new-fangled nonsense. Yet a conventional daily bath, even with hoist facilities, can, for a 70/80-year-old, prove utterly exhausting. In these circumstances a bed bath should be considered, perhaps alternating each day with normal bathing facilities.

When assisting patients who are bathing, the nurse should make doubly sure that they are able to dry themselves adequately. If not, she should do this for them gently and thoroughly. Problems can quickly result if moist skin surfaces are allowed to rub against each other when patients return to bed.

Meals

Nurses have little control over the actual ingredients placed before their patients. Nevertheless, it is the nurses' responsibility to ensure that the food is nourishing and adequate, to the patients' liking and attractively served so as to whet the appetite.

None of these attributes will be of consideration, however, if the meal is placed in front of the patient by a domestic (however well meaning) who then moves on to the next bed, leaving the patient gazing at a delicious meal that cannot be reached, or eaten, because of physical disability. Nurses must be acutely aware at all times of the rheumatic patient's physical limitations. The simple task of pouring water from a jug is often impossible because of the weight involved, even when the jug is only half full. Aids are supplied for home use and yet the patient is expected to cope while in hospital. Tasks which normal individuals take for granted are major problems for many rheumatic patients; because nurses are always busy, patients do not care to trouble them. It is up to the nurse to anticipate patient needs. Therefore, the nurse should be on hand to cut up food, move the table, stack the pillows and pour a drink, and of course, if necessary, assist the patient to eat, thereby ensuring that the patient has a satisfactory and enjoyable meal.

Diet

The dietician plays a prominent role in the overall care of patients, in particular by giving advice on weight reduction, which is a major problem for many osteoarthritic patients, especially preoperatively. Therefore, education on good dietary habits, started whilst in hospital, may well be of great value later.

Advice should be given to patients—particularly the elderly, who may be housebound—on the benefits of a high-protein diet. Also the patient with poor mobility should be advised of the benefits to be gained by including a high-fibre content in their daily diet in order to avoid constipation developing.

Patient Education

The subject of patient education is discussed fully in Chapter 7. At this point, however, it is worth stressing that patient education starts on admission, when patient and nurse first meet.

It has already been suggested that the patient experiencing an acute flare will also be suffering from emotional anxiety. It will be the nurse's fundamental task to alleviate this as quickly as possible. Once the nurse, with the cooperation of the patient, has compiled an individual care plan, the basis of a successful hospital stay will have been created. Formal education classes can be started as soon as it is considered appropriate, and the patient should be involved in all classes from which it is felt that ultimate benefit will be derived.

Physiotherapy

Admission to hospital can be seen not only as a means of receiving treatment but also as an opportunity for teaching and reinforcing the principles of physiotherapy. Treatment will naturally differ from patient to patient, and a more detailed account of the different types of treatment available can be found in Chapter 6.

The importance of physiotherapy in rehabilitation cannot be overstressed. The nurse should remember that it is her duty, as well as that of the physiotherapist, to motivate newly diagnosed rheumatic patients towards regular daily exercises (see Chap. 7) and to encourage patients suffering an acute flare through a gentle regimen of active assisted and isometric exercises until they too can gradually achieve a regular daily exercise programme.

The philosophy behind regular daily exercise is:

1. To maintain the normal range of movement in each joint
2. To improve and maintain muscle tone
3. To prevent deformity developing
4. To help reduce morning stiffness

Exercises are known to be painful, time consuming and boring. It is therefore extremely important for the nurse to understand these problems and to help patients come to terms with them by convincing them of the ultimate benefit to themselves.

Patients with ankylosing spondylitis (AS) benefit from a regimented exercise programme covering 2/3 weeks. Many hospitals now admit groups of

AS patients, who undergo intensive hydrotherapy and physiotherapy. The AS patient can actually feel and observe the benefits to be gained and consequently will be motivated towards a lifelong commitment to exercise, which is essential if prognosis is to remain good. The osteoarthritic patient can gain from being taught exercises which involve weight lifting and which can be continued at home after discharge.

Wax and arachis oil can be prescribed as treatment for painful and stiff hands or feet. Wax is more commonly used, oil being used if an allergy to wax should occur. Unfortunately, the oil has a pungent smell, which many patients dislike. Its advantage over wax is that both hands or feet can be exercised at the same time. Patients can also be prescribed wax for use in the home. However, the application of wax is expensive and time consuming, and can even be considered dangerous when used in the home. It is also impractical for a rheumatic patient living alone, because the sheer weight of a pan of wax can be an insurmountable problem. It must also be admitted that there may well be a large psychological element where some patients are concerned. The use of wax can be avoided, however, by educating the patient about the benefits of hot or cold soaks (see Fig. 4.2.).

Occupational Therapy

Once inflammation has subsided, referral to the occupational therapy department can result in a new lease of life for many patients. Assessment for the provision of aids to daily living (ADL) is the province of the occupational therapist (OT). Occupational therapists have the right to supply certain aids from source, or to recommend that they be supplied by a local authority. They also carry out domiciliary visits and can offer advice on structural alterations within the patient's home, particularly in the bathroom and kitchen areas, and outside in the garage and on paths and driveways, where the provision of ramps and rails can prevent a patient becoming housebound.

Education in joint protection is given priority. By supplying aids and teaching the correct method of their use much undue stress upon individual joints can be avoided, thereby preventing the recurrence of yet another 'flare' in the future.

As mentioned previously (see also Chap. 6, p. 168) splints—which after all are yet another form of joint protection—can also be supplied by the OT. These can be ready made, as in the case of Futuro wrist splints, or custom made, as, for example, when ulnar deviation is suspected.

Social Worker

Mainly because of the physical deformities which can develop in sufferers of rheumatic diseases, the medical social worker (MSW) is a very important member of the rehabilitation team. The problems she will be called upon to deal with once the patient is hospitalised include housing, pensions and home placements. She will liaise between other members of the primary health care team and will activate additional support systems on the patient's behalf, such as Meals on Wheels, home help, day centre placement, and many others (see Chap. 11).

Some medical social workers are also skilled sex counsellors and can be called upon to give advice in this context, should it be required. Certainly all patients for hip replacement, pre- or postoperatively, will require sexual counselling—a fact sadly neglected in some areas.

Rehabilitation

The patient admitted for rehabilitation may not be experiencing pain to the same degree as the patient suffering from an acute flare. Therefore, pain control and an extensive rest programme need not be given overall priority. Instead, the nurse elected to compile the individual nursing care plan can concentrate immediately upon methods of rehabilitation involving physiotherapy, occupational therapy, patient education and the instigation of a self-medication programme.

Patients admitted for rehabilitation fall into three catagories:

1. Patients newly diagnosed and therefore in need of a structured rehabilitation programme, including the instigation of new drug therapy.
2. Patients long since diagnosed who unfortunately have never been offered the benefits of rehabilitation. In fact they will probably have been told to 'go home and learn to live with it'. Reasons for admission may also include a review of drug therapy because of side-effects or lack of efficacy.
3. 'Wayward' rheumatic patients who, for various reasons, among which may be self-denial, have allowed their condition to deteriorate. They may have not been taking their medication regularly, or not attending for follow-up appointments, blood or urine tests etc.

Diagnosis

The patient who is admitted because his condition has not yet been diagnosed will obviously present a challenge to all involved in his care. Therefore, the nursing history obtained by the nurse, including her continual assessment of the patient's 'activities of living', will provide useful material which may help towards the final diagnosis.

Social Admission

Social admissions account for only a small percentage of all admissions and consist mainly of elderly patients sent in by consultants as an annual treat to help boost their morale or to enable relatives to take a holiday which would otherwise be denied them. Such admissions also allow annual assessments to be made.

Planning Patient Care by Use of the Nursing Process

The following case studies provide a descriptive account of the nursing process, including the initial assessment made by the nurse, followed by the care plan, evaluation and report of progress from admission to discharge.

Case Study 1

Interview and Identification of Problems

The patient, a young married woman aged 32 years, was admitted to the rheumatology ward diagnosed as suffering an acute attack of rheumatoid arthritis. She was able to give the nurse most of the information required; however, as she was obviously in pain, the nurse ensured that she asked only those questions relevant to the patient's present condition. The remainder of the information was obtained from the patient's medical notes and her husband, who visited later that day.

The patient's name was Patricia A., and she expressed a desire to be called Pat. She came from a city some 25 miles away and immediately showed her anxiety over the difficulties her husband would experience in visiting her because of the distance, and also over her two young boys aged 5 and 7, who would have to be cared for. Pat was well aware of the reason for her admission, having been referred from the outpatient clinic some 3 weeks earlier as an urgent case. Instead of being angry and upset at having to wait so long for admission, she said she was glad because it had given her time to make arrangements with friends and relatives to care for her children during her hospital stay. It soon became evident that the relationship between Pat and her husband was far from satisfactory, and she felt that the time lapse had also helped him to get used to the idea of her being away. The husband worked as a plumber for a large company and spent quite a lot of time working away from home. She did feel that the diagnosis of RA made just 3 years earlier had not helped an already strained marriage. As Pat was small, blonde and very pretty, and, despite her obvious pain and tired and drawn expression, was apparently of an exceptionally pleasing disposition, the nurse wondered what the problem could be. Though Pat believed in God she had no particular religious convictions. Her hobbies, since her diagnosis had been made, were limited, although she still enjoyed knitting and walking when her illness permitted.

She appeared physically to be in good condition. Her hair, naturally curly, was short and neat and caused her no problems. Her eyes, although she did not wear glasses, were giving her cause for concern, feeling heavy and tired. The sunlight bothered her and she had taken to wearing sunglasses much of the time. Her mouth was clean and she had all her own teeth with very few fillings. She did not smoke and had no apparent respiratory problems. Her skin, which was fair in complexion, was in excellent condition except around those joints which were acutely inflamed, mainly the ankles, right knee, both hands and wrists and the right elbow. In these locations the skin was hot, red and stretched tightly over the swollen joints. No obvious abnormality of any joints could be seen, with the exception of inflammation and extensive synovitis, which was present over all MCP joints and at the right wrist and right knee. Micturition and bowel elimination were normal, as were hearing and speech. Appetite was usually very good (she described herself as able to eat 'like a horse' when well), but recently her appetite had declined, mainly because she did not feel fit enough to cook, even though she had to force herself to do so because of the children. She thought her weight had dropped a little. Nights were a bad time for her, especially over the previous 6–8 weeks; and 'the tablets' were helping only a certain amount.

On examination there was no evidence of pressure sores, possibly because Pat had, until then, had little opportunity to take herself off to bed. Vital signs and clinical measurements pertaining to rheumatology were taken in order to establish a baseline to compare future measurements. The blood pressure (BP) was 98/70, temperature 36.4°C, pulse 84 beats/min, respiration rate of 18/min. Urinalysis showed a trace of blood (menstruation just finishing) with the remainder normal. Her weight was 44 kg and height 152 cm. Articular index (AI) was 31 with both wrists, all MCPs, PIP and the right knee recording 3. Right knee flexion with goniometer recorded 46°/64°; left knee recorded for comparison was 15°/120°. Grip strength was right hand 50 and left hand 60. Early morning stiffness (EMS) was 120 min. Pat's own pain assessment over the past week (on a score of 1–5) was 4. Mobility had been severely restricted over the past 2 months, although Pat had still managed to take the children to school and collect them in the late afternoon. Other than that she only managed essential shopping when her husband went with her to the supermarket.

Previous to the diagnosis of rheumatoid arthritis Pat had been perfectly fit and had never had an operation. She could remember suffering growing pains as a child, but that was all. As far as she knew she had no allergies to drugs or anything else. Rheumatologically, her right knee had been injected with a local hydrocortisone some 8 months previously with good results. Present medication consisted of indomethicin (Indocid) 25 mg t.d.s. and paracetamol 2 p.r.n. Past medication had been Nu-Seals aspirin 900 mg q.d.s., but this had been stopped when she experienced severe dyspepsia. A second-line drug had never been prescribed, although the doctor in clinic had mentioned the possibility. According to the medical notes, radiographs showed erosive changes evident in both feet and both hands.

The most recent haematological investigation, on a sample taken 3 weeks previously in clinic, showed an ESR of 68 mm/h and a haemoglobin (Hb) count of 10.2 g/dl. Findings from biochemical investigation were normal. Immunological investigation results showed rheumatoid factor positive, DAT 1:1000 and antinuclear factor negative.

When Mr. A. visited that evening he was able to furnish further information. They lived in a private three-bedroomed semi-detached house with gas central heating, situated on the outskirts of the city and close to school and shops. He said his wife was always cleaning and that the house was well kept. The paternal grandparents were evidently only prepared to help in the last resort. However, the maternal grandparents were willing and the children were with them now. The husband was obviously concerned more for his own comforts than for his wife, and he really could not see that she had much to complain of.

Assessment

An assessment of Pat's condition was then made by the nurse, based upon the information gained at the interview plus that taken from the medical notes and that gleaned from the husband. This encompassed the physical, psychological and social state of the patient; thus potential and actual problems could be identified and a nursing care plan developed, taking the patient's particular needs—and those of her family—into consideration.

The most obvious problem was pain, and this was reflected in Pat's inability to sleep at night or rest adequately during the day. The synovitis present in many of the joints, making them hot and swollen, resulted in limited mobility and therefore restricted routine personal hygiene. The high AI correlated well with these findings. Pat's weight was on the low side, but she had a small frame and a low weight was in her favour, placing less stress on her weight-bearing joints. Her complaint about 'heavy and tired' eyes did not sound like Sjögren's syndrome, nor did it sound like a side-effect to the drugs she was currently taking.

A potential nursing problem could arise if Pat were prescribed bed rest, as pressure sores could quickly develop. Careful and sensitive social investigations would need to be made into the problems Pat was experiencing within her marriage, and in addition the needs of two little boys would have to be considered. The diagnosis of rheumatoid arthritis had definitely resulted in a change of life style for Pat. She informed the nurse that prior to her illness she had been more outgoing, enjoying visiting and chatting to friends and attending night school for keep fit classes. Her physical disability at times restricted much of these pleasures, and even when she felt reasonably fit the children restricted her outside activities, as her husband was away so much. Nevertheless, if she could get rid of the pain, she insisted fairly cheerfully, she would be able to cope. The completed history charts for Pat are shown in Fig. 4.5a–c.

a

CONSULTANT: DR. H. A. BIRD
NAME: PATRICIA A.
ADDRESS:

D.O.B.: 4.3.51. AGE: 32
HOSPITAL NO.: 12345
DATE OF ADMISSION: 12.6.83 TIME: 10.15am
ADMITTED FROM: Home
RELIGION: C/E
MARITAL STATUS: Married

NEXT OF KIN:
NAME: Husband Tony A
ADDRESS: as above

TEL. NO.:
HOME: Leeds 45678 WORK: 910112 Bradford

G.P.: Dr. Jones
DISTRICT NURSE: Sr. White.
HOME HELP: No
DAY CENTRE: No
VISITORS: YES/NO
IF NO, WHY?:

GENERAL APPEARANCE/MENTAL STATE
Tired, a little anxious, pale, obviously in
pain, Excitable nature.

SOCIAL HISTORY
OCCUPATION: H/w
CHILDREN: 2 AGES: 5 and 8 years
OTHER DEPENDANTS: No
LIVES ALONE/WITH RELATIVE husband
HOUSE S.D. FLAT BUNGALOW
PART 3 SHELTERED
RESIDENTIAL CARE
TOILETS 1 BEDS 3
HEATING C/H Gas.

PAST MEDICAL HISTORY
OPERATIONS: No

PROSTHESIS YES/NO (See page 2)
HEALED GASTRIC/DUODENAL ULCERS No
CONCOMITANT DISEASE - SPECIFY
None

PSYCHIATRIC ILLNESS: No

VALUABLES HELD: £3.00.
REASON GIVEN TO PATIENT FOR ADMISSION:
Disease out of control. Admitted for rest,
physiotherapy and possible change of
drug therapy.
PROVISIONAL DIAGNOSIS:
R.A. "acute flare"
URINE: Trace of blood (menstruating)
Remainder NAD.
WEIGHT: 44 kg HEIGHT: 152 cm.

PRESENT MEDICAL HISTORY AND REASON FOR
ADMISSION
ACUTE FLARE ✓
REHABILITATION ✓
DIAGNOSIS
SOCIAL

RA	OA	AS	PMR
C. SPINAL			
OTHERS			

ANAEMIA YES/NO Hb 10.2.
CHEST Nil of note
ULCER YES/NO
GASTRIC DUODENAL

(pp. 98–100)
Fig. 4.5 a–c. Nursing history. Patient: Patricia A.

CLINICAL ASSESSMENTS ON ADMISSION

b

CONDITION OF:

MOUTH (GOOD) POOR
DENTURES   CROWNS
EYES (GOOD) POOR Photophobia last 8 weeks only
GLASSES   CONTACT LENSES
HEARING (GOOD) POOR
AIDS
SPEECH (GOOD) DIFFICULTIES

APPETITE Poor, last 6 weeks only.
DIET – (NORMAL) SPECIAL
SPECIAL DISLIKES Cabbage.
SLEEP PATTERN Poor, interrupted by pain, normally 7/8 hours good sleep.
BLADDER ✓
BOWELS nil
SMOKES nil
ALCOHOL occasionally

CONDITION OF PRESSURE AREAS
Norton Score 8

LEG ULCERS YES (NO)
WHERE

MOBILITY: GOOD (FAIR) POOR

AIDS:
WALKING STICK   CALLIPERS
ZIMMER   CRUTCHES
SPINAL COLLAR   NIGHT – DAY
WRIST SPLINTS:
RESTING   WORKING ✓ Future
SHOES ✓
OTHERS Requires A.D.L. assessment

Joints A.I.		Pain 0,1,2,3	Swollen	Prosthesis	Date	I.A.I.	Date	MORNING STIFFNESS HOURS MINS
Temporomandibular		—		Nil				120 mins
Cervical spine		—						
Sternoclavicular								
Acromioclavicular		—						T 36.4
Shoulder	R	— 1						P 84
	L	3	✓					R 18
Elbow	R	3	✓					
	L	3	✓					B/P 98/70
Wrist	R	3	✓					
	L	3	✓					FUNCTIONAL GRADE
M.C.P.	R	3						1
	L	1 3	✓					2 ✓
P.I.P.	R							3
	L	3	✓					4
Hips	R							5
	L	2						
Knee	R	1			R.Knee 8 months ago.			
	L	1						
Ankle	R							
	L	— 1						
Talocalcaneal	R							
	L							
Midtarsal	R	— 1						
	L							
M.T.P.	R							
	L							
Score		31						

GRIP STRENGTH

	R	L
1.	50	60
2.	50	70
3.	50	50
TOTAL	150	180
MEAN	50	60

GONIOMETER READING

	R	L
	46/64	15/20

PATIENTS ASSESSMENT OF PAIN ON ADMISSION

1   2   3   4 ✓   5

MEDICATION SHEET

PAST MEDICATION

	DATE
I.M. MYOCRISIN	
PENICILLAMINE	
HYDROXYCHLOROQUINE	No
PREDNISOLONE	
SULPHASALAZINE	
IMMUNOSUPPRESSIVES	

N.S.A.I.   No

ANALGESICS   Nu-SEAL ASPIRIN

OTHERS   No

HAS PARTICIPATED IN DRUG TRIALS

YES/NO

WHICH?

ADDITIONAL COMMENTS BY ASSESSOR

1) Problems within marriage, husband does not appreciate problems caused by Rheumatoid Arthritis.

2) Anxiety over leaving two small boys.

PRESENT MEDICATION

DRUG	DOSAGE	COMMENCED
PARACETAMOL	ii p.r.n.	
INDOMETHICIN	25 mg t.d.s.	

HAS PARTICIPATED IN SELF MEDICATION PROGRAMME   YES/NO

KNOWN ALLERGIES TO DRUGS

YES/NO - PLEASE SPECIFY

1.
2.
3.
4.
5.

KNOWN SIDE EFFECTS TO DRUGS

YES/NO - PLEASE SPECIFY

DRUG	S/E
1. Nu-Seals aspirin	dyspepsia
2.	
3.	
4.	
5.	

OTHER ALLERGIES - SPECIFY

No.

MEDICATION ON DISCHARGE

DRUG	DOSAGE
D-PENICILLAMINE	150 - 500mg daily
DISTALGESIC	i t.d.s.

FOLLOW UP SERVICES ON DISCHARGE

1. O.P.A.   ✓
2. DISTRICT NURSE   ✓
3. HOME HELP
4. MEALS ON WHEELS
5. TRANSPORT REQUIRED/ORDERED
6. SOCIAL WORKER (MEDICAL)   ✓
7. DATE OF DISCHARGE   7. 7. 83

WHERE TO: Home.

HAS HAD X-RAYS OF: DATES:

Hands and feet   1981

PATIENT EDUCATION CLASSES   YES/NO

Plan of Nursing Care

Having made the assessment the next step was to plan the nursing care. The most pressing problem to tackle was the pain that Pat was suffering, for unless this was brought under control it would prove impossible to implement other forms of treatment successfully. Intermittent bed rest was therefore prescribed, and this was to be reviewed daily. Pat would be encouraged to wear her day clothes and lie on top of the bed rather than in it if she wished. This would also allow her more freedom of movement should she wish to sit out in a chair for short periods, and thus relieve undue pressure on sensitive areas. While on the bed she would be advised to change her position frequently, taking into account her physical disability and resultant pain on movement. She would be allowed to use the toilet facilities, but would have to be taken in a wheelchair by a nurse.

Advice on the correct positioning of the involved limbs was to be given, and resting splints would be supplied for both wrists, with the instruction that only one be worn at a time, otherwise Pat would become totally dependent upon others for her simplest needs. Futura wrist splints would relieve this predicament, but they would not provide enough support for the MCP and PIP joints at this juncture.

Because fixed contractures can develop quickly, the right knee was to be observed carefully at all times. Meanwhile a pillow would be placed along the length of the limb and underneath the ankle to provide support and comfort. The possibility of providing a resting splint for this limb was also to be kept in mind should the slightest contracture of the knee be suspected. Goniometer readings of the right knee would be taken on alternate days. Pressure areas were to be attended to 4-hourly with the aim of retaining them in their present healthy condition until Pat was allowed to move around at will.

Analgesia, in this case Distalgesic two 4-hourly was to be prescribed, and Pat would be encouraged to take the tablets in order to control her pain and prevent it getting out of hand. Indomethacin was changed to piroxicam (Feldene) 20 mg daily.

An exercise programme would be instigated which would involve active assisted and isometric exercises only. Pat would be encouraged to perform the active assisted exercises at least twice daily with the help of the nurses, and to continue isometrics throughout the day.

Hot (hydrocollator) packs were to be applied to the knee, both wrists and hands, with the possibility of substituting ice if heat did not prove beneficial. This treatment could usefully be applied b.d. and should be reviewed daily.

Personal hygiene would be limited because of the restricted bed rest programme and also because of Pat's inability to use her hands with any real effect. A daily general bath or shower would be instigated under supervision. (The patient is taken to the bathroom in a wheelchair and placed in the bath using hoist facilities. As rheumatic patients benefit greatly from being allowed to soak for as little as 10 min in warm water, then a general bath or shower is preferable to a bed bath.)

Pat's reported inability to sleep at night was of great importance. (The rheumatology nurse must always be assured that the patient finds the bed comfortable and that the bedclothes and pillows are acceptable and adequate.) A cradle would be supplied for the right knee and a supply of small pillows would be available for placement between ankles and knees should Pat prefer to lie on her side. (Finding a comfortable sleeping position while keeping in mind the optimum position of all four limbs is not easily attained.) Pat would need help and reassurance from the night staff, particularly during the first few days of her hospital admission. Analgesics were to be made available for administration during the night should Pat require them, and night sedation (Mogadon) was to be offered initially before retiring, on the understanding that she would be under no pressure to take them should she not wish to do so.

Now that Pat would no longer be acting as chief cook and bottle washer, it was hoped that her appetite would quickly return. Attractive, nourishing meals were therefore to be served.

A decision was taken to refer Pat to the ophthalmologist for investigation of her eye complaint. Meanwhile she would be allowed to wear her dark glasses if she wished. Natural tears were also prescribed as a precaution and possible means of relieving her discomfort until the appointment with the ophthalmologist.

An assessment of Pat's AI and grip strength would be performed weekly by the nurse who had carried out the initial assessments. She would also use the same sphygmomanometer on each occasion. A daily diary card (DDC) was to be issued to Pat so that an ongoing assessment of pain, morning stiffness, and analgesic intake could be monitored. Some help would be required by the patient over the first few days in actually filling in the card because of difficulty in holding a pen or pencil. The completed nursing care plans for Pat are shown in Fig. 4.6a–c.

(pp. 103–108)
Fig. 4.6a–f. Nursing care plan. Patient: Patricia A. ▶

NURSING CARE PLAN

PATIENT NAME: PATRICIA A

HOSPITAL NO.:

a

Date	No.	Problem	Goal	Nursing Care	Review Date	Evaluation	Resolve Date
12.6.83.	1.	Generalized pain and stiffness due to hot swollen and inflamed joints caused by disease.	Decrease in inflammation and pain.	a) Intermittent bed rest at patients discretion. b) Correct positioning of involved joints using either pillows or splints c) Analgesia q.d.s. as prescribed. d) Application of heat/ice to affected joints b.d. e) Issue with D.D.C. to assess pain, Morning Stiffness, and analgesic intake.	daily daily daily daily	Patient experiencing less pain. Reduction in E.S.R. to 50. Lower A.I to 23. Analgesic requirements down to ii̲ t.d.s. D.D.C. score average 3.	17. 6. 83
12.6.83	2.	Personal hygiene restricted because of involvement of hands and elbows and bed rest programme.	Ability to wash and carry out all personal hygiene herself.	a) Assist patient with washing/bathing. Give daily general bath using hoist facilities or shower. Take in wheel chair.	daily	Patient experiencing less pain. Joints less stiff and swollen, therefore all movements less restrictive, patient now ambulant and able to wash herself.	21. 6. 83.
12.6.83	3.	Mobility reduced due to inflammation and prescribed intermittent bed rest.	Maintain normal range of movement unassisted in all joints. Start intensive physiotherapy.	a) Start passive/active assisted exercises b.d. with nurse or physio therapist. b) Start isometric exercises. Continue throughout day.	17. 6.83.	Normal range of movement maintained, patient now able to perform these unassisted but with supervision	17. 6. 83.

NURSING CARE PLAN

PATIENT NAME: PATRICIA A

HOSPITAL NO.:

Date	No.	Problem	Goal	Nursing Care	Review Date	Evaluation	Resolve Date
12.6.83	4.	Unable to sleep nights due to pain in involved joints.	Establish reasonable sleep pattern by relieving pain.	a) Check mattress and bed clothing suitable for patients comfort i.e. firm mattress, light covers, bed cradle. b) Supply resting splint and small pillows to place between ankles and knees. c) Administer analgesia during night if required. d) Give night sedation as prescribed if patient agreeable.	daily	Requesting analgesic only occasionally at night. Sleeping well most nights for 5/6 hours. Night sedation not requested up to now.	21.6.83.
12.6.83.	5.	Potential development of pressure sores due to disease and lack of mobility. NORTON SCALE 8.	Maintain healthy intact skin.	a) Intermittent bed rest - patient allowed to get off the bed and sit in chair at her own discretion to relieve pressure on vulnerable areas. i.e. buttocks, heels and elbows. b) While on the bed encourage patient to change position at least 2-hourly. c) Observe for signs of pressure 4-hourly maintaining hygiene as necessary.	daily daily daily	No development of pressure sores - skin intact - patient now up and about.	18.6.83.

NURSING CARE PLAN

PATIENT NAME: PATRICIA A

HOSPITAL NO.:

c

Date	No.	Problem	Goal	Nursing Care	Review Date	Evaluation	Resolve Date
12.6.83	6.	Potential development of fixed contracture of R. Knee due to disease, pain and lack of mobility	Prevent contracture developing.	a) Support R. Knee and foot on pillow ensuring limb lying in optimum position. b) Advise patient on importance of keeping limb straight whether in bed or chair. c) Supply resting splint at night. d) Can supply resting splint during day if patient has difficulty keeping knee straight herself. This will severely restrict her movement in and out of bed. e) Record goniometer reading of R. Knee alternate days.	17.6.83.	Patient experiencing less pain in R. Knee. Swelling and inflammation reduced. Actively moving R. Knee through normal range of movement without assistance. Right knee goniometer reading now 20°/100°. No fixed contracture observed.	17.6.83.
12.6.83	7.	Lack of appetite due to general ill health.	Regain patient's interest in food.	a) Provide with attractive small nourishing meals. b) Find out individual likes and dislikes from nursing history. c) Weigh weekly.	14.6.83	Eating very well. Has gained (2.1b) 1 kg.	15.6.83

d

NURSING CARE PLAN

PATIENT NAME: PATRICIA A

HOSPITAL NO.:

Date	No.	Problem	Goal	Nursing Care	Review Date	Evaluation	Resolve Date
12.6.83	8	Poor marital relationship resulting in lack of support both physical and emotional for patient (Problem expressed during interview).	Better understanding between husband and wife, hopefully improving marital relationship.	a) Arrange for husband to be counselled while visiting one day. If necessary without him knowing beforehand. b) Suggest husband joins Pat for some of the educational classes so that he will appreciate her problems better, also physiotherapy treatment so that he can help and encourage her to continue them on discharge.	After Counselling	Husband understands patient's problems better after counselling through optimum result not obtained as husband refused to attend education classes or physiotherapy. Medical Social Worker alerted to problem.	26.6.83
12.6.83.	9.	Anxiety at leaving 2 small children.	Relieve anxiety.	a) Reassure and allow open visiting for children at any time.	After first visit by children	Accepted situation after first visit by children, 7 days after admission.	19.6.83.
12.6.83	10.	Patient complained of photo-phobia over past 2 months.	To find cause of photo phobia.	a) Allow Pat to continue to wear dark glasses. b) Reassure until appointment with opthalmologist comes through. c) Administer "natural tears" as prescribed.	After opthalmologist appointment 19.6.83.	Opthalmologist appointment revealed no abnormality. Patient therefore reassured. Dark glasses to be worn only if patient wishes. Natural tears discontinued	20.6.83.

NURSING CARE PLAN

PATIENT NAME: PATRICIA A

HOSPITAL NO.:

Date	No.	Problem	Goal	Nursing Care	Review Date	Evaluation	Resolve Date
15.6.83	11.	Patient has poor control of disease due to lack of information on: a) disease process. b) drugs therapy c) reason for exercise d) advantages to be gained from a multi-disciplinary health care team.	Overall increase of knowledge of a,b,c,d, as listed under problem and thereby avoiding repeated "flares" of disease.	a) Educate by attendance at Patient Education Classes when fit enough to do so. b) Instigation of Self Medication Programme. c) Allay patient's fears about attending classes by suggesting a nurse accompanies her, at least initially.	After attending classes. After completing course. After first visit to classes.	Patient fully conversant with drug therapy following Self Medication Programme. Pre and Post questionnaires in connection with Patient Education Classes have yet to be analysed. However patient expressing a definite increase in knowledge and understanding following formal education classes.	22.6.83. 4.7.83.
18.6.83	12.	Poor mobility due to moderate inflammation still present in most joints	Reduction in inflammation and pain, increase in mobility.	a) Re-enforce correct positioning of involved joints in optimum position. b) Continue applying hot packs b.d. c) Encourage walking from ward to lounge at least b.d., more if she wishes. d) Start intensive physiotherapy e) Continue with analgesia.	23.6.83.	Patient experiencing less pain as shown by D.D.C. (2) on average. Analgesic intake down to one t.d.s. Reduction in E.S.R. to 35. A.I. down to 12. Mobility improved, now walking about ward without difficulty. Hot packs discontinued	23.6.83.

e

NURSING CARE PLAN

f

PATIENT NAME: PATRICIA A.

HOSPITAL NO.:

Date	No.	Problem	Goal	Nursing Care	Review Date	Evaluation	Resolve Date
19.6.83.	13.	Early morning stiffness – has shown no improvement since admission.	Reduction in minutes of Early morning stiffness	a) Advise warm shower first thing each morning before breakfast. b) Inform medical staff of problem if it persists with a view to changing drug therapy.	daily 22.6.83.	Reduction of Early Morning Stiffness to 30 min within 2 days of early morning showers being instigated.	23.6.83.

Implementation and Evaluation

Rheumatoid arthritis is a unique form of chronic illness—one in which the patient, though suffering severe disability and pain, is nonetheless mentally alert, is not acutely ill in the true sense of the word and certainly not sliding towards death as in many other forms of chronic illness. Consequently, they require a specific environment in which to overcome their individual problems. The degree of self-care which can be achieved and maintained is individual to each patient. However, the environment to which they will all eventually respond is similar. The patient should be admitted to a hospital where the pace is peaceful, leisurely and unhurried. Attitudes should be cautious, sympathetic and informed. Goals which are set should be realistic and gradually achieved. The creation of such an environment demands from the nurse every skill at her disposal, including manual, psychological, counselling, communication and teaching skills, with equal emphasis on each.

In Pat's case, over the following days and weeks, all of these nursing skills made a contribution. The result was that the pain she had experienced came under control by regular administration of Distalgesic and NSAIDs, combined with intermittent bed rest. After 5 days (Day 6) bed rest and attention to pressure areas was discontinued. Instead Pat was encouraged to walk from the ward to the lounge twice a day. She was also encouraged to eat at the dining room table. After a further 4 days (Day 10) Pat's condition had improved considerably and she was allowed complete freedom of movement about the ward. The right knee had been injected with a local corticosteroid on Day 3, when 30 ml of synovial fluid had also been removed, and it was now much improved. Because of this, and the established routine of the hot pads applied b.d. and the active assisted and isometric exercises, it was felt that the physiotherapist could be called in to start more intensive treatment of involved joints.

Personal hygiene became less of a problem as each day passed, and on Day 10 Pat was allowed access to the bathroom as she saw fit. Her hand involvement meant that she would always be slightly handicapped. Nevertheless she was much improved.

As had been suspected, Pat's lack of appetite appeared mainly to be due to her illness and the sheer necessity of having to cope at home. By Day 4 she was eating a normal diet, and continued to do so throughout her stay in hospital, eventually gaining 1 kg. Her discharge weight was 45 kg (7 st 1 lb).

After Day 4 Pat requested that a single duvet be brought from home for her own use, and this request was granted. She also had brought in a small pillow from which she derived great comfort when it was placed under certain troublesome joints at night. She had declined the use of a hypnotic and relied solely on Distalgesic and NSAIDs to control her pain. The change from paracetamol and indomethacin to Distalgesic and piroxicam had proved successful. Though never completely free from pain, by Day 10 Pat was sleeping fairly satisfactorily at night, only occasionally requesting analgesia. It was felt that, should she request it, a bath or shower during the night would now be permissible. Certainly, a shower or bath first thing each morning (as morning stiffness was still a problem) could be achieved alone.

On Day 16, after consultation between the medical staff, physiotherapist, nursing staff and Pat, it was decided to continue all treatment for a further 7 days and then review again. Second-line drug therapy had been started on Day 4. This was D-penicillamine in a gradually increasing dose regimen from 125 mg daily up to 500 mg daily. A patient self-medication programme (SMP) was started on Day 6, involving education of Pat by her primary nurse, once an established drug list had been drawn up. Pat was instructed in testing her own urine and was quite competent by Day 9. It took a little longer to achieve success with the medication programme as a whole, but by Day 11 Pat was fully conversant with her drug therapy. She was administering it confidently and understood and could quote from her drug information sheet with obvious enthusiasm.

Patient education classes had been delayed because of the prescribed bed rest. However, on Day 12 classes were started. Pat attended ten classes in all. She had initially agreed to go with some reluctance because of 'fear of the unknown' but became quickly integrated into the class and contributed enthusiastically.

The OT department had assessed Pat for ADL. Custom-made shoes were recommended. Erosions of the feet, evident on radiographs, were sufficient justification for this measure. An additional consideration was the fact that Pat spent the biggest part of the day at home on her feet in caring for her husband and two small children. Well-fitting shoes would eventually be of benefit by acting in a supportive capacity and thereby delaying the development of further deformity.

When not in the throes of an acute flare Pat could manage competently around her home. She had a walk-in shower already installed, and the kitchen fitments were well suited to her height and build. Nonetheless, OT were able to provide Pat with various small aids, for example for turning taps and peeling potatoes. Even more importantly, however, in the patient education class Pat learnt all about joint protection and how to plan and pace her day for when she was eventually discharged home. A home visit from OT was not considered necessary, but a home help was arranged to cover the first few weeks at home, after which a review was to be made.

Review time came again on Day 23, when a ward meeting of all disciplines discussed with Pat her stay in hospital and subsequent treatment. It was pointed out to Pat that clinically she had improved sufficiently to walk quite long distances on the flat and up and down stairs, while relatively free of pain. Her grip strength was still poor but had improved to right hand 80, left hand 100. EMS was still present but had dropped to 30 min, and AI measured that morning had registered 12, consisting of all 1s. Analgesic intake had dropped to just three Distalgesic tablets on average daily. Her pain score on the DDC showed over the past 7 days all 2s (mild) with only one 3 (moderate). Haematologically the ESR had dropped to 35 mm/h.

It was explained to Pat that these improvements, including the lowered ESR, could in the main be due to the rest and careful physical treatment she had received, rather than the drug therapy she was now receiving, though in the long term it was hoped the D-penicillamine would indeed show itself to be slowing down the progress of the disease. All in all Pat was very satisfied with her stay. Her husband had attended for counselling, albeit with reluctance. Afterwards, he appeared to appreciate Pat's problems better, although he refused to visit the physiotherapy department with her. It appeared that there had been sexual problems even before RA was diagnosed. An explicit booklet on overcoming sexual problems was given to Pat, but in the main it was not favourably received. It seemed doubtful whether the marriage would succeed, despite the counselling. The future could therefore be very difficult for Pat if she were left, as it appeared she might be, with two small children and rheumatoid arthritis to cope with. A medical social worker was therefore assigned to Pat to keep an eye on the situation and to step in when help was required.

Finally, the ophthalmologist's report was negative, but he wished to review Pat in 6 months' time. The completed daily progress sheets relating to Pat are shown in Fig. 4.7a–e.

(pp. 112–116)

Fig. 4.7a–e. Daily progress sheets. Patient: Patricia A. ▶

DAILY PROGRESS SHEET

a

Date		Signature
12.6.83.	Admitted at 10 a.m. alone. Reason for admission acute "flare" of rheumatoid arthritis affecting mainly R. Elbow, all M.C.P's, P.I.P's, both wrists, R. Knee and R. Ankle. Has 2 small boys 5 and 8 year, upset at leaving them. Husband has taken them to maternal grandparents. Initially put on bed rest. Has not been seen by Doctor or had nursing assessment done. Diet normal. Medication paracetamol 2 p.r.n. last given 10.15 a.m. on admission for severe generalized pain. Also, indomethicin 25 mg t.d.s. next due after lunch 12.30 p.m.	
12.6.83. 4 p.m.	Nursing assessment and care plan drawn up. Patient seen in conjunction with doctor. Medication changed to Distalgesic 2 t.d.s., piroxican 20 mg. daily.	
13.6.83.	1) Intermittent bed rest prescribed, patient has elected to change into day clothing. Resting splints supplied for both hands and wrists. Pillow supplied to support R. Knee and R. Ankle. Patient experienced relief of pain from application of hot packs applied to R. Knee, both hands and wrists this morning. 2) Continue care plan. 3) Not too happy with active assisted exercises because of resultant pain, but willing to persevere. Quite enjoys doing isometrics. 4) See Night report. 5 and 6) see No 1. 7) Has eaten all meals so far.	
13.6.83 Night report.	4) Disturbed night, slept intermittently only, because of pain, analgesia given. Hypnotic refused.	

Hospital No.	Name PATRICIA A	Consultant DR BIRD	Ward	Sex F

DAILY PROGRESS SHEET

Date		Signature
14.6.83.	Ward Round. No change in care plan. R. Knee aspirated. 30 ml. of synovial fluid removed. H.C.A injected.	
15.6.83.	No change in care plan, except for problem 7) patient eating very well. Gained 2 lbs in weight. D-penicillamine 150 mg. started today. Possible side-effects explained to patient.	
15.6.83. Night report.	Restless night. Appears uncomfortable, have suggested she brings in her own duvet.	
16.6.83.	Care plan continued 4) Request for own duvet, husband telephoned will bring in today. Goniometer reading R. Knee 30°/76°.	
16.6.83. Night report.	4) Slept well – No analgesia given. Obviously happy with own duvet.	
17.6.83.	1) Intermittent bed rest discontinued. Patient encouraged to walk from ward to lounge at least twice a day until she feels able to increase the distance. Future wrist splints supplied to be used in conjunction with resting splints. Hot packs continued b.d. 2) Coping better with personal hygiene. Supervised for bathing only. 3) Normal range of movement of each joint performed unassisted. Commence intensive physiotherapy programme tomorrow. Continue isometric exercises. 4) Sleep pattern much improved. Sleeping 5/6 hours each night. 5) and 6) see problem 1) 7) resolved. 11) Self-Medication Programme started. Also instructed in how to test own urine.	

Hospital No.	Name PATRICIA A	Consultant Dr. BIRD	Ward	Sex F

DAILY PROGRESS SHEET

Date		Signature
19. 6. 83.	Care plan continued. 9) Pat's children visited for the first time. As they appeared relaxed and happy she has lost her anxiety. A.I. 18, Grip Strength R.68. L.68. D.D.C. score for pain averaged over the week is 3 (moderate). Morning Stiffness averaged over the week 122 min, therefore not improving since admission. Suggest Pat takes a shower as soon as possible after waking each morning. Analgesic intake average over the week is 7. Goniometer Reading R. Knee 20°/100° Assessed by O.T. for A.D.L. Shoes ordered. 10) Ophthalmologist report negative.	
21. 6. 83.	Care plan continued. 11) Competent at testing own urine.	
21. 6. 83 Night report	4) Has slept well 5/6 hours without pain or disturbance for last four nights. Sleep pattern established	
22. 6. 83.	Ward Round. Care plan continued. 2) Able to bath unsupervised. Personal Hygiene therefore no longer a problem. 11) Self Medication Programme completed. Patient fully conversant with drug therapy. 12) Discontinue hot packs. May have complete freedom of movement about ward and adjoining rooms.	
23.6.83	Care plan continued. 11) Patient Education Classes started. 12) Early morning Stiffness reduced to 30 min. to continue with early morning shower.	

| Hospital No. | Name
PATRICIA A | Consultant
DR. BIRD | Ward | Sex
F |

DAILY PROGRESS SHEET

Date		Signature
26.6.83.	Care plan continued. 8) Husband counselled with reasonable result only. Refused to accompany Pat to physiotherapy or Patient Education Classes. Says he does understand the situation better however. (let us hope so). Medical Social Worker to be alerted. Weekly clinical assessments as follows: A.I. 12 au 1s, Grip Strength R. 76, L. 100. weekly average D.D.C. Score for pain is 2.2. Morning stiffness 38 min. Analgesic - intake 3 daily. Goniometer reading R. Knee 20°/110°	
27.6.83.	Ward Round. Continue care plan and review in 7 days.	
4.7.83	Ward Round. Pat expressed her satisfaction of the treatment she had received and said how much better she felt. Care plan continued with only problems 11 and 13 to be resolved. 11) Resolved today on completion of Patient Education Classes - hopefully will now cope far better with her problems so avoiding another 'flare' and possibly improving relationship between patient and husband. 13) Resolved after weekly clinical assessments had been made. As follows: A.I. 11 au 1s, Grip Strength R. 80. L. 100. Weekly average D.D.C. score of pain is 2 (mild) and early morning stiffness 30 min. Analgesic intake 3 daily. Goniometer reading R. Knee 20°/110° Weight is 45 Kg. This shows an increase of 1 kg. New shoes have arrived and the look on Pat's face says everything. It has been decided to organise a home help to cover Pat's first few weeks at home after	

Hospital No.	Name PATRICIA A	Consultant DR. BIRD	Ward	Sex F

d

e

DAILY PROGRESS SHEET

Date		Signature
	discharge and this is to take place in ? days' time. A follow up appointment at Leeds General Infirmary in 6 weeks' time. Meanwhile the G.P. informed and he will be asked to check blood in 1 month's time.	

Hospital No.	Name PATRICIA A	Consultant DR. BIRD	Ward	Sex F

Case Study 2

Interview and Identification of Problems

Mr. Thomas B. was admitted to the rheumatology ward as the result of an outpatient appointment some 3 weeks previously. After introducing herself, the nurse discovered that he was quite happy to be addressed as Mr. B......, though if she wished she could call him Tom.

The patient was 69 years old and a widower, his wife having died 3 years previously from cancer of the bowel. Her illness and death had all happened very quickly, and it had taken him a long time to adjust to his loss; however, now he had settled into a routine and was quite happy on his own. He lived near the centre of the city in his own small 'back to back' terraced house. He had an inside toilet but no central heating. As an ex-miner he enjoyed a free supply of coal and kept himself warm when the weather was bad, although the cold did not bother him unduly. Shops and a public house were within walking distance, but as many of the houses around him were being pulled down, the situation might change. He had one married son aged 45 and two grandsons aged 20 and 25.

Mr. B. was small of stature and immediately impressed the nurse with his quiet, pleasant nature. He was not in the least demanding, wishing only 'to do as he was told and get things sorted out'. He had been informed in the outpatient clinic that he was to have his knee examined inside, though he would not be put to sleep, and that he might be in hospital for around 7 days, although length of stay would be decided later. He was in no hurry to return home, having no dependants, but he knew he was going to miss his daily walk. Walking was his passion, and the problem with his knee had meant restricting this activity. This made him feel miserable, and he would therefore be glad if it 'could all be sorted out quickly'. Mr. B. mentioned that he always carried a walking stick and that this was a lifelong habit of his, although lately, he had found that he was using it as a support rather than for pleasure. He also revealed that, unfortunately, he always used his stick in his left hand because it was his left knee which caused him problems. He had no other hobbies, finding the housework and upkeep of his home a full-time job. He had actually just finished painting his house without assistance—he simply took his time. He was a member of the Church of England, although he only occasionally went to church. Should the hospital chaplin visit the ward he would be pleased to see him, as the church had been a great help when his wife died.

On the whole, Mr. B. looked a very fit man and young for his age. Soon after the interview had started the nurse realised that his hearing was slightly impaired, although no aid was worn. Speech was normal, but eyesight was not. Mr. B. had chronic glaucoma of the left eye and wore glasses with bifocal lenses. False teeth were worn and caused no problem. Appetite was very good, and he ate a normal diet with few dislikes. Bowel and bladder elimination were normal, with only the occasional nocturnal urgency of micturition. He did not smoke and usually drank two pints of beer at the weekend when his son took him out. Normally sleep was good, approximately 6 h a night, though lately he had been troubled with pain in the left knee, which naturally disturbed his sleep.

Mobility had been gradually reduced over the past 6 months since the patient had first experienced problems with his left knee. He could not remember having injured it, yet admitted stumbling occasionally while out walking. He agreed that he might have wrenched it, but could not remember. The nurse wondered if his history of being a miner might well have contributed. Personal hygiene was not affected; the patient could still manage to get in and out of his bath, though with increasing difficulty. Social services had never been involved with Mr. B. and he therefore did not receive Meals on Wheels or attend a day centre.

On examination, Mr. B.'s condition confirmed the nurse's impression as to his fitness. He had no skin problems or leg ulcers. His left knee was the only obvious abnormality. It was hot, red and swollen, and an effusion was present. Flexion, when measured with a standard goniometer, was only 15°/50°. The right knee, measured for comparison, was 10°/115°. Vital signs were taken to establish a baseline and were found to be as follows: temperature 36° C, pulse 78 beats/min, respiration rate 18/min, BP 138/98, urinalysis normal, weight 57 kg, height 160 cm, functional grade 3. The patient's assessment of his pain the previous day, based on a score of 1–5, was around 3–4 (moderate to severe).

The general practitioner's letter included in Mr. B.'s medical notes confirmed the patient's account of the problem. Initially the general practitioner had prescribed ibuprofen (Brufen) 400 mg t.d.s. This had helped for about 2 months, after which the condition of the left knee continued to deteriorate. Paracetamol two q.d.s., had been added, and a referral to the consultant rheumatologist had been made. Radiographs had revealed changes consistent with osteoarthrosis, although they were not conclusive.

Assessment

Overall, the patient was in quite good physical condition, his main problem centring upon his swollen and inflamed left knee. This had restricted his movements over the past 6 months, preventing him from taking his daily walk except for short distances. It had not prevented him from bathing himself or caring for his home, although unless it was attended to he felt that it might. Apart from his hearing being slightly impaired, the only other abnormality was his chronic glaucoma of the left eye, into which he instilled drops b.d. This condition did not appear to present a problem as Mr. B. obviously had it well under control. Pain, both day and night, bothered him, and certainly the medication he had been prescribed did not appear to be helping. Walking correctly was becoming a problem and the correct use of walking aids required attention. Also, the patient's knowledge of his condition was limited. Mr. B. appeared to be rather a stoical gentleman who would win through against all odds, preferring to ignore his disabilities in the firm belief that by doing so they might go away.

Plan of Nursing Care

As Mr. B. would be going to theatre for arthroscopy the day after admission, it was decided to delay compiling the nursing care plan until after his return to the ward.

On the patient's return from theatre, pain in the left knee was still the most pressing problem. Therefore rest, though not in bed but sitting in a chair with the left leg supported, was advised. Mr. B. was instructed not to place any weight on his left leg for at least 24 h. Crutches would be supplied. (Alternatively a wheelchair could be used whenever the patient wished to visit the toilet.) Hot or ice packs were to be applied b.d. to the left knee, and knee flexion measured using a standard goniometer on alternate days. It was suggested to Mr. B. that he took the paracetamol regularly (i.e. two tablets 4-hourly instead of p.r.n.), in an attempt to control his pain more successfully. Indomethacin was to be continued as prescribed. A DDC would be issued to monitor closely the patient's pain and analgesic intake. Physiotherapy would start after 24 h. Alerting the night staff to Mr. B.'s problem of severe pain would ensure that his physical comfort and analgesic cover was adequate. Since the problem of slightly impaired hearing could cause problems of misunderstanding, all members of staff, including other disciplines, would be informed of the problem.

Mr. B.'s obvious lack of knowledge regarding his disability had soon become apparent to the nurse. Therefore patient education classes and a self-medication programme would be included in the patient's overall treatment. The OT department would be contacted to assess for ADL and the medical social worker would be alerted. Fig. 4.8a–c shows the completed nursing care plans for Mr. B.

Implementation and Evaluation

Because of the patient's changing circumstances following arthroscopy, continued reassessment of his condition was made and new nursing care plans were drawn up to cater for any new development which arose.

On Day 3 Mr. B. was much relieved that the arthroscopy was over; indeed he declared that it was not as bad as he had feared, thus confirming the nurse's previous impression of his stoical nature. Although he had been keeping all weight off his left knee, pain was still a major problem and was not relieved by paracetamol. Distalgesic two t.d.s. was prescribed and the ibuprofen was changed to naproxen (Naprosyn) 500 mg b.d. The application of hot packs were continued twice daily. Physiotherapy was started on Day 4 and this included weight-bearing exercises and walking practice, and also instructions on the correct use of walking aids. By the time of his discharge Mr. B. was using his stick in the correct right hand, and was well motivated towards daily exercise.

(pp. 120–122)
Fig. 4.8a–c. Nursing care plan. Patient: Tom B. ▶

a

NURSING CARE PLAN

PATIENT NAME: THOMAS B.

HOSPITAL NO.: 78910

Date	No.	Problem	Goal	Nursing Care	Review Date	Evaluation	Resolve Date
10.8.83	1.	Pain in left Knee due to inflammation. Not relieved by arthroscopy carried out yesterday (9.8.83)	Decrease in inflammation and pain.	Allow patient to sit in chair and a) Support left leg on firm pillow. Advise patient not to perform any weight-bearing activities for at least 24 h.	24 hours	Patient experiencing less pain. D.D.C. registers 3. Analgesia reduced to one tds	12.8.83.
				b) Provide crutches so that patient can still use toilet facilities independently or take him in a wheel chair.	24 hours	L. Knee flexion improved 20°/70°	12.8.83
				c) Apply hot packs to L. Knee twice daily or ice if poor result from heat.	daily	Hot packs continued see problem 6.	
				d) Administer analgesia and N.S.A.I as prescribed.	daily		
				e) Measure flexion of L. Knee using standard goniometer alternate days.	16.8.83		
				f) Give D.D. Card to monitor pain and analgesic intake	16.8.83.		
10.8.83	2	Unable to sleep at night, due to pain in L. Knee.	Establish sleep pattern by relieving pain.	a) Ascertain patient comfortable in bed by providing bed cradle and support under L. Knee.	daily	D.D.C. score 2 sleeping 5/6 hours without analgesia	18.8.83
				b) Administer analgesia for pain as prescribed.			

NURSING CARE PLAN

PATIENT NAME: THOMAS B.

HOSPITAL NO.: 78910

Date	No.	Problem	Goal	Nursing Care	Review Date	Evaluation	Resolve Date
10.8.83	3	Slightly impaired hearing which may result in misunderstanding	Prevention of misunderstanding.	Inform all disciplines of patients problem thereby circumventing any embarrassment or misunderstanding taking place	daily	No problems arose during hospital stay.	
10.8.83	4	Poor knowledge of management of disease relating to L. Knee problem.	Overall increase in knowledge resulting in better management.	To attend Patient Education classes relevant to his problem.	on completion of classes.	Attended two classes, one on osteoarthritis and one on exercise and joint protection. Pre and post questionnaires to be evaluated	20.8.83.
10.8.83	5.	Potential mismanagement of drugs therapy due to lack of information.	Clear understanding of drug therapy.	Will take part in Patient Self-Medication Programme.	on completion of programme	Now conversant with drug therapy including eye drops for GLAUCOMA. Could selfmedicate by	15.8.83.
12.8.83	6	Reduced mobility due to mild degree of pain and inflammation of L. Knee.	Reduction in pain and inflammation resulting in increased mobility.	a) Apply hot packs b.d. to L. Knee. b) Start physiotherapy to include weight-bearing exercises and walking practice. c) Administer analgesia and N.S.A.I. as prescribed	daily	Effusion of L. Knee developed. Also increase in pain. D.D.C. Score 4. Hot packs continued see problem 8.	

NURSING CARE PLAN

PATIENT NAME: THOMAS B.

HOSPITAL NO.: 78910

c

Date	No.	Problem	Goal	Nursing Care	Review Date	Evaluation	Resolve Date
15.8.83	7.	Intra-articular injection of HCA and aspiration following effusion of L. Knee.	Prevention of complications developing following I.A.I.	a) No weight-bearing for 24 h following injection. b) Observation of L. Knee for increased pain, swelling and redness. c) Provide crutches or take patient to toilet in chair.	24 h	No sign of complications.	16.8.83
15.8.83	8.	Pain in L. Knee following development of effusion, cause unknown.	Relief of pain.	a) Continue hot packs b.d. to L. Knee. b) Administer analgesia and N.S.A.I as prescribed.	daily	Patient experiencing less pain. D.D.C. registering 2 each day. Patient walking about freely Started physiotherapy again	18.8.83

On Day 5 the doctor informed Mr. B. that there was no evidence of RA in the synovium of the left knee. No crystals were found and all findings therefore suggested an inflammatory osteoarthritis. He would continue with physiotherapy, also exercising other joints involved in walking, so as to strengthen and stabilise them as they might well have to take additional strain while his left knee was causing problems.

Day 5 also saw the commencement of the self-medication programme. As Mr. B. had only two drugs plus his eye drops to deal with, he quickly learnt the facts and was allowed to self-medicate entirely unaided by Day 7.

By Day 7 an effusion had developed once more in the left knee, and an intra-articular injection (IAI) of hydrocortisone acetate (HCA) was prescribed following aspiration of 15 ml of synovial fluid.

Relevant patient education classes were held on Days 8 and 10 and Mr. B. attended both of these. They contained useful information on osteoarthritis, covered the philosophy behind exercise and explained the essentials of joint protection and the use of hot and cold packs at home.

Hot packs were discontinued on Day 11, and, as Mr. B. had become more ambulant than he had been for some months, he was therefore allowed out into the hospital grounds to walk about. The length of time spent there was to be left to his own discretion. Mr. B. enjoyed this 'treat' so much that it was repeated each day during the remainder of his stay, even to the extent of allowing him to venture into the town. Left knee flexion was measured on alternate days with a standard goniometer and showed an improvement over the 11 days from 15°/50° to 12°/90°.

A ward round was held on Day 11, when the doctor, physiotherapist and nurse discussed with Mr. B. his present condition and future treatment. It was decided to discharge the patient 2 days later into the care of his general practitioner. He would continue his exercises on returning home and it was hoped that he would maintain much of his regained freedom of movement.

The social services in Mr. B.'s area were alerted because of his age and the fact that he was living alone. The completed daily progress sheets relating to Mr. B. are shown in Fig. 4.9a, b.

(pp. 124–128)
Fig. 4.9a,b. Daily progress sheets. Patient: Tom B. ▶

DAILY PROGRESS SHEET

Date		Signature
9.8.83	Admitted 10 a.m. alone. Reason for admission diagnostic arthroscopy on L. Knee. To be performed tomorrow 10.8.83. at 2 p.m. under local anaesthetic. Patient informed. Appears relaxed and unconcerned. Seen by Doctor. May have oral diazepam 5 mg t.d.s. today only should he appear anxious. Otherwise give diazepam 10 mg. orally 1 hour before arthroscopy plus pethidine 50 mg I.M. Appears to be a fit, pleasant elderly gentleman, whose only other problem apart from slightly impaired hearing is chronic glaucoma of L. eye which he seems to have under good control instilling eye drops tinia daily. Present medication for problem with L. Knee paracetamol ii p.r.n., and ibuprofen 400 mg t.d.s. Diet normal. Nursing care plan delayed until after arthroscopy. Meanwhile hot pack to be applied to L. Knee tinia daily.	
9.8.83. night report.	Disturbed night due to pain. Analgesia given.	
10.8.83.	10 a.m. Hot pack applied to L. Knee with good result. Returned to ward 2.45 p.m. following arthroscopy of L. Knee. Has 2 stitches in situ. Nursing Care Plan drawn up.	
10.8.83. night report.	2) Disturbed night D.D.C. registers 4., analgesia given.	
11.8.83.	1) Pain continues without relief. Medication changed to Distalgesic ii t.d.s. and naproxen 500 mg. b.d. D.D.C. registers 4. L. Knee flexion 20°/50°. Continue with no weight bearing on L. Knee for a further 24 hrs. Hot packs relieved pain for approximately 1 hour.	

Hospital No.	Name	Consultant	Ward	Sex
78910	THOMAS B.	DR. BIRD	1	M

DAILY PROGRESS SHEET

b

Date		Signature
12. 8. 83.	1) Patient experiencing less pain. Knee flexion 20°/70°. D.D.C registers 3. May walk to toilet unaided. Started physiotherapy.	
13. 8. 83.	Care plan continued. 5) Self-Medication Programme started. Doctor has informed patient, no evidence of R.A. in synovium of L. knee or crystal deposits. Findings suggest inflammatory osteoarthritis. Present treatment therefore in keeping with these findings. O.T. have assessed for A.D.L.	
15. 8. 83.	6) Care plan continued. Has developed effusion of L. knee. Pain and swelling increased. D.D.C. registers 4. Stop physiotherapy. Seen by Doctor. I.A.I. of HCA prescribed preceded by aspiration. 15 ml of synovial fluid removed. 7) and 8) Treatment as care plan.	
16. 8. 83.	7) No sign of complications, may therefore start weight bearing again. Two stitches removed from L. knee. Wound has healed well. 8) Hot packs continued with good results. Knee flexion 20°/70°.	
18. 8. 83.	Care plan continues. 4) Started Patient Education Classes on osteoarthritis. Physio. re-started.	
18. 8. 83. night report	2) Sleeping 5/6 hours. Good sleep pattern therefore established.	
19. 8. 83.	Ward Round. 8) Hot packs discontinued. D.D.C. score averaging 2. Analgesic intake one b.d.. Knee flexion 120/90°. Patient allowed out walking in hospital grounds.	
21. 8. 83.	Patient discharged into care of G.P. Medical Social worker alerted because Mr. B. lives alone. No follow-up appointment made.	

| Hospital No. 78910 | Name THOMAS B. | Consultant Dr. BIRD | Ward | Sex M |

Summary of the Implementation of the Nursing Care Plan

In order to assist the reader to understand the daily progress sheets, one or two points require clarification.

On the nursing care plan for Case Study 1 (Fig. 4.6a) it can be seen that problems have been allocated numbers. On the daily progress sheets these same numbers are used when each problem is reported on. For example, on the nursing care plan problems are identified as follows:

1. Generalised pain and stiffness etc.
2. Personal hygiene restricted etc.
3. Mobility reduced due to inflammation etc.

On the daily progress sheet (Fig. 4.7a) for Day 2 (13.6.83) it reads:

1. Intermittent bed rest prescribed etc.
2. Continue care plan.
3. Not too happy with active assisted exercises etc.

This procedure simplifies reporting on all counts, and makes it very easy for new staff or junior staff to understand each patient's individual situation at a glance.

Nursing Aspects of Investigative Procedures

The following is a glossary of the investigations (partly covered in Chapter 2) in which the nurse will be involved on a rheumatology ward. An important part of her role will be to give psychological support to patients undergoing such investigation, both before and after the procedure.

Arthroscopy—examination of the interior of the knee using an arthroscope
  Problem:
    1. Suspected inflammation of the synovium or crystal deposition
    2. Pain following trauma
  Reason for investigation:
    1. Examination of joint cavity as an aid to diagnosis
    2. Collection of synovial fluid
    3. Biopsy of synovium
    4. Collection of crystal deposits
    5. Therapeutic lavage
  Method:
    The knee can be examined under either local or general anaesthetic. A greater freedom of movement of the arthroscope is possible under

general anaesthetic. Nevertheless, a good, if restricted, examination can be made under a local anaesthetic

Local anaesthetic:

The patient is given an oral sedative e.g. diazepam (Valium) 10–20 mg (to allay anxiety) plus IM pethidine 50–100 mg 1 h preoperatively for relief of pain.

Normal preparation as for theatre, not forgetting thick theatre socks. No special skin preparation required

General anaesthetic:

As local, except that the patient is starved for 6 h preoperatively. IM diazepam 10 mg is given 1 h preoperatively

Special treatment:

In either case the patient may return from theatre with one or two sutures in situ. These are left in for 5–7 days and then removed. An Elastoplast dressing may have been applied, or a pressure bandage if internal bleeding is suspected. Patients often remain in bed for 24 h following the procedure. Temperature pulse respiration and BP should be recorded after a general anaesthetic only. Any sign of increased pain or bleeding should be reported immediately. Discharge after 24–36 h

Endoscopy—examination of the stomach by use of a gastroscope

Problem:

Suspected gastric ulcer following complaints of nausea, loss of appetite, flatulence, epigastric pain or a low Hb (less than 9.0), especially if the patient is taking NSAID or aspirin

Reason for investigation:

Confirmation and location of gastric ulcer and hiatus hernia

Method:

After starving for at least 6 h, the patient is given an IM or IV injection of diazepam (Valium). The endoscope is then passed into the stomach and observations are made. A biopsy may also be taken at the same time. The whole procedure should take 20 min

Side-effects:

Drowsiness. As this investigation is usually done on a day admission, patients are requested to bring an escort with them and not to drive or drink alcohol until the following day

Intra-articular Injections—of corticosteroids within the joint capsule

Problem:

Inflammation of joint (synovitis) causing pain. May not have responded to physiotherapy

Reason for injection:

1. Pain relief
2. Removal of synovial fluid
3. Introduction of corticosteroid

Method:

Strict aseptic technique must be observed. Any effusion (synovial fluid) must be removed first by aspiration.

The drug used can be one of many. At Leeds we favour the use of triamcinolone hexacetonide 20–40 mg, which has a long-lasting effect.

Possible side-effects:

1. Infection introduced at the time of injection. Very rare if strict aseptic technique is adhered to, and NO TALKING rule observed during administration of injection. Increased pain or swelling after injection must be reported
2. Steroid arthropathy (damage to cartilage) can occur if injections are given too frequently into one site, especially weight-bearing joints. It is not certain what causes this damage but it could be either local action of the steroid or scarring of the cartilage by the administrator's needle
3. Possible systemic side-effects may occur, even after only one injection, in the case of pituitary-adrenal suppression

Special precautions:

Patients are advised that weight-bearing joints which have been injected should not be used for at least 24 h. Joints in the upper limb should also be treated with caution, and heavy lifting should therefore be avoided for a similar period of time

Myelogram—radiograph to visualise the spinal cord

Problem:

Suspected nerve route or spinal cord compression, or central disc prolapse

Reason for investigation:

1. As an aid to diagnosis—the dye should define the site of neurological involvement
2. As a visual aid should surgery be demanded

Method:

A lumbar puncture is performed and an oily radiopaque dye (iodized oil) is injected into the subarachnoid space. This will clearly outline any structural abnormality within the spinal canal, for example a prolapsed intervertebral disc or tumour.

Side-effects and treatment:

1. Severe headaches—may be due to leakage of cerebrospinal fluid from lumbar puncture site. Patient should therefore be placed in a bed with the head raised for at least 6–12 h following procedure
2. Arachnoiditis—a reaction to the dye. BP and TPR should be recorded as a matter of routine.

Radiculogram—as myelogram, but the technique is restricted to the examination of the lower lumbar and sacral nerve roots

Method:

Patient is kept upright (standing or sitting) during examination, and the patient remains sitting for approximately 6 h afterwards

Side-effects and treatment:
As the solution is a water-soluble radiopaque dye it cannot be removed. Hence the patient must remain upright in an attempt to prevent headaches occurring. Nausea and vomiting may occur. Antiemetics may be given

References

Joint Consultants' Committee Meeting (1983) Nursing process criticised. Br Med J 287: 439
Luker KA (1979) Teaching the nursing process. Nursing Times 75(35): 1488–1490
McFarlane JK, Baroness of Llandaff and Castledine G (1982) A guide to the practice of nursing using the nursing process. Mosby, St Louis, Appendix 1, p. 135
Thurtle OA and Cawley MID (1983) The frequency of leg ulceration in rheumatoid arthritis: a survey. J Rheumatol 10: 507–509
United Kingdom Central Council (1982) Working Group 3, Education and Training. The development of nurse education. Discussion document I. (Government publication)

Further Reading

Carlson JH, Craft CA and McGuire AD (1982) Nursing diagnosis. Saunders, Philadelphia
Elliott M (1979) Nursing rheumatic disease. Churchill Livingstone, New York
Hunt JM and Marks-Maran DJ (1980) Nursing care plans. HM & M, Aylesbury
Kratz CR (1979) The nursing process. Baillière Tindall, London
McFarlane JK, Baroness of Llandaff and Castledine G (1982) A guide to the practice of nursing using the nursing process. Mosby, St Louis
Panayi GS (1980) Essentials of rheumatology for nurses and therapists. Baillière Tindall, London
Roper N, Logan WW and Tierney AJ (1981) Learning to use the process of nursing. Churchill Livingstone, Edinburgh

5

Surgical Nursing

Introduction

Although rheumatic diseases are generally thought of as a medical problem, no book on the combined care of the rheumatic patient would be complete without a chapter on surgical intervention. Indeed, many hospitals now hold combined clinics where orthopaedic surgeons and rheumatologists see patients together to discuss the surgical management of their patients' disease.

In the case of the rheumatic patient, surgery is usually an elective procedure which is carried out for one, or a combination of the following reasons:

1. To diminish pain
2. To increase function
3. To prevent deformity
4. To maintain independence

Major advances have been made in the surgical field, the most dramatic being the total hip replacement in patients suffering from diseased hips. As a result of this treatment many patients who for years endured misery and pain are now enjoying a new lease of life. If must be stressed, however, that surgery is not a cure for arthritis, but it can be a valuable supplement to medical treatment.

This chapter is divided into two sections. The first part deals briefly with the surgical procedures currently available; the second discusses the nursing management which is specific to the rheumatic patients undergoing surgery.

Surgical Procedures

Synovectomy

Synovectomy is the excision of the synovial membrane, usually performed in cases of rheumatoid arthritis. In cases of severe synovitis which rest and medication have failed to resolve, synovectomy may be beneficial. When it is performed at an early stage in the disease process, it can help to relieve pain and prevent progressive deformity. It is usually performed on joints which have an easily accessible synovium such as the metacarpophalangeal joints, the elbows and the knees, all of which have a good chance of success. However, there are some joints in which it is less successful such as the ankle, hips, wrists and interphalangeal joints.

Unfortunately, synovectomy can ultimately lead to loss of movement due to postoperative immobility and adhesions, and frequently the synovitis re-occurs when the synovium regenerates. Postoperative physiotherapy and exercises are very important following synovectomy to prevent the formation of adhesions, but if these are not successful within 3 weeks, then it may be necessary to manipulate the joint under anaesthetic.

Entrapment Neuropathies

An entrapment neuropathy occurs when a peripheral nerve is subjected to excess pressure in a confined space. Several types of entrapment neuropathy are found in rheumatoid arthritis, the most common being the carpal tunnel syndrome. This occurs when tenosynovitis of the surrounding tendons compresses the median nerve underneath the flexor retinaculum in the carpal tunnel. It is often an early feature of rheumatoid arthritis and is experienced by approximately 20% of patients at some time. The patient complains of burning paraesthesiae of the thumb, index and middle finger, which worsens at night or after exercise. In severe cases there is wasting of the thenar eminence. For patients suffering from arthritis the consequences can be particularly incapacitating, as it can prevent the use of walking aids.

Diagnosis can be confirmed by the use of nerve conduction studies. Symptoms can be reproduced by using local pressure at the site of the entrapment. This is known as Tinel's sign.

Mild cases of carpal tunnel syndrome are treated by rest, night splinting and injections of corticosteroids into the carpal tunnel, but persistent cases usually need decompression surgery. This simple surgery consists of the division of the transverse carpal ligament and synovectomy of the flexor tendons. Patients usually make an uneventful recovery, and full function and sensation are quickly restored.

Less common sites are:

1. The lateral popliteal nerve at the knee
2. The ulnar nerve behind the medial epicondyle of the humerus

3. The posterior tibial nerve behind the medial malleolus (tarsal tunnel syndrome)

All respond well to surgery.

Tendon Repair

Spontaneous rupture is not uncommon in patients suffering from rheumatoid arthritis. It usually involves the extensor tendons of the fingers. This is due to abrasion of the tendons where they pass over the dorsum of the distal ulna. The tendon is repaired and the underlying cause removed, in this case by excision of the ulnar head.

Tenotomy

Tenotomy is used to correct flexion deformities, often of the hand or knee.

Osteotomy

Osteotomy is the surgical division of a bone which is then allowed to re-unite. Although this used to be a fairly common operation on the hip, it has been largely superseded by replacement arthroplasty. Its main use now is on young patients with osteoarthritis whose range of movement is still good but whose pain demands surgical relief. In rheumatoid arthritis it is used relatively rarely. In osteoarthritis of the hip McMurray's osteotomy (Fig. 5.1) is still carried out occasionally in young people. It consists of intertrochanteric division of the femur with medial displacement of the femoral shaft to below the acetabulum. Early osteotomy has the advantage that later it can be converted to a total hip replacement if necessary.

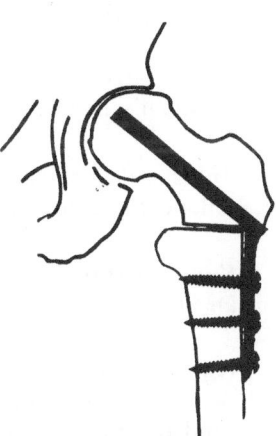

Fig. 5.1. McMurray's osteotomy of the hip. [Wright V and Haslock I (1977) Rheumatism for nurses and remedial therapists. Heinemann Medical, London]

The knee is the most common site for osteotomy, which is usually combined with re-alignment surgery such as that for severe varus or valgus deformities. Tibial defects are the usual cause of varus malalignments, whilst valgus deformities are due to lateral femoral defects. Single osteotomies can be carried out across the upper part of the tibia or at the lower end of the femur. When both procedures are carried out at the same time, it is a double osteotomy, known as Benjamin's operation.

Spinal osteotomy is occasionally carried out for marked kyphosis in ankylosing spondylitis, but this is a hazardous operation because of the proximity to the spinal cord and its roots. Advances in the early medical management of this disease have all but eliminated the need for this operation.

Arthrodesis

Arthrodesis is the fixation of a moveable joint by a surgical operation in which the diseased joint is excised and fusion of the bone ends is allowed to take place. If the fusion is sound, this results in a pain-free joint in the correct position, but at the expense of complete loss of movement.

Whilst this operation can be beneficial in some circumstances, it is rarely used because of the development of arthroplasty. In rheumatoid arthritis its usefulness is severely limited, because (1) success depends on bone fusion, which is difficult to secure in porotic bones, and (2) an immovable joint places extra loads on adjacent joints, which are likely to be diseased and incapable of withstanding additional stress without further damage.

Despite its disadvantages, however, arthrodesis can be useful in joints requiring stabilisation but where loss of movement is acceptable.

Radiocarpal Joints.   Arthrodesis of the radiocarpal joints is a very successful operation in the treatment of the rheumatoid hand, resulting in a pain-free, stable joint and an improved grip strength, with very little loss of function. Some surgeons determine the optimum positioning of a joint before arthrodesis with the aid of splints. These are applied to the wrist, for example, before surgery to ascertain if the joint is in its most functional position to suit the patient's needs.

Ankle and Tarsal Joints.   Arthrodesis of the ankle and tarsal joints is an excellent procedure, provided there is sound fusion.

Knee.   Arthrodesis is not the preferred surgery in the knee but can be used if an arthroplasty fails.

Hip.   Arthrodesis of the hip is used only in young adults with osteoarthritis whose knees and other hip are fully mobile. Older patients are usually treated by total hip replacement.

The Spine.   Atlantoaxial subluxation causing compression of the spinal cord and neurological symptoms is treated by fusion of the atlas to the axis to give stability. This may occur due to ligamentous instability in rheumatoid arthritis.

Arthroplasty

Arthroplasty is the term used for the surgical reconstruction of a joint. There are two types of arthroplasty: (1) excision and (2) replacement.

Excision Arthroplasty

Excision arthroplasty is the excision of the ends of one or both articulating surfaces to leave a gap which subsequently fills with fibrous tissue. The joint is left pain free, and deformities can also be corrected, but the operation results in limited range of movement and poor joint stability, which makes it unsuitable for surgery of the large weight-bearing joints.

The most common use is at the metatarsophalangeal joints where the metatarsal heads are trimmed and the bases of the proximal phalanges are excised in a procedure known as Fowler's operation (Fig. 5.2).

Pain under the metatarsal heads can be successfully relieved by a combination of excision arthroplasty and division of the extensor tendons. The toes and forefoot are then re-aligned giving the foot a more normal appearance. This may enable some patients to wear normal well-fitting shoes, which can be a great morale booster to the more fashion conscious.

It is possible to re-align the fingers with the metacarpal heads from dislocated metacarpophalangeal joints. Unfortunately, the formation of postoperative adhesions can cause stiffness and subsequent loss of function.

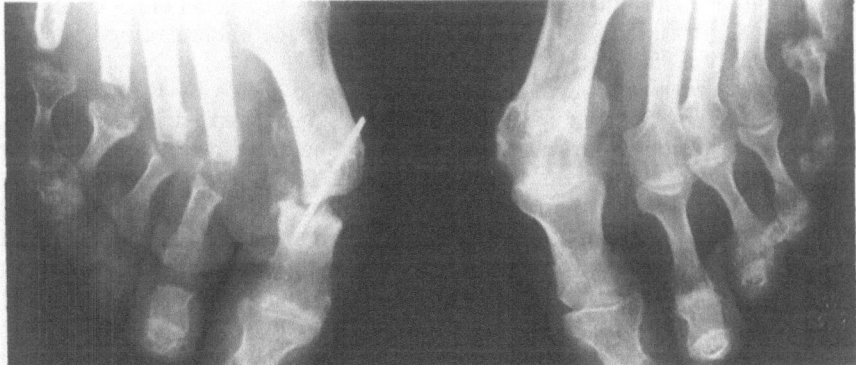

Fig. 5.2. Fowler's operation on the feet. The operation has been performed on the right foot in this picture. The metatarsal heads have been removed and a pin inserted in the big toe. The left foot remains unaltered.

Excision of the ulnar head at the wrist can give great relief from pain. This can be combined with arthrodesis of the radiocarpal joint to increase the range of pain-free supination and pronation. At the elbow the radial head can be excised with a resulting relief of pain but leaving an unstable joint.

Girdlestone arthroplasty of the hip is contemplated when other procedures fail. It is used in patients who are in considerable pain and are confined to a wheelchair or bed. The femoral head and proximal femoral neck are removed. The patient has to remain in a wheelchair because of the instability of the joint but is relieved of pain.

Replacement Arthroplasty

Replacement arthroplasty is the replacement of the whole or part of a joint by synthetic substitutes. It is carried out to relieve severe pain, restore function, re-establish joint stability and to maintain independence. The success of the operation depends on the successful attachment of the prosthesis to the existing bone. This requires that (1) there is sufficient healthy bone to provide a strong anchorage and (2) that the prosthesis can be permanently and rigidly fixed in place.

Metal to metal and metal to plastic joints have been used. Today the metal to plastic joint is the most common because its low friction reduces the possibility of the prosthesis becoming loose.

There are arthroplasties available for hips, knees, elbows, shoulder and metacarpophalangeal joints. Of these the hip is by far the most successful and commonly used.

Total Hip Replacement. The surgical procedure of total hip replacement involves the replacement of both the femoral head and the acetabulum by synthetic substitutes. It is used in patients with either osteoarthrosis or rheumatoid arthritis and has the most dramatically beneficial effect of any of the surgical procedures carried out in the field of rheumatology. It has approximately a 95% success rate.

The operation was first introduced in the early 1960s by Prof. Sir John Charnley of Wrightington Hospital in Wigan. The Charnley prosthesis has been refined over the years and today remains one of the most widely used. It consists of two components, a stainless steel femoral replacement and a high-density polythene (polyethylene) cup. These components are bonded into position using polymethylmethacrylate cement. This substance is not a glue but a cold curing cement with excellent void-filling properties, which, when hardened, forms a ridged mechanical key between the bone and the prosthesis. Providing the bond is secure, the joint will be pain free and mobile almost immediately after surgery. However, full stability will not be achieved for a number of weeks because the surrounding muscle requires time to recover from the trauma of surgery. A number of commonly used prostheses are shown in Fig. 5.3.

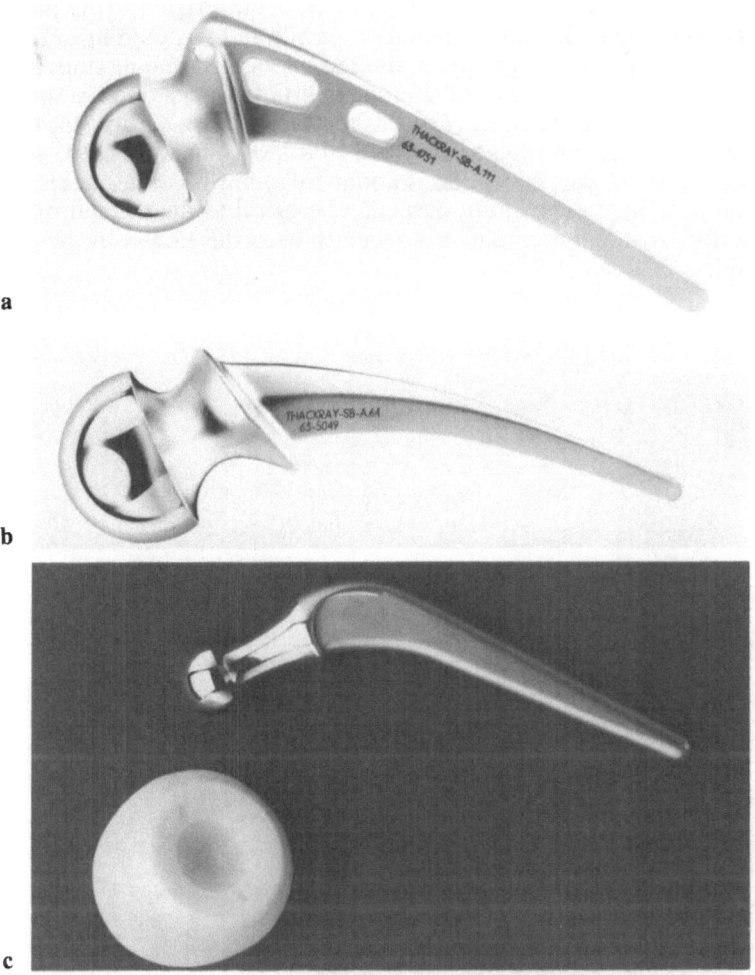

Fig. 5.3a–c. A selection of hip prostheses. **a** Austin Moore prosthesies; **b** Thompson prosthesis; **c** Charnley extra-heavy flange prosthesis and flanged standard cup. (Courtesy of Chas. F. Thackray Ltd., Leeds)

Until recently total hip replacement has been reserved for older patients because predictions of the joint life were uncertain. As the number of artificial joints in use has increased and as the design of the joints has developed, so confidence in their durability has grown to the point where they are now considered appropriate treatment for some younger patients. In this instance it is more successful in osteoarthrosis with its increased bone density and slower progression than in rheumatoid arthritis, which is a more rapid destructive process.

The Knee.   The development of the hinge-type arthroplasty for the knee has proved to be far more difficult than that of the ball and socket joint largely because, unlike the hip joint, which is stabilised by its surrounding muscles, the knee joint must not only have inherent stability, but must allow a small degree of rotation as the knee flexes. For this reason it is at an earlier stage of development than is the hip replacement and so is less commonly used. The current success rate for this operation is about 50%, but it is reasonable to expect a significant increase as joint design and surgical techniques improve with experience. A new knee joint has recently been developed by bioengineers working in Leeds.

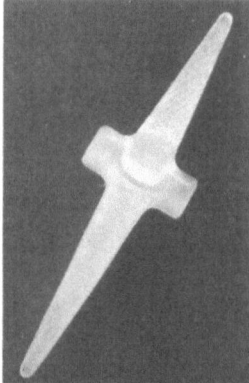

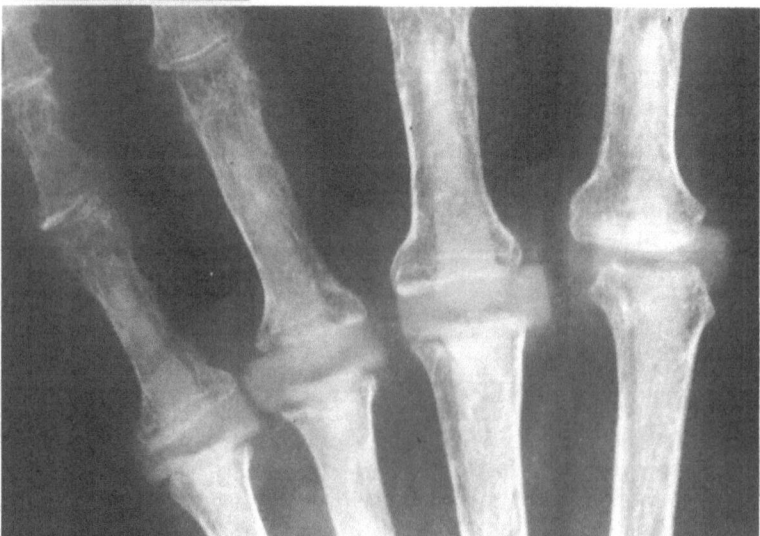

Fig. 5.4a,b. Finger joint replacement. **a** Silastic spacer used to replace deformed metacarpophalangeal joints in rheumatoid arthritis (magnified). **b** Radiograph showing successful insertion of interphalangeal joint prostheses (same patient as in Fig. 2.2).

The Elbow. Like the knee the elbow is a hinge joint, and therefore replacement arthroplasty is fraught with the same problems of instability. So far the results have proved disappointing.

The Shoulder. Although the shoulder is similar to the hip in that it is a ball and socket joint, replacement arthroplasty is still at an experimental stage. The reason is not only because the shoulder is less frequently affected by arthritis, but also because the shallower ball and socket joint and smaller volume of bone at the joint make replacement difficult.

The Hand. For some years now surgeons have been replacing the joints of the fingers. So far, the most successful has been a spacer made of Silastic (Fig. 5.4), which is inserted at the metacarpophalangeal joints to prevent the bone ends coming into contact. This allows pain-free mobility of the fingers and thus function is restored. Many surgeons would regard the success of this technique as now second only to the success of hip arthroplasty.

Nursing Management

It is not our aim to give a detailed account of orthopaedic nursing. For that, readers should refer to an orthopaedic textbook such as *Orthopaedic Nursing and Rehabilitation* by Mary Powell (1982). Instead, this part of the chapter will focus on the aspects of care which are particularly relevant to the surgical nursing of rheumatic diseases. As rheumatoid arthritis is the most common of the inflammatory arthritides it will be used as a model.

Most rheumatic patients requiring surgery will be treated in a general orthopaedic ward. For the outcome of surgery to be successful it is necessary for the nurse and related health professionals to have a clear understanding of the nature of the disease and of the particular difficulties that this can create.

Rheumatoid arthritis is a chronic, inflammatory, systemic illness which has periods of exacerbation and quiescence. It is characterised by a synovitis which causes painful, hot, swollen joints, which in turn lead to deformity and loss of function. Patients complain of fatigue and loss of appetite, and many have severe morning stiffness.

Since rheumatoid arthritis is a systemic disease, the patient is not merely suffering from joint disease but is in general ill health. Systemic manifestations include anaemia, vasculitis, scleritis, episcleritis, pleural effusions and pericardial effusions. Rheumatoid nodules can also be present when the disease is severe. They are usually found at areas of pressure but can occur in the lungs, brain and heart. As the disease progresses, the skin becomes thin and fragile and so is very easily damaged. Ulcers frequently develop at the ankles and on the lower limbs.

In patients suffering from rheumatic disease, surgery is normally an elective procedure and only rarely needs to be performed as an emergency. Consequently, the decision to operate can be taken over a period of time after tripartite discussion between the physician, the surgeon and the patient. Sometimes patients are admitted for conservative treatment prior to their surgery so that they may be at their optimum fitness. This will prepare them to cope both physically and mentally during their postoperative period.

Patients' Expectations and Motivation

With the possible exceptions of early synovectomy and release of entrapment neuropathies, surgery in rheumatic diseases is normally contemplated only if medical treatment has failed to relieve the suffering of chronic pain and the subsequent deformity and loss of function. As a result many patients regard surgery as a last chance, and this attitude may have a danger of unrealistically high expectations. It is therefore essential that patients are fully informed of the expected outcome of their surgery, for if their high hopes are not realised the postoperative depression and loss of motivation which result can be devastating. The nurse is the health professional who has more contact with patients than the other members of the multidisciplinary team. She should make it her responsibility to educate patients about the proposed surgery and also—because patients sometimes hear only what they want to hear—to make sure that the goals which patients set for themselves are realistic and can be achieved.

It cannot be stressed too strongly that only if patients are positively motivated will they be able to cope with the demands made upon them both physically and mentally, during the essential pre- and postoperative physiotherapy programme. This is important as the success of the physiotherapy will largely determine the amount of mobility and function that they will eventually regain.

Environmental Needs

In a few hospitals rheumatic patients needing surgery are treated directly from a specialised rheumatology unit. This benefits both staff and patients. The staff gain valuable surgical experience and breadth of knowledge, whilst the patients are cared for by a knowledgeable multidisciplinary team with whom they are already familiar. The specialised unit is also likely to be adapted to the patients' environmental needs. In a general ward rheumatic patients can be deprived of their independence by lack of facilities and ignorance of the disease process on the part of the staff. By contrast, orthopaedic wards will usually have some items of equipment suitable for the rheumatic patient such as toilet rails, high toilet seats and bathroom hoists, be able to accommodate wheelchairs and be in possession of specialised orthopaedic seating. Items which are less likely to be available are lightweight crockery, specially adapted cutlery, tap turners and specialised door handles. However, it must be emphasised that the best equipped unit and the most skilled surgeon will not result in successful surgery without the education of the patient and the multidisciplinary team responsible for his or her care.

Contraindications to Surgery

Contraindications include not only the usual medical contraindications to surgery but also psychological problems.

Psychological Problems. Patients who are severely depressed are not good candidates for surgery. It is much wiser to treat their depression first and leave decisions about their surgery until their mental state has improved. If the nurse becomes aware that her patient is severely depressed, she should inform the surgeon, who may defer surgery if he thinks this appropriate.

Similar problems arise with abnormally overanxious patients; if it is not possible to alleviate this state over a period of time with careful counselling, a successful outcome will be in doubt, as these patients may be unwilling to comply postoperatively.

Medical Problems. Many arthritic patients are elderly and, although being elderly is not in itself a contraindication to surgery, such patients who are also suffering from pulmonary or cardiac complaints would have difficulty in participating in the rigorous postoperative rehabilitation regimen.

Patients unable to tolerate a general anaesthetic are also excluded. However, minor procedures such as surgery to relieve carpal tunnel syndrome can be carried out under local anaesthetic, and occasionally more major procedures are performed under local nerve block.

Skin. The skin of the rheumatic patient can present great problems to the surgeon as it is thin, fragile and slow to heal, particularly if the patient has been receiving steroids. For surgery to be successful the skin must be intact, in good condition and free from infection over the proposed surgical site prior to any surgery being carried out.

Vasculitis. If the patient is suffering from vasculitis the chances of the wound healing can be very poor indeed because of the decreased blood supply and lack of nutrition. Some surgeons believe active vasculitis to be a contraindication to surgery and prefer to defer surgery until the vasculitis has been controlled by medical means, particularly if surgery on a limb is contemplated.

Infection. Local or systemic infections are definite contraindications to replacement surgery. If a prosthesis becomes infected, experience has shown that the chances of saving it are less than one in three.

Patients receiving corticosteroid therapy should be monitored carefully as steroid therapy masks infection. A raised white cell count or elevated temperature preoperatively should always be investigated.

Preoperative Management

Rheumatoid arthritis is a systemic illness; therefore it must be recognised by the nursing team that rheumatic patients will need rest and must be encouraged to take it. Patients should have been taught how to pace themselves and so not become overtired. It should be remembered that they may have been awake since the very early hours because of their pain and stiffness. Many rheumatic patients habitually rise a few hours before other members in the household so that they can exercise, have a warm bath to relieve their pain and stiffness and so be ready to face the day at the same time as other members of their families.

Bed cradles should be supplied, and a lighweight cover on the bed is essential. A bedside stool may be necessary to facilitate getting in and out of bed independently.

Rheumatic patients may need help with their personal toilet and with dressing but may be able to maintain their independence with the help of simple aids. It is important that these are supplied if the patient fails to bring their own into hospital.

Meal times can become an acute embarrassment if the nursing staff fail to notice the patient in difficulty with their eating implements or unable to cut up their food.

As mentioned previously, the skin of the rheumatic patient is very thin and fragile and will bruise easily. This can be due to the disease process or as a drug induced side-effect if the patient is on steroid therapy. There is also the risk in these patients of subluxation, dislocation and even fracture if the nurse is overzealous in her ministrations. It is very important that the skin is intact and free from infection over the operation site; therefore, particular care must be taken by the nurse when in contact with these areas as even the slightest excess pressure can cause bruising or abrasion of the skin.

Anaemia

Many patients suffering from rheumatoid arthritis become anaemic. The anaemia can be the simple hypochromic microcytic iron deficiency anaemia which results from drug-induced gastric bleeding or the normochromic normocytic anaemia which occurs when the disease is active. If it is the latter, the anaemia will usually disappear as the disease comes under control, but if it is the former the patient may need a preoperative blood transfusion.

Medication

Medication plays a large part in the lives and treatment of rheumatic patients and is covered elsewhere in this book (see Chap. 2). Many patients are on a multiplicity of drugs, some of them highly toxic; therefore it is important to be aware of drug interactions and the side-effects that can occur.

Non-steroidal Anti-inflammatory Drugs. Most patients suffering from arthritis will receive NSAIDS. The timing of the administration of these drugs is of the upmost importance as most of them are gastric irritants and therefore should be given with food or milky drinks. Many patients are used to having their NSAIDs immediately upon waking to help relieve their pain and stiffness or alternatively a suppository or a slow-release NSAID just before retiring at night.

Patients taking phenylbutazone may be at risk if they require lower limb surgery as this drug and its derivatives cause fluid retention. These patients are also more susceptible to congestive cardiac failure, particularly if elderly.

Second-line Agents.   If the patient is taking one of the long-term agents such as gold or penicillamine, weekly urine testing is indicated as these drugs can cause kidney damage. They also cause blood dyscrasias, and therefore a full blood count including white cells and platelets should be carried out prior to surgery.

Steroids.   Patients receiving systemic steroid therapy will need a boost of hydrocortisone to prevent collapse from adrenal insufficiency during surgery and postoperatively. This can be given either intravenously or intramuscularly, according to the wishes of the surgeon and anaesthetist.

Antibiotics.   The results of postoperative infection can be disastrous, and therefore many orthopaedic surgeons prescribe a course of prophylactic antibiotics. This is particularly important if the patient is to receive a prosthesis. The antibiotic given, the mode of administration and the duration of the course will be determined by the surgeon.

Anticoagulants.   Prophylactic anticoagulants are used by some surgeons to decrease the risk of postoperative deep vein thrombosis and pulmonary embolism. However, it is of interest that the rheumatic patient may be less at risk than patients with other diseases, in spite of the relative thrombocytosis which, as part of the systemic manifestations of rheumatoid arthritis, might have increased the risk of thrombus formation.

Patients taking high doses of salicylates and who are subsequently given anticoagulants must be observed carefully for signs of bleeding, as the action of anticoagulants is potentiated by salicylates.

Preoperative Patient Education

Preoperative patient education is an essential nursing function, carried out to ensure that patients understand the proposed surgical procedure, to help them to set down achievable goals and teach them how to achieve these goals. A patient who is taught in this way is far more capable and willing to comply postoperatively than one who is left uneducated. This programme of education is described in more detail in Chapter 7.

Figure 5.5 shows a sample preoperative teaching sheet which can be used. The nurse and the patient discuss its contents together, and the patient's acceptance and understanding can be evaluated. This helps the patient to set realistic goals and then achieve those goals.

SUBJECT	PATIENTS UNDERSTANDING	NURSES EVALUATION
SURGICAL PROCEDURE		
EXPECTED OUTCOME OF SURGERY		
PATIENTS OWN GOALS		

PREPARATION FOR SURGERY
    Skin preparation
    Patch tests		

IMPORTANCE OF PHYSIOTHERAPY
    Pre-op.
    Post-op.
    Restrictions		

DRUGS		
VITAL SIGNS		

POSITIONING
    Abduction
    Elevation
    Cervical Precautions		

IMPORTANCE OF INFECTION
    General
    Wound		

LENGTH OF HOSPITALISATION		
SEXUAL COUNSELLING		
OTHER		

Fig. 5.5. Preoperative teaching sheet.

Patients requiring major surgery such as a total hip replacement should be taught what to expect and how to cope with their postoperative regimen a few days before their surgery. It can be appreciated that immediately after surgery is not the most appropriate time to try to educate anyone! They should also be encouraged to practise everyday functions. Lying in a supine position with legs in abduction and with one arm in a splint due to IV infusion is not the most advantageous position in which to eat, use a bedpan or carry out one's personal toilet, but all these activities are possible if they have been practised preoperatively. Similarly, for patients requiring hand surgery, it can be useful to immobilise one arm before surgery to enable them to practise eating, dressing etc. and so relieve some of the postoperative burden.

Preoperative Physiotherapy

The physiotherapist plays a major role in the rehabilitation of patients undergoing surgery. She will visit such patients preoperatively to make an assessment of their physical condition and teach them about their postoperative physiotherapy regimen. Deep breathing and coughing will be taught to facilitate venous return and prevent hypostatic pneumonia. Depending upon the area of the surgery, exercises such as quads and gluteals drill and plantar and dorsiflexion of the ankle will also be taught to maintain function and aid circulation. If the patient will need to use crutches after surgery these are usually provided beforehand and instructions given on their correct use. Monkey poles can be a valuable aid to mobility whilst the patient is bedridden, but it should be noted that patients suffering from rheumatoid arthritis may have great difficulty in their use if their hands and arms are affected. Patients suffering from cervical problems must be warned not to use their head and neck as a pivot whilst lifting with the aid of a pole, as they put themselves at risk of atlantoaxial subluxation. It is advisable for this group of patients to wear a collar at all times.

Preparation for Surgery

Rheumatic patients are prepared for surgery in the same way as any other group, but special care must be taken when shaving patients if they are receiving steroid therapy because of the fragility of their skin and low resistance to infection. Theatre staff should also be made aware of the special care required when handling this group of patients.

If the patient has neck involvement or stiffness of the temporomaxilliary joint the anaesthetist should be informed, as intubation may be difficult and serious airway problems can occur. A cervical collar should be worn to the operating theatre to remind all concerned that this patient could be a special risk.

Postoperative Management

A detailed account of postoperative nursing care is outside the scope of this book. Instead, a brief outline of general principles specific to rheumatoid arthritis will be given.

It is essential to realise that each surgeon will have his or her own likes and dislikes, and that each patient is an individual and needs to be treated as such. Consequently, it is not possible to lay down rigid rules for the nursing care of these patients. However, the emergence of the nursing process and its individual care plans provide an ideal framework in which general nursing principles can be tailored to meet the individual requirements of each patient and their efficacy can be evaluated.

Upper Limb Surgery

On return from the operating theatre the patient should be nursed with the limb in an elevated position. The simple orthopaedic rule of elevating the hand higher than the wrist, the wrist higher than the elbow and the elbow higher than the shoulder should be followed assiduously. This will aid venous return and prevent gross oedema. Elevation may be achieved by placing the limb on a firm pillow or suspending a sling or pillowcase from a drip stand. If a plaster cast or posterior splint has been applied the phalanges must be left exposed and easily visible so that signs of circulatory impairment can be observed. Postoperative analgesics are given in adequate amounts to keep the patient comfortable. For the first 48 h temperature, pulse and respiration are observed 4-hourly and then, providing they remain within normal limits, recorded twice daily.

Patients suffering from rheumatoid arthritis are confined to bed for as short a period as possible. Providing no adverse reactions occur, the patient will be allowed out of bed in the evening of the same day as surgery. The limb must remain in an elevated position when the patient is ambulant. If a drip stand is used to elevate the limb, it can be wheeled about by the patient. A triangular bandage may also be used, as it is less cumbersome than a suspended sling. However, some patients suffering from cervical problems may find this bandage uncomfortable, and it can be dangerous as it is usually tied at the neck and can therefore cause atlantoaxial subluxation. If this is the case, a sling which passes over the shoulder on the unaffected side and under the shoulder of the surgical side can be used. Being able to use one hand will have been taught preoperatively, but the patient will still need extra help with dressing, washing, feeding etc. during the first 24-h postoperative period.

Surgical dressings should be observed for signs of infection, and patients are advised to keep their dressings dry. A plastic bag can be used to cover the dressing when the patient is bathing or showering.

Exercises will begin according to the appropriate regimen and will be taught by the physiotherapist. However, it is the responsibility of the nurse to ensure that the patient complies with the exercise programme when the physiotherapist is not in attendance.

Lower Limb Surgery

Lower limb surgery can include arthrodesis, excision arthroplasty and replacement arthroplasty. Rather than giving a detailed description in each case, the postoperative care specific to a rheumatic patient who has undergone a total hip replacement will be used as an example. The nursing management of the total hip replacement can be adapted to the other surgical procedures, but for a detailed account of orthopaedic nursing and physiotherapy, the reader is referred to the useful textbook by Powell (1982).

When patients return from the operating theatre they are nursed in a recumbent position until fully conscious and then in a semirecumbent position for the first 24 h. A blood transfusion or intravenous infusion will be in situ and a drain will be inserted into the wound and attached to a suction bottle to remove any serosanguineous exudate and prevent the formation of a haematoma. As with all patients undergoing major surgery, vital signs should be monitored frequently until they become stable and then 4-hourly. Patients who are receiving steroid therapy must be treated with special care when a sphygmomanometer cuff is being applied as ecchymosis can easily occur. The toes of the affected limb should be checked for sensation, warmth and capillary refill. To minimise the risk of dislocation, the patient's legs are kept in a moderate degree of abduction, and external rotation is avoided by the use of a firm wedge such as a Charnley pillow placed between the malleoli.

Adequate analgesia must be given, but many patients are surprised to find that, except when moving or being turned, the degree of pain experienced in the joint operated upon is much less than they had anticipated. However, patients suffering from rheumatoid arthritis can quickly become very stiff as a result of the enforced positioning and immobility. Heat or cold can be applied to the affected joints, and passive movements of the limbs can bring great relief.

If the patient has an intravenous infusion in situ the arm will be placed on a splint and held with a crepe bandage; this should be released every few hours, as the arm can become very stiff. If the patient has fragile skin, care must be taken when re-applying the splint so as not to cause abrasions or ecchymosis. Pillows should be arranged with great care and must never be placed beneath the knees, as contractures can occur within 24 h.

During the first few days after surgery rheumatic patients will need much encouragement and assistance from the nursing staff to help them to adjust to their new situation. Nursing staff must be at hand in adequate numbers. A minimum of two nurses, and preferably three, are required to lift the patient on and off a bedpan and carry out the care of pressure areas. The patient may be turned, but the legs must be kept in abduction at all times and rotation should be avoided. This rule will apply throughout the whole of the patient's hospitalisation. When such patients are more mobile about the bed and able to carry out their own personal toilet, they must be advised to avoid extreme flexion of the affected hip. For example, they should be told not to sit upright at a 90° angle, as this could lead to subluxation. A visit from the occupational therapist can be very useful at this time as she can provide aids to enable patients to reach without the need for excessive flexion of the hip.

Early mobilisation of rheumatic patients is essential as they suffer greatly from morning stiffness and inactivity stiffness. The rapidity at which this is carried out will vary according to the preference of the surgeon and the individual patient's condition. As soon after surgery as the patient is able to comply, physiotherapy commences with deep breathing exercises and passive limb movements. Usually, by the second postoperative day quads and gluteals drill and more active exercises will commence under the supervision of the physiotherapist. When the drains have been removed, and if the patient's general physical condition allows, weight bearing is encouraged. The rate of ambulation will be decided by the surgeon, who will be advised by the physiotherapist. Many patients are able to take short supervised walks using some form of walking aid within 1 week of their surgery. To prevent flexion contractures patients need to lie completely flat for an hour a day. This is normally divided into two half-hourly sessions for patients suffering from rheumatoid arthritis, to avoid inactivity stiffness.

Surgical dressings can be left untouched if they remain clean and dry, but should be changed if they become soiled. Infection is the greatest enemy of replacement arthroplasty and so a constant watch for this must be made. Patients receiving steroid therapy should be particularly closely observed as these drugs mask the signs and symptoms of infection. Sutures are usually removed between the 12th and 14th day, but should be left in place longer if the patient is taking steroids, as healing is delayed. When the sutures have been removed and the wound has healed, the patient may take a bath or shower. Because of the possible consequence of infection, patients must be advised to report to the nursing staff any tenderness, redness or swelling of the incision site.

Postoperative Complications

In addition to the complications of surgery in general, such as deep vein thrombosis and pulmonary embolus and hypostatic pneumonia, a specific though rare complication of total hip replacement is the hypotension which can lead to cardiac arrest shortly after the insertion of methylmethacrylate bone cement. If the bones are porotic, fractures can occur when the patient is being transferred to and from the operating table. Dislocation of the prosthesis can occur, but the most common source of prosthetic failure is infection.

Preparing for Discharge from Hospital

Before being discharged from hospital, patients should visit the occupational therapy department, where they can be assessed in their ability to cope with daily living and instructed in the use of aids. Because the patient will not be allowed to bend down to tie shoe laces or put on slacks or stockings, as this involves extreme flexion, instruction will be given in the use of dressing aids. It can be useful if the patient's relatives are also present at these sessions so that they will be aware of the situation and will know what assistance the patient will need when at home. Some hospitals encourage patients to take weekend leave under the care of the district nurse. This enables the patient, relatives and health professionals to assess the degree of help which will be necessary for the patient to maintain an independent and meaningful life-style. An instruction sheet, as shown in Fig. 5.6, should be issued to rheumatic patients before discharge stating what they may and may not do. This will serve as a 'back-up' to what they have already been taught during their hospital stay.

Sexual counselling is a topic that many doctors and nurses avoid, feeling that it is an embarrassing subject, but it is very necessary; once the subject has been approached, the barriers tend to lift. Counselling should be offered to all patients regardless of age. Younger age groups tend to think that sexual activity stops when pensions start, but we are assured by our older patients that this is not so! Sexual intercourse should be avoided for the first 6–8 weeks after surgery, and, when recommenced, any position which involves extreme hip flexion is contraindicated. The most sensible position is supine with legs in abduction.

Patients are usually discharged about 3 weeks after surgery with some form of walking aid. The progress of the patient is then followed in the outpatient clinic.

DO'S

1. Wear well fitting shoes, when walking.
2. Keep legs in abduction — place a pillow between your legs when in bed, use it when turning over in bed.
3. Use walking aids until your next out-patients appointment.
4. Watch for signs of (a) General Infection
                          (b) Wound Infection
Report to your Doctor if symptoms appear.
5. Use aids to daily living, to avoid excessive flexion.
6. Do avoid extreme positions during sexual activity.

DON'TS

1. Avoid excessive hip flexion — do not bend more than 90°.
Use aids when dressing etc.
2. Do not cross your legs when sitting.
3. Do not sit (a) In low chairs
              (b) On low toilet seats — use a toilet raise
              (c) In low bath — use a plank or plastic seat.
4. Do not sit for long periods, get up and walk around every hour.
5. Do not drive or play sports until advised by your surgeon.

Fig. 5.6. General home instructions for total hip replacement.

Conclusions

Surgery may not be a cure for arthritis but it is a valuable addition to conservative medical treatment. When surgery is carried out on the right patient, who has the right mental attitude and who has achievable expectations, it can improve immeasurably the quality of life.

In the case of rheumatoid arthritis it must be recognised that this is a systemic illness which in itself gives rise to many complications. The drug therapy used in its treatment can give rise to further complications. Because of these complexities the surgical nursing care of rheumatic patients is particularly demanding, both mentally and physically and can only be carried out to a high standard if the nurse has a thorough knowledge of the disease process and its treatment. If rheumatic patients are to achieve the maximum possible benefit from surgery they must be cared for by a knowledgeable multidisciplinary team that understands the difficulties which are specific to the surgical treatment of rheumatic disease.

Education—of those providing as well as of those receiving care—is the foundation on which a successful outcome is built.

Reference

Powell M (1982) Orthopaedic nursing and rehabilitation, 8th edn. Churchill Livingstone, Edinburg

6

Physiotherapy and Occupational Therapy in the Management of Rheumatic Diseases

Introduction

In the past the treatment of rheumatic diseases in the United Kingdom was provided in spa towns. Here, in addition to hydrotherapy (or balneotherapy), other physical treatment could be used, including various applications of heat such as mud and wax, electrotherapy using light or electrical stimulation, and manipulation and massage. From this variety of treatments arose the specialty of 'physical medicine', and many present-day rheumatologists received their initial training in this field. Subsequently 'rheumatology' has emerged within the field of general internal medicine as a clinical specialty in its own right, incorporating the expertise of specialties such as immunology and clinical pharmacology in relation to rheumatic diseases. Since the development of 'rheumatology', rehabilitation medicine has grown as a speciality in its own right. It embraces the subspecialties of physiotherapy and occupational therapy and provides management for a wide variety of disorders as diverse as surgical amputation, neurological abnormalities and rheumatic diseases. This chapter will concentrate on rehabilitation medicine as applied to rheumatic diseases.

Physiotherapy

A large proportion of physiotherapy time is devoted to the management of rheumatic diseases, and physiotherapy departments in rheumatic disease hospitals specialise in this aspect of physiotherapy alone.

The aims of physiotherapy can be summarised as:

1. The relief of pain
2. The prevention of deformity
3. The correction of existing deformity
4. Increasing the mobility of joints
5. Improving muscle strength
6. Encouraging independence in the home or hospital environment

A large variety of specialist techniques are available in physiotherapy departments. At the ward level both doctors and nurses should be familiar with the 'first aid' of managing a flare of arthritis.

Management of a Flare of Arthritis

Management of a flare includes rest followed by mobilisation (see also p. 81). Almost all patients will respond well to rest; pain relief is produced by adequate medication and achievement of an effective dosage of anti-inflammatory drugs. If a flare-up is severe, maximal inactivity can be obtained by combining bed rest with splintage of all affected joints, usually in plaster of Paris rest splints made for each individual patient. It may be sensible not to splint one arm so that patients can continue to feed themselves; this helps their morale. After an initial short period of frustration, most patients find that the lack of need to move painful joints produces profound relief from stress. The bed used should have a firm mattress and bed-boards may be placed under the mattress. No pillows should be placed under the knees, as their presence would encourage the formation of flexion deformities at these joints. Flexion deformities at the hips can be minimised by asking the patient to lie in a prone position at least once each day with the feet over the end of the bed. Foot rests may be used to provide ankle alignment at 90°. Static exercises are taught to patients even while they are in their splints. Passive movements may be of less value than active movements, and a few physicians prefer to avoid them altogether. Immobilisation for up to 3 or 4 weeks rarely produces permanent loss of movement, if bed and chair are used alternately. In practice, however, immobilisation will usually be for a shorter period and will be accompanied by static exercises.

Once pain relief has been achieved, mobilisation should follow gradually. Increasing pain and subsequent stiffness as the patient mobilises are warning signs that too much exercise is being provided. Periods of activity lasting 5 or 10 min at 1- or 2-hourly intervals are likely to be better tolerated than more intensive sessions of exercise once or twice daily. Performance of exercises may be preceded by a period of warmth provided by heat lamps or warm water or analgesics, although some patients find ice packs preferable in providing more counterirritation. Heat and cold may be applied at times other than physiotherapy periods. Physical activity is gradually increased in a stepwise pattern, and, as this is done, the splints can be removed for increasing periods. When the muscles are strong enough, weight bearing can be introduced; appropriate walking aids will be available in the first instance to give graded weight relief. At a later stage exercise routines such as washing and grooming are practised, possibly with the aid of the occupational therapists. Subsequently the ambulant patient is assessed in the occupational therapy department for appropriate aids and appliances that might be fitted with benefit in the patient's home; this aspect of management is considered later in the chapter.

Relief of Pain

If patients fail to respond to a simple therapy with warm water or hot water bottles, a variety of alternative methods of relieving pain are available in physiotherapy departments. These can be summarised as follows:

1. Electrotherapy—e.g. Infrared radiation
                        Shortwave diathermy
                        Ultrasound
                        Microwave therapy
2. Hydrotherapy—e.g. Undercurrent douche
                        Vichy massage and douche
3. Wax and oil bath for hands and feet; mud packs for larger joints
4. Ice packs
5. Massage, usually following infrared radiation or other heat treatment

Infrared Radiation (IRR). This relieves pain and relaxes superficial muscle spasm whilst increasing a superficial blood supply. A non-luminous generator of electromagnetic wavelength 4000–7700 Å is used, and shorter wavelengths in this spectrum penetrate to 1–10 mm. A period of treatment lasting 20–30 min is normally prescribed daily.

Shortwave Diathermy (SWD). This relieves pain by inducing muscle relaxation and increasing vascularity. Wavelengths of the electromagnetic spectrum are used at a frequency of 27 Mc/s with a wavelength of 11 m. This is capable of full body penetration and produces the greatest heating effect in fatty tissue. The dosage prescribed varies according to the size of the patient and the chronicity of the condition. Metal in the patient's tissues (e.g. an artificial joint prosthesis) and cardiac pacemakers are both contraindications for this sort of treatment, since the metal absorbs heat to a greater degree than surrounding tissue (according to its specific heat) and may cause local tissue burns. In addition, electrical malfunction of a cardiac pacemaker may occur; all patients who have cardiac pacemakers should be instructed to inform the physiotherapist of this fact if ever they enter a physiotherapy department. The duration of treatment is usually 10–20 min.

Ultrasound (US). This form of acoustic vibration is used to remove oedema, increase blood supply and reduce pain. The frequency of vibration is

0.81 Mc/s with a wavelength of 1.5 mm. The depth of penetration varies considerably according to the nature of the tissue. For acute conditions a 3-min period of therapy might be used; for chronic conditions longer periods of therapy are given.

Microwave Therapy. This is used for increasing the circulation, reducing muscle spasm and raising the threshold of pain nerve endings. Wavelengths of the electromagnetic spectrum are used at a wavelength of 12.25 cm, which allows for a depth of penetration of 3 cm. Unlike shortwave diathermy, which appears to heat up fat, the greatest heating in microwave is produced in the vascular tissues. A 10–13 min period of therapy is likely to be given daily at a strength of up to 200 w.

Hydrotherapy. This treatment may only be available in certain departments that possess a deep pool. Warm water produces muscle relaxation in its own right, and early weight bearing can be encouraged as the body is supported by the buoyant effect of the water. A series of graded exercises can be given in the warm water. If the pool is deep enough a set of steps can be provided for practice on stair-climbing. Patients are supported by the use of appropriate floats that are strapped onto the body so that even non-swimmers can benefit from this treatment. There is probably some psychological benefit by reinforcing hydrotherapy with an underwater douche in which water at a slightly higher temperature is played onto the body through an underwater hose to cause additional relaxation of affected areas. The temperature of water in a standard hydrotherapy pool is likely to be between 34°C and 37°C. An underwater douche uses water at a temperature around 40°C. A Vichy massage is performed while the patient lies on a firm surface under an apparatus that sprays water from a needle-point spray over the whole body at a temperature of up to 40°C. A physiotherapist massages the patient under this fine spray of water.

Heat Therapy. Wax provides a local heat when the hands are dipped into it. The use of arachis oil at 50°C provides an alternative, if the patient is allergic to wax. The wax is heated in a metal heating bath to a temperature of 50°C, at which point the solid wax becomes liquid. At this temperature the hands or feet can be placed in the wax and then removed when it solidifies gently around the patient's joints, thus providing local heat at the site where it is most required. As the wax begins to cool, further larger amounts can be moulded into the shape of a small tennis ball and patients can then undertake active movements of the hand to mould this into different shapes. This activity exercises the small muscles of the hands while the wax, with which the hands are in constant contact, keeps these joints warm and supple. It may be convenient for a large group of patients to participate in this sort of therapy simultaneously in a 'wax class'.

Mud provides an alternative. It is warmed in a special warming container and scoops of it can then be wrapped in towels which are draped around the patient's larger joints such as the knee and elbows. There is no intrinsic therapeutic property in the mud but it provides a physical effect similar to wax and may be cheaper and more manageable for larger joints. However, although some patients can continue with wax therapy at home, they are unlikely to be able to do this with mud therapy.

Cold Therapy. It is interesting that although a majority of patients with rheumatic diseases derive pain relief from the use of heat, a minority are undoubtedly helped by cold therapy and may even be made to feel worse by warmth. Experimentally it can be shown that a brief cutaneous cooling initially stimulates nerve tissue, but a longer period of cooling diminishes sensation (5–7 min). If nerve tissue is cooled for 20–30 min, there is a reduction in muscle tone and nerve conduction velocity and this may account for the pain relief that is obtained from this. In addition, there is the effect of vasoconstriction, which is likely to ameliorate oedema; often heat treatment, which tends to cause vasodilatation, will accentuate oedema for a short period of time. The metabolic rate of the tissues may be reduced by cold therapy and inflammation may be similarly retarded. Muscle tone may be increased, however, so that the muscles become harder to exercise after a period of cold than after a period of heat. Care should be exerted in the treatment of ischaemic tissue or extremities of the body with poor circulation. The methods of application vary. A cold pack is a cellophane bag or pillow filled with crushed ice (a packet of frozen peas may be easier for the patient to use at home.) This can be wrapped around large joints such as the knee and elbow or smaller joints such as the hands. An alternative treatment for the hands and feet is to immerse the limb in a bath of cold water. Ethyl chloride spray can be used for the relief of localised muscular sprains, where it probably works by counterirritation in addition to reducing local blood supply. Finally, patients sometimes benefit from 'contrast baths', whereby periods of cold treatment are alternated with periods of heat treatment.

Skin Rash. We have seen skin rashes occurring in patients submitted to physiotherapy, usually pool therapy, if large amounts of chemicals have been added to the water to prevent cross-infection. These skin rashes usually settle with conservative treatment and, if a barrier cream is subsequently used, do not necessarily form a contraindication to physiotherapy. Patients with infectious diseases or severe skin rashes can still participate in physiotherapy pool sessions if the department has a Hubbard tank, which allows patients to have individual physiotherapy. This is also of use for incontinent or epileptic patients.

Prevention and Correction of Deformity

The main factors in the prevention of deformity are:

1. Use of splints
2. Use of collars for the cervical spine
3. Re-education of muscles at all joints including the lumbar spine

4. Provision of walking aids
5. Attention to chiropody
6. Provision of made-to-measure footwear
7. Measurement of true and apparent leg length and the correction of inequality of leg length, thus preventing strain on joints in the lower limbs

Exercises to increase muscle power and to re-educate muscles are clearly the province of the physiotherapist. On the whole we prefer exercises that increase muscle power to the use of supports such as a corset in the lumbar spine, although occasionally patients may benefit from the immobilising effect of a corset which produces pain relief. The manufacture of splints may be performed in the physiotherapy department or in the occupational therapy department. The materials from which they are made are discussed in more detail later in the chapter. Walking aids are likely to be ordered by the physiotherapist. In the early stages of rehabilitation, patients may use a Zimmer frame, progressing to callipers and crutches at a later stage and finally to the use of a walking stick or no walking aids at all. One problem with patients who have rheumatoid arthritis is that the wrists are frequently involved and this makes the use of a Zimmer frame difficult. Gutter crutches, which are supported not by the hand alone but along the whole length of the forearm, are to be preferred. As patients improve they are likely to discard these for a simple walking stick which is held on the side *opposite* to the worst involved joint. Inequality between leg length should always be corrected with an appropriate raise on the shoe or boot. This inequality in leg length may vary with time as a cartilage in the joint wears away and the bony surfaces telescope upon each other. Leg length should be re-assessed at 6-monthly or annual intervals. Prevention of deformity is particularly important in patients

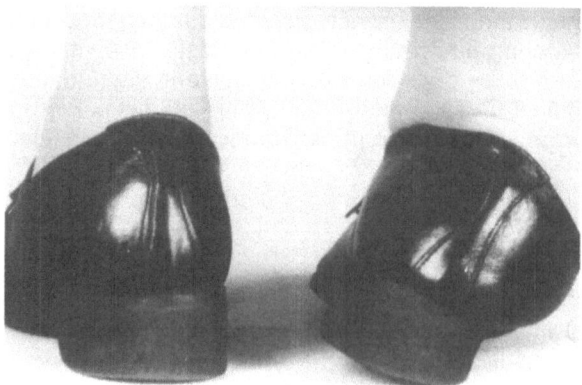

Fig. 6.1. Inappropriate footwear. These surgical shoes are badly worn on the right. A wedge support (or even a T-strap iron) is needed here to allow easier walking and to prevent further strain on the joints of the lower limbs.

with rheumatoid arthritis. Figure 6.1 demonstrates the provision of a raise on a shoe to allow balanced walking. Figure 6.2 shows a patient with rheumatoid arthritis who has been provided with rest splints that rest the joints in the positions of maximum function. For further details the reader is referred to the book by Downie and Kennedy (1981).

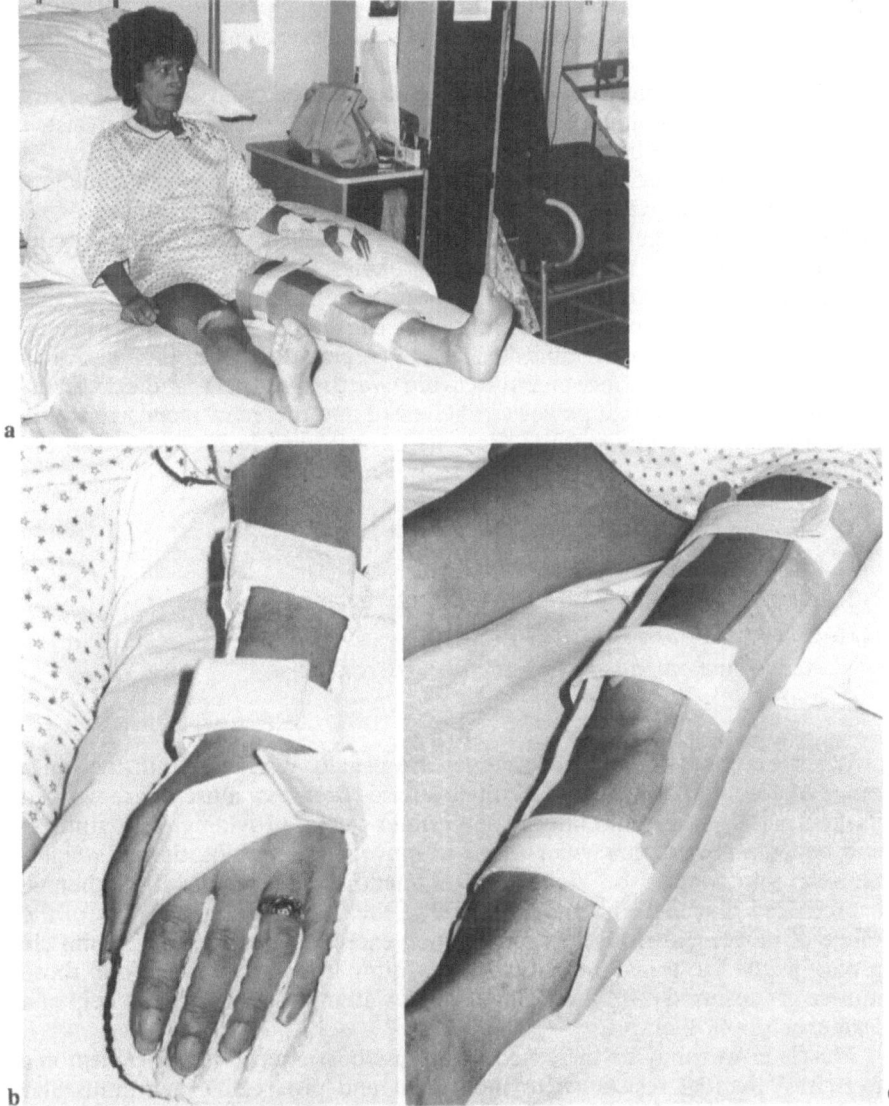

Fig. 6.2a–c. Resting splints. **a** The patient is sitting in the position of maximum function. The body is supported by pillows. The wrists and knees are splinted and the ankles are dorsiflexed. **b** A wrist splint rests the joints in the position of maximum function. **c** A firm knee splint guards against flexion deformity at this joint.

Maintenance of Joint Mobility and Improvement of Muscle Strength

It is important in the management of all patients with rheumatoid arthritis, once pain relief has been obtained, to maintain joint mobility and improve muscle strength. It is especially important in the very early stages of the treatment of ankylosing spondylitis, particularly the spinal involvement in this condition, and in the spinal involvement of related seronegative spondarthropathies.

Although ultrasound and some other electrical treatments may accelerate the improvement of joint mobility, pool therapy and progressive resisted exercises remain the basis of treatment. Although it is hard to quantify the relief in pain produced by physiotherapy (except by the use of visual analogue scales), serial measurements of the range of joint movement which are likely to improve with regular exercise provide a useful incentive to encourage patients to complete their exercise programmes.

Each patient should be taught to perform exercises correctly, and an exercise programme is tailor made to suit each individual patient's needs. Patients are told how many times they should repeat the exercises and advised on the correct speed of movement to avoid overtiring muscles and exacerbating inflammation. Muscle power can be tested and recorded according to the Oxford scale. With this method the state of each muscle is recorded on the following scale:

0. No contraction
1. Flicker or trace of contraction
2. Active movement with gravity counterbalanced
3. Active movement against gravity
4. Active movement against gravity and resistance
5. Normal

When exercises commence, muscles are usually worked within the inner range of accepted movement. As the exercises progress, muscles are worked in their middle range and later at their outer range, providing pain, stiffness and oedema permit this wider range of movement. Mobilisation of weight-bearing joints must be done in conjunction with muscle-strengthening exercises so that there is enough power in the muscle groups to control the range of movement. Muscle-strengthening exercises are given to the muscle groups needed to transfer a patient from sitting to standing and also to those muscle groups used during walking, even if walking is done with the help of a frame or physiotherapist.

Muscle power may be increased by the use of isometric exercises, isotonic exercises, manual resistance to movement and progressive neuromuscular facilitation. In this last method joints are moved to the full extent of their range and held there. The muscle group that limits movement at this point is then contracted against resistance for a few seconds. In the relaxation phase that follows, the range of movement can be extended further. Springs and weights may assist physiotherapy, and malleable resistances and underwater resistance provide alternatives to graded exercise programmes. To increase muscle endurance, isotonic exercises or progressive resistant exercises are used. A variety of aids are available, including the static bicycle and the rowing machine. Some of these can be purchased and incorporated in the patient's home. Finally, muscular activity is coordinated with exercises which concentrate on transfers and stabilisation, progressive neuromuscular facilitation to the limbs and balance and writing exercises.

In the management of ankylosing spondylitis we have found it of value to admit patients to 'spondylitis exercise classes'. Patients are graded according to their disease severity. If fusion of the spine has occurred, exercises are likely to be modest; if the patients are young with very early disease, exercises are likely to be strenuous. We have found that the competitive atmosphere of these spondylitis classes encourages patients to continue at home with the exercises they have learnt in hospital, and the classes provide an ideal opportunity for imparting patient education.

Encouragement of Independence

Once the arthritis is quiescent and muscle power has been built up and coordination taught, patients progress to graded functional programmes that will maintain their independence. Examples include the complex upper limb movement required for dressing, washing and using the toilet, and the complex of lower limb movement for negotiating stairs and steps. At this point the physiotherapist is likely to be working in conjunction with an occupational therapist, who will provide appropriate aids in order to make these goals more easily attainable. Subsequently it may be of value for a physiotherapist and occupational therapist to make a combined visit to the patient's home after discharge from hospital in order to confirm that the advances made as a result of hospital treatment have been retained and consolidated in the patient's home background.

Research Aspects of Physiotherapy

Physiotherapy techniques, like many procedures in other branches of medicine, have not always been subjected to the most rigorous scientific scrutiny of controlled trials. In the marketing of a new drug the manufacturer is forced by government regulations to submit that drug to a comprehensive programme of clinical trial testing in which the drug is evaluated both against placebo compound and then against proven comparator products. This must be performed in every disease for which it is proposed to market the drug. By contrast, a new physiotherapy technique is not submitted to such close scrutiny before it is applied to patients. Admittedly the technique may be relatively non-invasive compared to the possible side-effects of a drug (hydrotherapy has not to our knowledge ever killed anybody!), but it would still be reassuring for health service economists to know that some of the treatments that are time honoured in physiotherapy are more efficacious than the masterly inactivity of leaving the patient at home without any such treatment. What are the precise benefits, for example, of shortwave diathermy over a hot water bottle?

General physiotherapy is only of value for a short period of time after it has been given. It is therefore important that physiotherapists educate their patients in the routine continuation of the exercises they have learnt in hospital when they return home. This may also mean the education of relatives who will assist the patient with the home exercises. The help of a relative will have to be enlisted if wax treatment has been prescribed in the home and the patient has extensive hand and wrist involvement that prevents him or her from lifting the saucepan in which the wax has been heated.

Recent research by Dr. Anne Chamberlain and her colleagues in the Rehabilitation Unit in Leeds has compared physiotherapy for osteoarthrosis of the knee given both in hospitals and at home. The results suggest that home physiotherapy was almost as effective. This has serious implication for the already overstretched physiotherapy services. If patients can be sent home with a set of instructions on the correct exercises after a period of appropriate tuition in hospital, the need for regular attendances in the department is circumvented. Physiotherapists are thereby released to give greater attention to the more complex physiotherapy problems of rehabilitation in which they have received special training. (Physiotherapists who wish to evaluate their own work in this critical fashion will find advice on trial methodology in Chapter 12.)

Physiotherapists should perhaps liaise more closely with engineers and biologists in the design of equipment. A recent survey of exercise bicycles by a bioengineer working in Leeds suggested that many models currently available were not as efficient as they might be in subjecting muscles to progressive incremental increase in work in their optimal physiological position.

Occupational Therapy

Functional Assessment

Functional assessments require some particularly close liaison between the occupational therapist and the patient. Functional assessments rely partly on questioning by the therapist (a check list of daily activities is likely to be used) and partly on the therapist's observation of the performance by the patient of relevant daily living activities.

The purpose of a functional assessment is:

1. To help the patient achieve the maximum level of independence permitted by his or her disability in relation to age, personality and home environment

2. To provide adequate help and instruction to whomever assists or supervises at home a person who is unable to reach full independence

The activities of daily living on which the patient is likely to be evaluated can be classified as follows:

1. Personal care: feeding, dressing, bathing, toilet and incidental activities
2. Domestic care: cooking, housework, laundry, shopping
3. Child care (where appropriate): feeding, dressing, bathing, nappy changing, toilet training, lifting
4. General and recreational: e.g. sewing, mending, knitting, gardening
5. Mobility and outdoor activities: steps, stairs, traffic, public transport, private transport

Activities of Daily Living Assessment

The patient for whom a physician has requested an activities of daily living (ADL) assessment will be given an appointment or a series of appointments in the occupational therapy department. The ideal department is constructed so as to resemble the inside of a house, with a series of small rooms. One of these will be a bathroom, one a toilet, one a bedroom, one a lounge and one a kitchen. Patients pass from room to room under the observation of the occupational therapist and are evaluated on simple daily tasks. The department is likely to be provided with a full range of adaptations. Thus the kitchen may have a sink of adjustable height so that the exact height of a sink for optimum function for each individual patient can be measured. There will also be a selection of kitchen appliances designed, for example, to enable the patient to lift saucepans full of hot water off a cooker or open tins.

A typical check list of aids and appliances that are most likely to be supplied as a result of this assessment is as follows:

1. Bath aids—bath seats, non-slip mats, safety handles
2. Toilet aids—commodes, raised WC seats, hand rails and hoists to enable the patient to use the WC
3. Eating aids—plates and cups of the non-slip variety, adapted cutlery
4. Dressing aids—elastic shoelaces, shoehorns with long handles, stocking aids, adapted clothing
5. Walking aids—sticks, walking frames, callipers, plastic splints
6. Household gadgets—gardening tools, pick-up stick, kitchen gadgets, cooking gadgets, etc.

Information will also be given on joint protection, and appropriate splints will be provided (see p. 168). These compensate for weak muscles and diminished range of movements and protect joints. Key and tap turners increase the leverage of weak and painful upper limbs. Figure 6.3 shows a variety of the types of aid that are available.

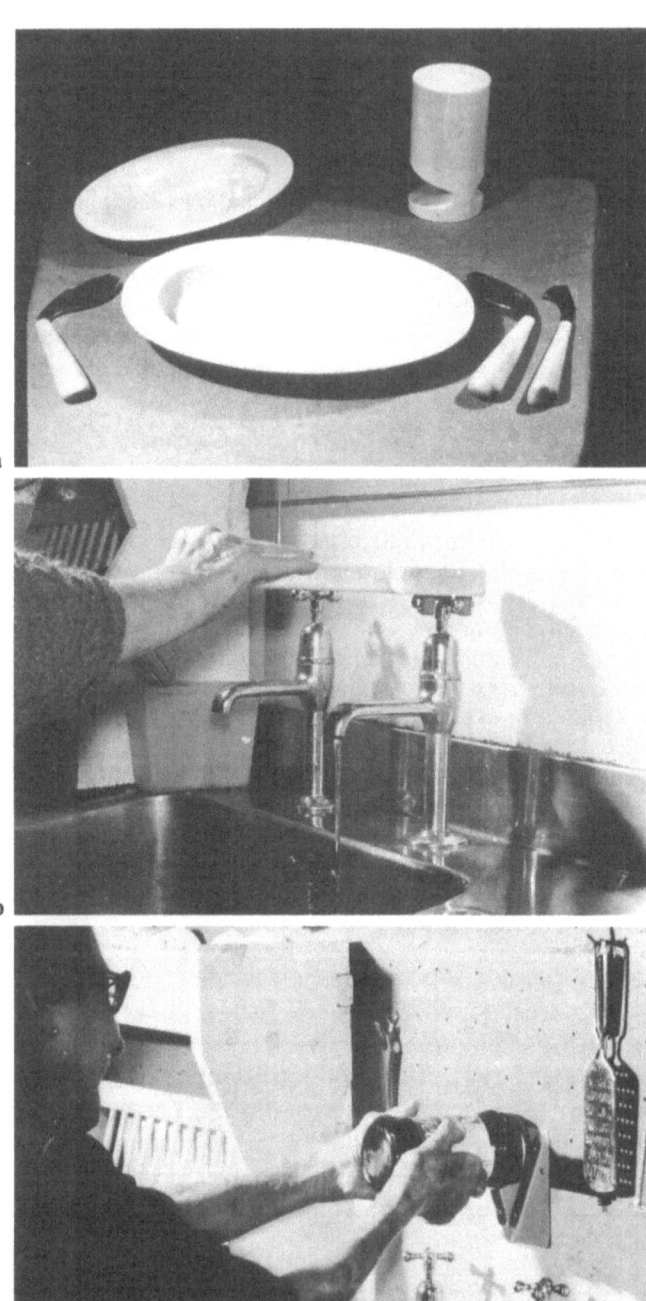

Fig. 6.3a–c. Aids to independence. **a** A table setting for the patient with rheumatoid involvement of the hands. **b** Aid to turning taps. **c** Aid to assist in the opening of jars.

If the patient is more severely disabled additional appliances will need to be considered as well as those mentioned above. These include:

1. Beds—mechanical, electrical and tilting
2. Hoists—portable or ceiling tracked
3. Wheelchairs—self-propelled, attendant-propelled or electrically propelled
4. Kitchens—adapted equipment and/or specially designed working surfaces
5. Chairs—adapted with ejector seats or special design
6. Reading aids—talking book library, book-rests, page-turners
7. Writing aids—electric typewriters
8. Intercommunication devices—call system adapted telephones

The most severely incapacitated patients may need the patient-operated selector mechanism (POSSUM) system to enable them to retain control over their environment.

Specific Programme for Joint Mobilisation

In coordination with the physiotherapist, the occupational therapist may design a series of activities that are appropriate for each joint. For example, basketry, weaving and needlework performed at home will encourage flexion and extension of the fingers. Weaving and basketry involve coarser movements which are needed to fully exercise the wrists. Large basketwork, carpentry and rug weaving may help to keep elbows and shoulders mobile. Foot-operated sewing machines or the use of a bicycle will encourage mobilisation of the ankles or knees. Patients may prefer to set aside a short period of time each day to put their joints through a series of regular graded exercises. These may be simple physiotherapy exercises, though more interest can be added if they are linked to socially acceptable or recreational pursuits. Moreover, practising a recreational pursuit (such as basketry) in the evening will consolidate the improvement that has been obtained by the regular physiotherapy exercises performed at intervals during the day. Patients who have to remain at home all day because of unemployment may find the mental stimulation provided by the constructive diversion of their craft work into money-making ventures most acceptable.

The most sophisticated form of this assessment, activity analysis, grades various activities in terms of their value to the patient. Thus dressmaking scores highly for creativity and concentration but scores low for initiative, intricacy and repetition. By contrast typing is said to score highly for concentration, repetition and structured activity, but involves no creativity and little initiative. Different occupations can thus be matched to a patient's needs according to whether there is a rheumatological, neurological or psychiatric disability. In relation to the elbow joint, for example, a progressive plan of skills of increasing severity that develop flexion and extension of this joint can be given to the patient. Thus sanding and tapestry require minimal flexion and extension; however, once these skills have been accomplished patients may progress to sawing or stool-seating. Once a wide range of flexion and extension of the elbow joint coupled with good muscular power has been achieved, patients can indulge in gardening, darts or even archery.

If there is a specific problem of muscular function, possibly caused by loss of a nerve, activities can be designed to exercise each muscle group governed by that nerve. For example, the median nerve controls pronators of the forearm, flexors of the wrist, flexors of the fingers and thumb and intrinsic muscles of the hand. A coordinated programme for rehabilitation after a median nerve injury (which is perhaps due to compression arising from rheumatoid synovitis) would include weaving for pronators of the forearm, basketry or typesetting for flexors of the wrist, typing or piano playing for flexors of the fingers and thumb, and basketry or mosaic work for the intrinsic muscles in the hands.

Aids Centres

Many rheumatology units are now designated as official rehabilitation centres, and an outpatient aids centre is often linked to such units. A spare building in the hospital grounds may have been converted into a 'display shop' which demonstrates the wide variety of different aids and appliances that are available for incapacitated people. Members of the public are invited to telephone for an appointment (a necessary procedure since demand inevitably outstrips supply with current health service finances) and can attend to compare the various appliances that are available. A recent survey in Leeds showed that a majority of the patients who order special arthritic chairs for their homes have never seen the models before ordering them, let alone tried them out for size. Most chairs are ordered in response to newspaper advertising or personal recommendation. Only if all the different models are displayed in a single room can patients discover the best piece of equipment to match their particular circumstances. Very few individuals would buy a suit or dress, for example, without first trying it on.

Research Aspects of Occupational Therapy

As in the field of physiotherapy, research is a somewhat neglected area of occupational therapy. Because there is a wide spectrum of disability among the patients involved, it is often impossible to recommend a single best appliance, as can be done in relation to drugs or physiotherapy procedures. Rational research in occupational therapy is directed towards providing adequate information for making a choice and encouraging manufacturers to improve their product so that the more useless sorts of appliances are no longer to be found on the market.

However, there is still scope for simple projects that have been neglected in the field of occupational therapy. Mrs. Janet Stowe, a Research Occupational Therapist working in Leeds, recently visited all the bathrooms and toilets of one of the city's principal teaching hospitals. She was amazed to find that very few of these toilets allowed access for wheelchair patients or patients with incapacity, and the bathrooms had similar design faults. Admittedly, the need for wheelchair access may not be great in acute surgical wards, but this is not so on medical wards, where many patients have neurological conditions that result in poor coordination and where many patients are convalescing from strokes. We suspect that the problem is not confined to the particular hospital that was selected for evaluation. Nursing sisters in charge of wards should take individual responsibility for ensuring that all toilet and bathing facilities on their ward are suitable for even the most disabled of their patients. They should agitate for more funds to be diverted by health service administrators to effect these simple but important changes.

Aids to Mobility

It should be the aim of therapists to get patients as fully mobile as possible unaided. Nevertheless, in many instances this may be impossible. Aids to mobility can be arranged in a logical progression according to the substitution for normal walking which they provide. Aids can be divided into:

1. Partial weight-relieving aids—sticks
                                         crutches
                                         walking frames
2. Complete weight-relieving aids—patient-propelled wheelchairs
                                          attendant-propelled wheelchairs
                                          powered wheelchairs
                                          outdoor vehicles

Partial Weight-relieving Aids

The simplest aid is a walking stick. This is usually used in unilateral lower limb disease. It is carried in the hand opposite to the lower limb joint involved. The use of two sticks enables the patient to walk more efficiently and achieve even greater weight relief. The handle of the stick should be adapted to the shape of the patient's hand. Although a curved handle is preferred by patients with strong hands, a straight handle may be more suitable for patients with rheumatoid arthritis. The handle can be made soft to touch by covering it with sorbo rubber or plastic foam, and some sticks are available with moulded plastic handles that are individually moulded for the patients hands. Greater support can be provided by a three-legged (tripod) or four-legged (tetrapod) stick. These are demonstrated in Fig. 6.4.

The traditional underarm crutch (axillary) is only used for short-term use. Elbow crutches or gutter crutches are normally more suitable for patients with rheumatoid arthritis. A selection of crutches is shown in Fig. 6.4.

Walking frames are unsatisfactory for widespread rheumatoid disease because their use involves weight being borne through the hands and wrists in a position anterior to the body, thus putting undue strain on these joints, and because a normal walking pattern in rheumatoid arthritis is often not possible. A housebound trolley may be a solution for a disabled housewife since it provides a carrying surface as well as conferring stability to the patient, particularly if gutter crutches are fitted for its use (Fig. 6.4).

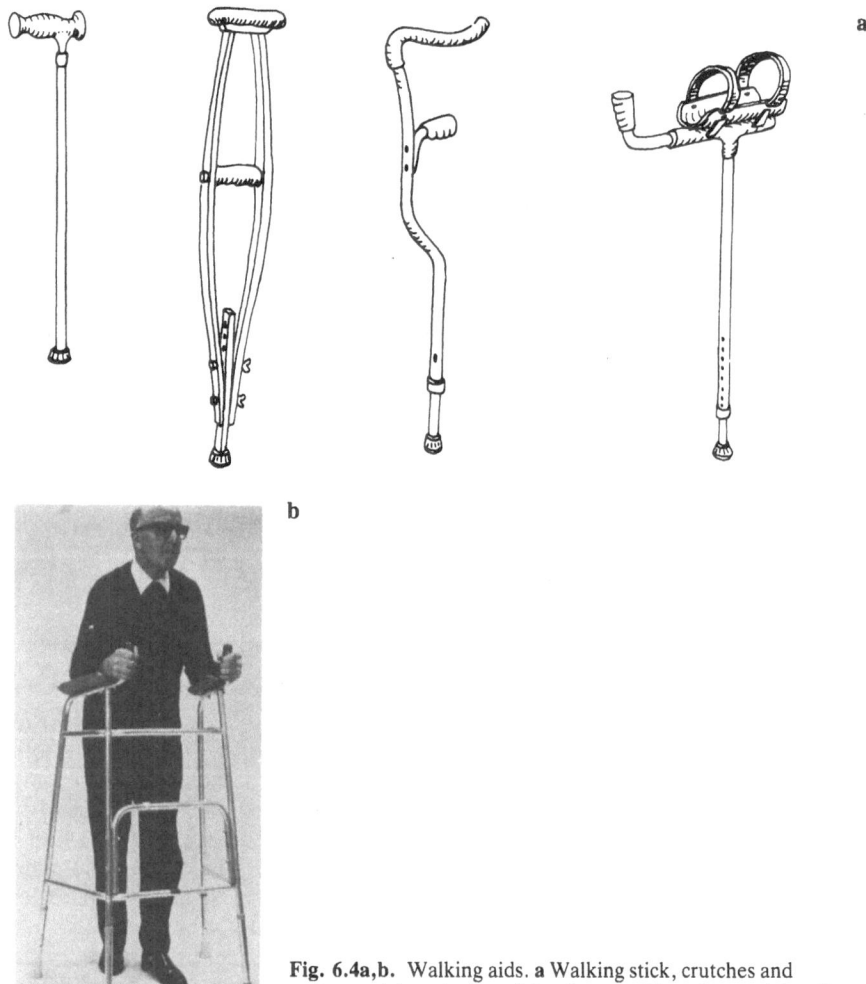

Fig. 6.4a,b. Walking aids. **a** Walking stick, crutches and gutter crutches. **b** A walking frame with gutter crutches for patients with arthritic wrists.

Complete Weight-relieving Aids

Many patients with rheumatoid arthritis can benefit by provision of a wheelchair, although some have a psychological barrier in its initial acceptance. A self-propelled wheelchair implies adequate function of the upper limb joints. This is not normally the case in rheumatoid arthritis, for which a self-propelled wheelchair with a small motor is likely to be more suitable. However, two alternative techniques for propelling a wheelchair may be assessed before placing an order for a motorised wheelchair. In one method two sticks are used to 'punt' the chair along. In the second method the patient's legs are used to 'walk' a chair forward. Suitable castors are needed on chairs if these methods are adopted. In addition, before ordering the chair the type of cushioning, brakes, foot rests and arm rests all need to be considered in relation to each individual recipient.

The design criteria for an outdoor wheelchair that is used in conjunction with family and friends are quite different to the criteria for an indoor chair that is used around the house. The latter has to be more manoeuvrable and capable of turning tight corners. As a result, comfort may have to be sacrificed.

The most useful type of wheelchair may be the standard lightweight transit chair (DHSS model 9L or 9LR in the United Kingdom, the latter model having a folding back). These are light and enable patients to be pushed out of doors; they are also small enough to be used in a large house. In cramped circumstances the standard size lightweight wheelchair (DHSS model 8L) may be appropriate, although many rheumatoid patients prefer an ultra-light self-propelling wheelchair (DHSS model 8BL), manipulating it around corners with their feet and elbows. In addition to the official NHS aids described above, a variety of alternative aids are available from private manufacturers.

Electrically powered wheelchairs are also available but may compromise on manoeuvrability. Those in which the leading castor-wheels are driven by the motor have greater manoeuvrability than those in which the back wheels are driven. In deciding on the best model for a particular patient there is no substitute for a practical trial of 2 or 3 days, preferably in the home itself.

If a patient requires a wheelchair, they may also require hoists at appropriate points in the home. There are four main types of hoists:

1. Overhead hoists fixed to the ceiling joists. They run on a fixed track, but if this is judiciously placed the hoist can be used in both bedroom and bathroom.
2. Hydraulically operated hoists which are mobile and therefore can do duty in different places. Often these take up too much space in small modern houses, and the overhead hoist is likely to be more appropriate.
3. Bath hoists that are operated by water pressure. These are safer than the standard electrical hoist used in bathrooms.
4. Car hoists that can be fitted inside a car or on the roof of a car to enable the patient to manoeuvre into one of the front seats.

On occasion a physician may feel that the patient merits assistance with outside transport. In the United Kingdom such cases should be referred directly to the Regional Artificial Limb and Appliance Centre where they will be examined by an appliance medical officer. Estimation is made of the patient's fitness to control a powered vehicle on a public highway. Eligibility is usually confined to amputees, those patients who to all intents and purposes are unable to walk and to slightly less disabled patients with very limited walking ability who need personal transport to get to and from work. If these conditions are met, powered vehicles (which may be petrol or electrically driven) may be provided by the Department of Health and Social Security (DHSS). Certain categories of patients may be eligible for a car in place of a three-wheeled vehicle, but this provision is usually confined to persons who have to look after a child, who live with a blind relative or who have haemophilia.

The various allowances for which disabled people may be eligible are listed in Appendix C (see p. 146).

Splints and Splinting

There are four main types of splints used in rheumatology:

1. Supportive splints—these may be plaster of Paris casts to provide complete rest for an acutely inflamed joint. Lighter removable splints fashioned from one of a variety of modern plastic materials are less heavy and equally rigid and may, for example, prevent movement at a painful wrist joint while allowing some freedom to elbow and finger joints.
2. Corrective splints—flexion deformities of the knee can be treated by serial plaster of Paris splints, each one bringing the leg slightly straighter. Once the joint is straightened, plastic night splints may be substituted.
3. Restrictive splints—these are used where some movement is unavoidable but it is desired to reduce the range. Examples are plastic collars used in cervical spondylosis and the various surgical belts to treat lumbar disc lesions.
4. 'Lively' splints—these are mobile contraptions that include springs or elastic bands in their design and are used sometimes to treat the hand deformities caused by arthritis.

There is an increasing variety of materials from which splints can be made. Polyethylene, Orthoplast, fibreglass and leather all combine lightness, strength and durability with ease of construction and use. Plastazote possesses some of these qualities but lacks strength, although its lightness may compensate for this. All are preferable to plaster of Paris splints, which are heavy for daytime use. Velcro or similar simple fastenings should be used, and care should be taken to ensure that the fastenings are placed at sites where patients can use them without the help of a relative.

The splint is fitted in the position of optimum function for the joint. For the elbow this is likely to be 90° of flexion. This enables the patient to eat, wash their face and comb their hair—tasks that would be quite impossible if the elbow joint was fixed in an extended position. The wrist should be held at 10° of extension with the thumb left free and finger flexion allowed for optimum function. The knees should be splinted in the extended position to counteract the tendency for flexion deformities. Ankles are held at 90° to keep the foot at the most efficient walking position in relation to the extended leg.

Feet and Footwear

The foot may be involved at an early stage both in osteoarthrosis and rheumatoid arthritis. In osteoarthrosis degeneration occurs at the base of the big toe, leading to hallux valgus. As a result a bony protuberance appears on the medial aspect of the forefoot which chafes against the shoe leather on the medial side of the shoe, leading to pressure ulcers and callosity formation in some cases. In rheumatoid arthritis the early disease involvement is at the metatarsal heads. Patients feel as though they are walking on marbles or pins, and a firm pad or metatarsal insert needs to be provided to increase the depth of padding between the jagged metatarsal heads that take the weight of the body and the ground on which the foot is walking. In more advanced rheumatoid disease other problems may occur. The lateral toes dislocate at the metatarsophalangeal joint and pressure lesions develop on the underside of the feet as the normal supporting plantar arch is eroded away by the disease. Hammer toe and claw toe may occasionally occur.

Drugs have only a limited role to play in the management of arthritic foot problems; however, if there is a large amount of oedema, the use of a diuretic may help. The footshape undergoes progressive change once arthritis is established. This is more marked for rheumatoid arthritis than osteoarthrosis. Patients have severe difficulty finding 'high-street' shoes that fit them, and specialist shoes will be required. In providing these, particularly in rheumatoid arthritis, the physician may opt for a rapid succession of shoes with limited life to accommodate the changing footshape rather than an expensive single pair of shoes that is intended to last for 10 years. The National Health Service (NHS) provides—free of charge on the prescription of a consultant— surgical shoes for those with crippled feet, but the quality of the service varies. Ideally shoes should be light in weight, attractive to look at, cushioned at tender areas and provide room for deformities; wear, rain resistance and style are not so important. A shoe is wasted if the footshape has changed significantly during the time that elapses between prescription and delivery. If chiropody is envisaged, this should be provided before the new shoes are fitted.

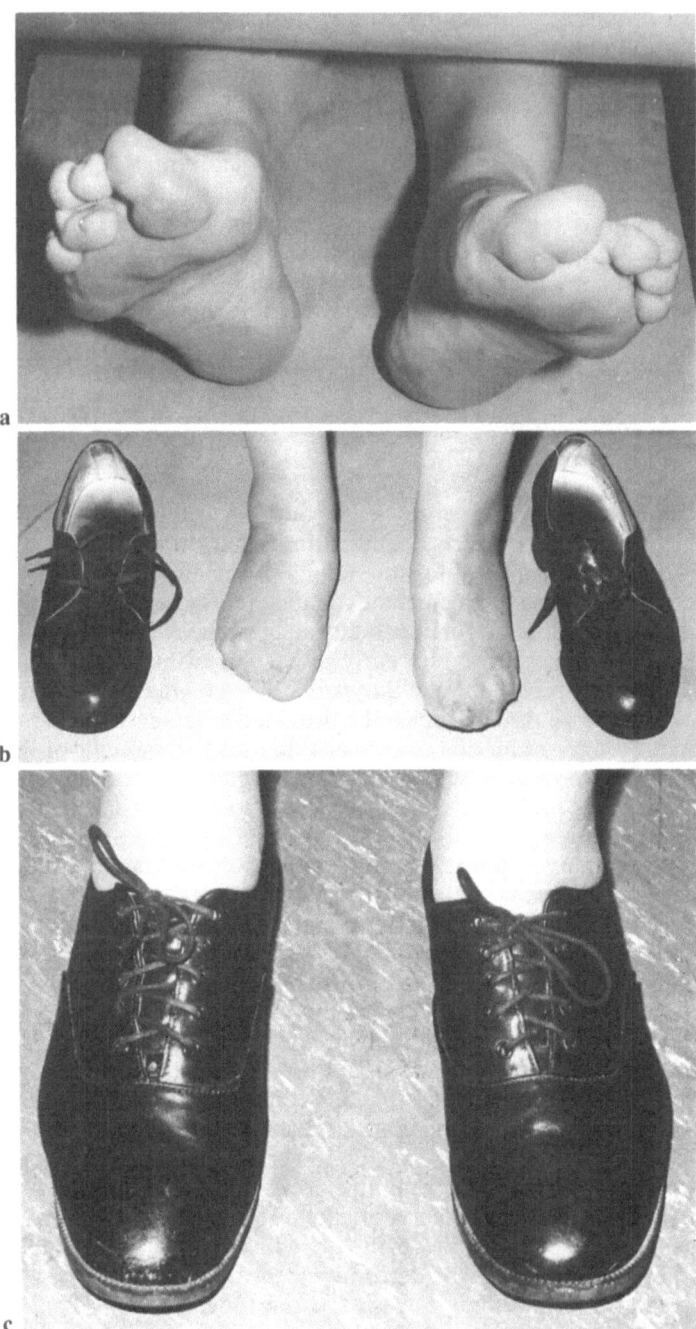

Fig. 6.5. a Rheumatoid feet showing typical deformities. Conventional shoes will not fit such feet. b and c Examples of shoes custom made for a patient with a foot involvement.

The shoes available include:

1. Traditional handcrafted surgical shoes. These are made to measure, often requiring several intermediate fittings, but are very expensive and are often too heavy for many patients.
2. 'Depth' shoes, which are provided from a large stock. They resemble conventional shoes in appearance and normally have wide uppers to accommodate a majority of foot sizes. An individually made Plastazote or cork insole is moulded to the sole contour before the shoes are provided. This method of provision is quick and relatively inexpensive, but is not always suitable for patients with severe deformity.
3. Shoes made specially from plaster casts taken of the feet. The cast is posted to the manufacturer who makes a positive replica of the foot, adapts this as a last on which he makes the shoe, using soft leather and modern microcellular rubbers and plastics. The foot is 'packaged' for maximum comfort, and the method is quick, cheap and needs no intermediate fittings. A majority of patients find the shoes comfortable, though they are not always stylish. Shoes are delivered by post to the patient's home address.

A variety of shoes available for arthritic feet are shown in Fig. 6.5.

Reference

Downie PA and Kennedy P (1981) Lifting, handling and helping patients. Faber & Faber, London.

7

Patient Education

Introduction

Patient education is an emerging discipline, based largely upon a counselling process which helps to convey relevant information to the patient. In the past this information was rather limited in both quality and quantity, probably because of the prevailing attitude, 'The doctor knows best' (Fig. 7.1). Fortunately, with the evolution of a more enlightened society, where social prejudice and moral obligation have become open to discussion, the barrier created by such an attitude has been largely broken down.

Education or, more correctly, the imparting of information, on a one-to-one basis has been the accepted practice for many years in hospitals. Not only doctors and nurses, but all disciplines who have personal contact with patients have employed this method of communication. Patient education is not therefore a new invention or revelation. What *is* new is the way the subject is

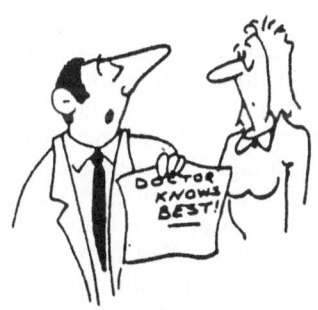

Fig. 7.1.

'I find this is the only patient-information leaflet I need!'

approached. Today patients are eager for information about their medical problems, and provided that medical facts are explained in a way that lay people understand, the result must be beneficial to all concerned. A recent trial (L. Wallace 1983, personal communication) suggests that patients who are well informed preoperatively do significantly better than those given only a little information or no information at all. Our own practice in Leeds of informing patients extensively about their drug therapy has been evaluated as resulting in 98% compliance.

In many countries, among them the United States, Canada and Australia, centres with interests as diverse as coronary care, diabetes and cancer care, as well as patient health education, pharmacology and preoperative education have conducted research in an endeavour to determine the benefits or otherwise of patient education. Most have proved conclusively that this form of patient care can no longer be ignored. We present a small sample of their findings.

In one study a total of 256 cancer patients were interviewed (Cassileth et al. 1980). It was found that the younger the patient, the more closely the patient conformed to the well-informed standards of patient behaviour; the older the patient, the more likely the patient was to prefer the older non-participatory patient role. Patients who wanted to be involved in treatment decisions were significantly more helpful than others. In a hypertensive study (Watson 1979), it was found that patient failure to comply with the appropriate medical regimen was the major obstacle to recovery from many disease states. In a study in patient education in ambulatory care (Smith 1977), improved educational theory and staff teaching skills demonstrated improved compliance rates, a decrease in hospital re-admissions and decreased morbidity.

The diabetic, of course, has long been the recipient of excellent patient education. The reason for this is clear: Diabetes is a life-threatening disease, and failure to educate the patient about his condition and treatment would result in the patient's death. Other chronic diseases have fared less well. There is a vast reservoir of rheumatic patients who have been only partially educated under the old system. Surely the necessity and responsibility for educating them to a much higher degree lies with those working in the specialty of rheumatology. Some of the patients newly diagnosed will be condemned to years of chronic medical care. They deserve something better than to continue to be educated as in the past.

Fortunately, rheumatic patients rarely die of their illness. Even so, their lives may be changed dramatically by a cruel and debilitating disease. Although this disease may not cause their death, it may well deny them their freedom of mobility, which to most people is the very essence of life.

How can such patients be helped? The aim must be to do everything possible to alleviate the patients' mental and physical anguish, to help them come to terms with their individual problems, and to live as pain free and as mobile an existence as possible. In order to achieve these aims there is a need for a method of education superior to that conventionally used. This chapter will discuss various forms of education suitable for different situations. These are:

1. Outpatient education
2. Outpatient group sessions
3. Inpatient education
4. Self-medication in hospital

Realistically, only suggestions can be made here for the reader to build upon. However, with a good foundation much can be achieved.

There are two possibilities as to who should be the educator—the doctor or the nurse. The merits of each will be discussed later in the chapter. However, for the time being and for ease of description the term 'counsellor' will be used.

Outpatient Education

We shall consider one patient with rheumatoid arthritis. After giving a brief outline of her medical and social history we shall proceed towards a method of education considered as a series of steps in which each problem is identified and the appropriate intervention sought. This method can be applied to all rheumatic diseases, adapting to the individual situation accordingly.

Case Study

Mary S. is 55 years old, married with four children and working part time as a school cook. For some weeks she has been experiencing pain in her hands and shoulders, and as this is causing her problems at work she decides to visit her general practitioner. Indomethacin 25 mg t.d.s. is prescribed, and Mary is sent for blood tests and radiography of the hands and feet. Her next appointment is given for 1 month's time.

The test results show ESR 45 mm/h and rheumatoid factor positive 1:64. The radiographs show no obvious abnormality. Because of the raised ESR and the positive rheumatoid factor, her general practitioner decides to refer Mary to a rheumatologist. Meanwhile Mary's hands have become even more painful and swollen. Her shoulders feel a little less stiff.

At the local hospital Mary is seen by the rheumatologist, who, after taking a comprehensive medical and social history, performs a complete physical examination. All blood tests are repeated, with the addition of liver function tests, electrolytes and full blood count. Her weight is taken and urine is tested routinely. The rheumatologist asks Mary to return in 3 weeks' time when he will have more results on which to base his diagnosis. Meanwhile he tells Mary that she may be developing a mild form of arthritis, particularly of the hands.

After 3 weeks, at her return appointment, Mary's results read as follows: Hb 10.0 g/dl and ESR 45 mm/h; rheumatoid factor positive 1:256 and antinuclear factor negative. All remaining results were within normal limits. The biochemical results, coupled with the physical examination—which revealed painful wrists, together with hot, swollen and painful MCPs and PIPs of both hands, restricted movement of both shoulders and a painful left elbow—confirm the rheumatologist's previous suspicions, Mary is informed of the diagnosis—rheumatoid arthritis. For the present the indomethacin is increased to 50 mg t.d.s. and in addition paracetamol two p.r.n. is suggested.

Traditionally it is at this stage that a patient would expect an explanation of the diagnosis. However, we would like to suggest than in addition to the doctor's explanation, every patient should be given the opportunity to participate in a concise patient education programme based on the following format:

Problem No. 1: **Mental State (Anxiety)**
Intervention: **Counselling**

At this early stage the counsellor will need to assess the patient's mental attitude and decide how much information to give. Should the patient's physical condition necessitate admission to hospital, the education programme can take place there.

A subjective assessment can be made by listening to the patient's description of the illness, how it started and how it is progressing, and also the extent to which the patient's life has been altered because of it. Some patients will be both receptive and talkative; others will be in a state of mental shock and prove incapable of understanding anything said to them. In the latter case, the whole situation will need to be approached very carefully and tentatively, and at this juncture education may well only consist of encouragement and support for the patient and the patient's family from the hospital staff and the medical social worker.

After the initial interviewing the counsellor decides that Mary is both anxious and apprehensive; nevertheless, she appears well motivated and eager for help and information. As the education programme is to take place in the outpatient department, encouragement should be given for a relative or friend to accompany the patient for all or some of the education vists. This can be of enormous benefit to the patient and ultimately the whole family.

Problem No. 2: **Lack of Medical Knowledge**
Intervention: **Description of Disease Process**

Having assessed Mary's mental state and decided that she is receptive, the counsellor begins by giving a brief and uncomplicated description of rheumatoid arthritis. For example:

We do not know the cause, but it is an inflammatory process which can affect all the joints, though usually not all at the same time. This inflammation causes the joints to become hot and swollen. The drugs that we give you will help to reduce this inflammation, and the swelling will gradually subside.

Questions should be answered as they arise, without being too concerned at this stage as to the amount of information actually being understood or retained. Next, the description should be backed up with hand-outs, such as the booklet *Rheumatoid Arthritis*, produced by the Arthritis and Rheumatism Council (ARC)[1]. These can be useful, but an alternative would be to produce one's own booklet, which need not be expensive but which may be more comprehensive.

The counsellor asks Mary to read the booklet at home and advises her of the benefits to herself and her family if they can also be persuaded to read them. The counsellor suggests that she underlines in pencil anything which is not clear so that it may be discussed at her next visit.

Problem No. 3: **Drug Compliance**
Intervention: **Drug Information Sheets**

Drug information sheets (DISs) are indispensable. They are of enormous advantage both to the patient and the counsellor. DISs can be drawn up by the pharmacy, the medical staff or a combination of both. There should be a DIS produced for every drug dispensed to rheumatic patients, including all drugs on the periphery and likely to be dispensed, e.g. anticoagulants, antidepressants, diuretics etc. Figure 7.2. shows an example of a DIS. Each sheet should contain the following information:

Name of drug—both generic and trade
Reason for taking drug
Directions for taking drug
Description of drug
Dosage of drug
Possible side-effects
Special instructions
Additional information

The responsibility for updating these information sheets should lie with the pharmacy.

It is widely understood that wastage of medication results from misuse on the part of the patient. This can almost always be directly attributable to lack of information. As the patient is confused, abuse occurs, resulting in underdosing or overdosing. Another danger is that the patient may stop taking medication for fear of imagined or actual side-effects. By educating each patient and giving concise instructions, the results could be dramatically improved. (Drug therapy is discussed in more detail under the heading 'Self-medication in the Hospital Setting', see p. 194.)

---

[1] Arthritis and Rheumatism Council, 841 Eagle Street, London WC1R 4AR. Telephone number: 01 405 8572.

PATIENT EDUCATION, LEEDS UNIVERSITY.

DRUG INFORMATION SHEET.

INDOCID (Indomethacin)   NAME:

I. WHY YOU ARE TAKING THIS MEDICINE:

This is an anti-inflammatory drug used to reduce joint
swelling and pain, to decrease morning stiffness, and to delay
the time of onset of fatigue. Improvement in the way you
feel may take from 1 to 2 weeks, and is maintained as long as
you are taking this drug.

II. HOW TO TAKE THIS MEDICINE:

Indocid is taken in divided doses throughout the day. It may
be prescribed as a one-a-day dose taken at bedtime.

Indocid should be taken with or after meals during the day
and with food or milk at bedtime. Never take Indocid on an
empty stomach.

III. DESCRIPTION:

25 mg. — ivory capsule marked Indocid "25" MSD.
50 mg. — ivory capsule marked Indocid "50" MSD.

IV. SIDE EFFECTS THAT HAVE OCCURRED IN SOME
PATIENTS TAKING THIS MEDICINE:

1. Headache, dizziness.   4. Blurred vision.
                                 5. Fluid retention in hands
2. Upset stomach.   and legs.
3. Skin rash.   6. Disorientation.

If any of these side effects occur, bring them to your doctor's
attention.

V. ADDITIONAL INFORMATION:

Whenever possible, Indomethacin should not be taken at the
same time as other drugs, as it may alter the effect of drugs
that lower blood pressure and drugs that alter mood swings.

Fig. 7.2. An example of a DIS.

As mentioned previously, indomethacin 50 mg t.d.s. and paracetamol two
q.d.s. have been prescribed for Mary. Therefore, she should be supplied with
DISs relevant to both these drugs. Having given Mary her DISs and having
discussed them with her in detail, the counsellor stresses that, as more visits
are to follow, she should not expect to absorb all the information in one day.

Problem No. 4: **Living with the Disease**
Intervention: **Planning, Pacing and Priorities**

The counsellor explains to Mary that if she learns to plan her day carefully she will eventually derive increased benefit from doing so.

With the cooperation of an employer, patients who are at work each day can learn to plan their workload so that periods of physical activity are followed by periods which are more sedentary. In many instances this can be accomplished with help from an occupational therapist and social worker. They could visit the patient's place of employment and advise accordingly. In these days of increasing public awareness of the disabled, much can be achieved.

Patients at home must also plan so that periods of physical activity (of perhaps 2 or 3 h) are followed by periods of rest. Housework, for instance, may only be continued if the patient feels sufficiently rested. By this method patients will achieve a regular workload with which they can cope, thereby preventing undue physical strain and mental stress from developing. Once patients realise that in this way they are able to achieve positive results (a tidy house and a cooked meal), they will also benefit psychologically.

The counsellor should suggest to patients that they ask themselves what it is they wish to achieve that day. For example, do they wish to shop or visit friends in the evening. If so, they must accept that routine jobs be left undone, thereby conserving their energy for their alternative activities. Remind them that they do not have to stop living but simply adjust to their shortcomings, and life will become more bearable. By planning their day ahead, pacing their activities and by asking themselves what their priorities are, they should find that they are able to derive more pleasure and satisfaction from life.

In Mary's case, working 4 h each morning, Monday to Friday, and having to cope with her home and family, life is not going to be easy. Assuming that she wishes to remain in work (and we would not suggest that she leaves if she is happy there), she should be advised to share all the responsibility for running the home with the rest of the family, including sharing the cooking, cleaning and shopping. Should her family prove uncooperative then counselling them may help. Alternatively, she might consider reducing her hours of work.

Problem No. 5: **Development of Disease Activity**
Intervention: **Daily Exercise with Physiotherapy**

There is controversy over the precise value of regular daily exercise. Indeed, studies designed to evaluate the extent to which exercise might prevent disability are hard to perform and evaluate. Nevertheless, we certainly feel that they do, and the following few examples may help to prove our hypothesis.

Dedicated athletes spend hours in daily exercise in order to increase muscle tone and to strengthen muscle power. These healthy young athletes find their performance is improved when they exercise regularly, and reduced when they fail to do so. Footballers, sprinters, gymnasts and many other athletes fall into this category. The swimmer, although he has chosen a discipline which is a complete form of exercise in itself, will add weightlifting to his activities in order to improve his performance. In the case of the rheumatic patient, it is known that daily exercise will help to maintain the normal range of movement of each joint.

For at least 10 years the treatment of ankylosing spondylitis has consisted of regular daily exercise. Consequently, it is a rare occurrence to observe anyone within the normal population who is obviously suffering from this disease. Previously, treatment consisted of bed rest for weeks at a time, which sadly resulted in 'poker back'. Treatment of Still's disease over the past 4 or 5 years has also consisted of regular daily exercise. The photograph on the right in Fig. 7.3. clearly shows the benefits.

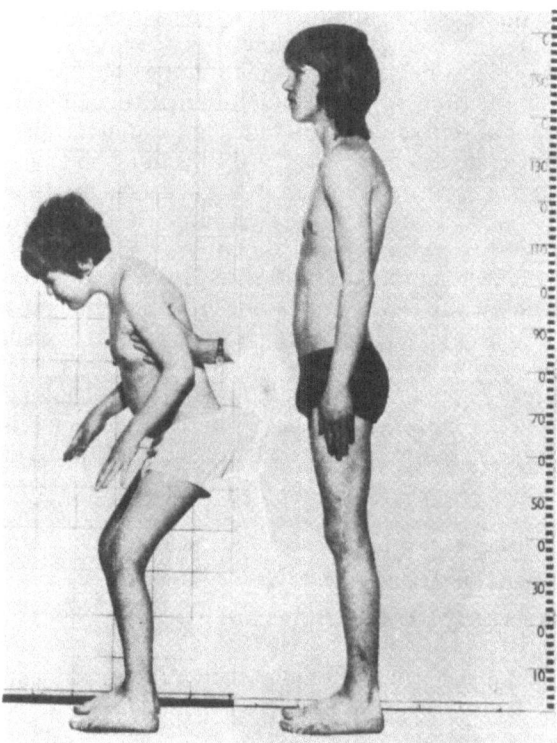

Fig. 7.3. The value of physiotherapy. A patient with juvenile polyarthritis before (*left*) and after (*right*) physiotherapy. Lapse of 3 years between the two photographs. (Courtesy of Dr. B.M. Ansell and the ARC)

Newly Diagnosed Rheumatoid Arthritis Patient

A patient suffering from rheumatoid arthritis will undoubtedly develop painful joints. These joints may become inflamed and eroded. Understandably the patient will use the involved joint as little as possible, resulting in muscle wasting, loss of muscle power and a reduction in the normal range of movement. In the long term, deformity may develop until eventually the disease may burn itself out. Meanwhile, the patient is left with a whole series of useless joints and has become physically impaired.

Immediately the patient is diagnosed, therefore, the counsellor must contemplate the introduction of a series of exercises which cover every joint, and emphasise that they should be carried out daily whenever humanly possibly. These exercises must not take too long to perform, otherwise the patient will not be motivated. The main purpose of these exercises will be to maintain a normal range of movement within each joint. This in turn will help to sustain a strong supporting muscle and improved muscle tone.

The counsellor should instruct the patient, that in the event of a 'flare' advice and encouragement will be given to continue with the exercises, but in a modified form which involves active assisted and isometric exercise only. As the 'flare' subsides (as they always do in time), then the exercises should be continued as before.

Daily Exercise Sheet.   The counsellor should formulate a Daily Exercise Sheet in her own unit in conjunction with the physiotherapy department. Ideally, an appointment should be made to see a physiotherapist at the same time as the sheet is handed out; a patient can then be fully assessed by a chartered physiotherapist and also instructed on how to perform the exercises correctly. Information on active assisted and isometric exercises should be included on the daily exercise sheet.

A long-term controlled trial would be needed to evaluate whether daily exercise alters the course of rheumatic disease. At present, bearing in mind the flexion deformities that occur if joints are not regularly exercised, it would seem prudent to advocate exercise.

Mary is given an exercise sheet and an appointment with the physiotherapy department. Any problem which develops in relation to these exercises can be discussed at her next visit and if necessary a second referral made to the physiotherapy department.

Problem No. 6: **Physical Inability to Cope with Day-to-Day Tasks, Including Personal Hygiene**
Intervention: **Assessment by Occupational Therapy Department, Including Other Specialists**

Once diagnosed, all rheumatic patients should be referred to the occupational therapy department. These patients have problem joints and require help immediately before deformity has developed.

Splints

The occupational therapy (OT) department can supply splints for every joint, either ready made or made to measure. The department also specialises in 'aids to daily living' (ADL).

Mary may be newly diagnosed, but it would be reasonable to assume that she is having difficulty in opening jars, turning taps on and off and peeling vegetables. Also, because her painful shoulders restrict movement, she may be having problems with personal hygiene. Many aids can be supplied to help alleviate this problem. She would certainly be well advised to wear wrist splints while working. She uses her hands a great deal as a cook, carrying many heavy pans and dishes. Therefore, the support gained from wearing splints will be beneficial. Plastic, waterproof splints can be prescribed for use while cooking, so enabling her to use water as she requires.

Futura splints can be supplied for use around the house, plus another pair to wear while sleeping. So often patients complain that their hands are painful in the morning, mainly due to the unnatural position in which the hands lie during sleep. Splints worn during sleep will help to alleviate much of this problem. The counsellor should remind the patient to put the splints on *before* starting work, and not to wait until pain in the hands has developed. The splints will limit movement and provide support—the main principle of joint protection.

One further point worth mentioning is that splints are regarded as ugly and 'unfeminine'. For this reason alone many female patients reject them. Once the patient has been convinced of their usefulness, the counsellor should assure her that she need not wear the splints on social occasions.

It is important that patients are referred to OT early in treatment. By supplying aids immediately, as little stress as possible will be transferred to painful and inflamed joints when they are most vulnerable to damage. Occupational therapists will pay domiciliary visits to advise on custom-made aids (see Chaps. 4 and 6).

Footwear Specialist

Had a radiograph of Mary's feet revealed evidence of erosions, then undoubtedly she would eventually require specialised footwear. In the United Kingdom custom-made shoes are available on prescription. Although they are expensive (approx. £150–£200), they can be supplied completely free of charge to patients who are unable to purchase ordinary shoes which provide the necessary comfort and support. Mary's radiographs did not reveal erosive changes. Had they done so, persistent standing, as is involved in her job as a cook, would certainly aggravate the condition. Early detection of erosive change in the feet should prompt the supply of correct footwear immediately and not after deformity has developed. The shoes may be shop bought, rather than custom-made, providing they fulfil the criteria laid down for correct footwear: Shoes must be deep and wide, made of a soft malleable material—

preferably leather, with a low comfortable heel, and incorporating a fastening which is easy for the patient to manipulate.

Ensuring that correct footwear is worn, may help to delay the development of foot deformity. Shoes, after all, are simply another form of splinting. Should the cost of custom-made shoes appear prohibitive, the counsellor should compare it with the cost of foot surgery and also consider the pain and discomfort to the patient caused by foot deformity. One important point to consider is that unless the patient is motivated towards wearing custom-made shoes, considered by many, particularly the young, as 'invalid shoes', then there is little point in prescribing them. Instead, the counsellor should suggest that the patient visits the shoe specialist and asks to be shown exactly what can be offered, before a decision is made. Once the female patient has been convinced of the long-term benefits of wearing the correct footwear, the counsellor should also tell her to wear her prettiest fashion shoes (if she is able) when out with her husband or friends. Providing she does not stand around in them, both she and her husband will benefit psychologically.

'Hand clinics' are an integral part of many rheumatology departments; it is encouraging that more departments are also establishing 'foot clinics'.

Problem No. 7: **Poor Diet**
Intervention: **Refer to Dietician**

While Mary is working as a cook she is inclined to nibble the food as she prepares it. Even the diagnosis of RA has not resulted in her losing weight; in fact she is overweight. Fortunately, at least for the present, no weight-bearing joints are involved. Nevertheless, the gaining of excessive weight is a definite disadvantage. An appointment with the dietician should be made so that the correct advice can be given.

Problem No. 8: **Elderly Dependent relative**
Intervention: **Medical Social Worker**

Mary is fortunate in that she has a family which is supportive, and there are no financial problems, even if she decides to stop working because of her physical disability. There is, however, an elderly female relative living close by who depends upon her for daily support and companionship. By referring this problem to the medical social worker a solution can be sought. It is doubtful whether the relative would wish to leave her home. Therefore the district nurse, Meals on Wheels and other community services can be contacted, so that much of the physical burden, which has fallen on Mary in the past, can be relieved.

Problem No. 9: **A 'Flare'**
Intervention: **Specific Treatment, Including Analgesic, Ice, Heat, Rest**

A 'flare' is the term used by both the professional and the lay person to describe an acute attack of inflammation in one or more joints. Since a 'flare-up' is described in one dictionary as a 'burst into blaze or anger' this is indeed an apt term: Unless a 'flare' is quickly brought under control it will very soon get out of hand—as can a burst of anger.

Development of a 'Flare'

Pain is usually the first symptom a patient is aware of. A quick examination of the painful site will reveal a hot, swollen and stiffening joint. Gradually, unless preventive measures are taken, the pain will increase, the joint will become hotter and more swollen, and the stiffness will result in almost complete immobilisation of the involved joint and consequently of the whole limb. If more than one joint is involved the result can be traumatic for the patient, sometimes out of all proportion to the apparent physical disability involved. If pain is not brought quickly under control a vicious circle develops. The pain, anxiety, tension and depression lead in turn to more pain, which becomes increasingly more severe as each hour passes.

Treatment of a 'Flare' in the Home

Analgesia/Anti-inflammatory Agents. As soon as a 'flare' develops, the patient should immediately take additional analgesia and/or anti-inflammatory agents (provided this does not exceed the maximum dose as advised by the physician), whichever helps to control the pain. The patient should continue to take extra medication every 3–4 h until the 'flare' is brought under control. The usual medication will be continued as before.

Heat. The patient should apply heat to the painful area(s) using either moist or dry heat. This therapy should be continued until the pain begins to ease.

Cold. Some people find cold (ice) more beneficial than heat. It is simply a matter of personal preference. The cold therapy should be administered as for heat.

Rest. The affected joint or joints should be immobilised in the optimum position either by bed rest or splinting, or a combination of both. However, active assisted and isometric exercises can be continued.

Once the patient is convinced of the positive benefits of implementing this regimen, natural anxiety and tension will be lessened. Depression will not readily gain a hold, and the vicious circle will have little chance of developing. By gaining control of the 'flare' in this way, the possibility of hospitalisation becomes increasingly remote.

The education of the patient's family, is also important for successful 'flare' control. The members of the family can help to reduce much of the tension by administering the heat or cold, encouraging the patient to rest, or simply by providing cups of tea at frequent intervals. The family will also benefit from the knowledge that they have helped the patient to remain at home, within a loving and caring environment, thereby avoiding the stress normally placed upon families when one member becomes hospitalised.

Patients living alone will obviously find the possibilities of success with this treatment regimen somewhat lessened. They may have no one to provide the hot water bottle or the tea and paracetamol, and therefore rest becomes more of a problem. Sadly, they may also have no one to give encouragement or sympathy. Nevertheless, by following the suggested method of coping with a 'flare', they should eventually succeed, though it may take a little longer.

Problem No. 10: **Decreased Sexual Activity**
Intervention: **Sexual Counselling**

The medical social worker is an indispensable health care team member, who, apart from dealing with financial and social problems, may also have trained in sexual counselling and can be called upon in this capacity. However, the very important subject of sexual activity can be tackled very successfully by the patient's counsellor. Providing the subject is not discussed until rapport has been developed between them, much can be achieved. One excellent way of approaching the subject is to offer the patient the booklet *Marriage, Sex and Arthritis*, which can be supplied by the ARC. Although this booklet is good in many ways, it has been felt by patients to be not explicit enough. The counsellor should consider compiling an alternative booklet, possibly a little more explicit. If the information given to the patient is concise and covers all aspects of sexual problems for both single and married people, there will probably be little need for further discussion. An explicit booklet is far less embarrassing for everyone. Moreover, it can be taken away and read by the patients and their partners, preferably when they are together in the privacy of their own homes. Many patients benefit from sexual counselling when it is offered, yet initially they may never *dare* to enquire.

It is the young, newly diagnosed rheumatic patient, male or female, who may appear reticent when sexual problems are discussed, yet their need may be greater than most. Any existing sexual relationship may still be immature, when suddenly they find themselves having to cope with a disease which may well remain with them for the rest of their lives and which will surely have a lasting effect upon any future sexual activity. The problem is compounded if the patient is a young mother with toddlers, and is lessened in middle age when the patient may well have an older, caring partner.

The female patient can find a change in bodily image becomes increasingly hard to accept. Hand deformities, whether nodules or ulnar deviation, cause much anxiety. Most of the body can be disguised by clothing, but the hands, unfortunately, remain exposed unless gloves are worn, and this is impracticable. Other bodily changes occur which she suspects will reduce her sexual attraction—as indeed they may. Recognition of her anxiety by all the disciplines involved in her care is vital.

Summary of Outpatient Education

Providing patients have actively participated in the educational sessions they should at this stage:

1. *Have an understanding of the disease process.* This information should help the patients to adjust mentally to their illness. They will now be aware of their individual expectations and will more readily cope with their new-found limitations.
2. *Understand their drug therapy.* All the important facts concerned with their medication will have been explained. The common fears concerning drug therapy, particularly the side-effects, will have been alleviated, and compliance will now replace reluctance when medication is due. Should second-line drug therapy be introduced, patients will be ready to accept responsibility for themselves by not only checking their urine and ensuring their blood is taken, but also being aware of the significance of these tests and understanding the results.
3. *Be motivated towards exercising.* Exercises may well be resented because they are time consuming and often painful to perform. Now, however, patients will appreciate why they are necessary. This understanding will not make the exercises more enjoyable or less painful, but each exercise will acquire a more beneficial long-term aspect which will encourage patients to consider them worthwhile.
4. *Be able to cope with a 'flare'.* Hospitalisation will no longer be the first thought of patients when the disease is at its most intense, and instead of fearing the approach of a flare they will appreciate what is happening and respond accordingly, thus ensuring that the vicious circle of pain, tension and depression will not develop.
5. *Have developed a better sexual understanding.* They will acknowledge the need for a completely new approach to sexual activity between themselves and their partners.
6. *Have a knowledge of other disciplines beneficial to them.* They should know how to contact by name and telephone the occupational therapist, medical social worker, dietician, shoe specialist, psychologist, physiotherapist and pharmacist.

The Counsellor — Who Will Adopt the Role?

Obviously each unit must decide for itself who is to adopt the role of counsellor. As mentioned at the beginning of this chapter, both the doctor and the nurse, and indeed most other disciplines, already educate the patient; however, the degree to which they are able to do so is severely limited by time, which is very short, and the number of patients, which is very high. The doctor's main role is to diagnose, and therefore a large proportion of the time allocated to the doctor is already committed. The nurse, however, is in a different situation and she could be the ideal counsellor. Consideration should be given to the possibility of having a nurse whose main role would be educational counselling. She would hold her own clinics, consisting of patients referred directly to her from the doctor after the initial diagnosis has been made and appropriate drug therapy introduced. The number of educational visits would depend on the patients' individual needs. Specially trained nurses, called Clinical Nurse Metrologists or Rheumatology Nurse Practitioners, have been in existence for some time at the Leeds General Infirmary. Their role is a little more specialised than that outlined above and will be fully described in Chapter 10.

A majority of self-respecting physicians will wish to take full responsibility for patient education themselves. This may be a counsel of perfection. When, for financial and historical reasons the proportion of physicians to patients is poor, patient education by paramedics provides an alternative solution — and one which is often preferred by the patients. Nurses at the bedside are in full-time direct contact with patients; their transposition to an outpatient role is simply a logical progression.

Outpatient Group Sessions

The suggestions which have already been made should be easy to implement in most rheumatology units, for the majority of facilities mentioned are already available in all NHS hospitals. However, the second form of educational provision we propose is not readily available, and its implementation will therefore require organisation and cooperation from all disciplines, including the hospital authority.

If all rheumatic patients, when first diagnosed, were able to avail themselves of the facilities mentioned previously, there would be no need for outpatient group sessions. Unfortunately, however, a vast number of patients suffering from various rheumatic diseases are ignorant of the basic medical facts. In order to reach as large an audience as possible outpatient group sessions should be held.

The educational group sessions can be directed towards one disease only, for example osteoarthritis or rheumatoid arthritis, although discussion of a variety of diseases may well prove more practical. They can be held as frequently as is feasible. If a 2-hourly session, on 3 consecutive weeks, four times a year could be arranged, this would be a major breakthrough. Whenever possible they should be held in the evening, so that relatives can accompany the patients. Not only does this provide the opportunity to educate relatives, but it also solves another major problem—transport. Most relatives can supply this fairly easily in the evening after work.

Each session may last from 1 to 2 h, bearing in mind that patients suffering from rheumatic diseases cannot sit for lengthy periods without experiencing much pain and discomfort. It should also be remembered that these patients may be feeling ill or depressed; therefore, a session lasting too long will achieve little except stiff limbs and a sense of frustration.

The decision as to who should give the lectures will be made by the individual unit and will depend upon the disease in question. All disciplines should be involved, and often the disciplines may overlap. (The importance of each discipline knowing exactly what is being taught by their colleagues will be discussed more fully later.) Obviously the list of lecturers should include nurses, occupational therapists, physiotherapists, medical social workers and doctors where possible. As these members of staff may be giving up their own free time to run the classes, the workload can be more easily spread by the recruitment of as many disciplines as possible. A further useful suggestion is to include a known and willing patient as a speaker. The cardinal rule in a situation like the one presented is to have a strong group leader. This person must be capable of keeping the group directed towards the subject and must not be afraid to bring group members into line should they stray from the point. It could be all too easy for a group of vocal patients or relatives to take over. Time for discussion should always be allowed at the end of a session, and participants should be informed of this at the start, as naturally they will wish to contribute and to ask questions. Provision of a cup of tea or coffee is very necessary at some point in the evening.

Sessions can be held anywhere with heat, light, water and suitable toilet facilities. The special needs of the disabled must be taken into account. An adapted toilet should be available if at all possible, and of course easy access into the building itself via ramps or lifts is essential. One suggestion, apart from the obvious one of approaching the local hospital authority for the use of a room, is to contact the local branch of the ARC. It will probably have a room which is regularly used for members' meetings and which will meet all the necessary requirements.

Because sessions are held in the evening most staff are willing to give their time free, and it is possible, as already mentioned, that the local hospital authority will be only too pleased to allow the use of a hall or room free of charge. The ARC can also be approached for funding. One of the aims of this council is to support education in relation to rheumatology; therefore, funding to cover hand-outs, tapes, video equipment etc. and other expenses incurred can be applied for. Consideration can also be given to approaching the drug companies. In return for a discreet display of their company name a generous contribution may often be forthcoming. Whilst patients are the ones who will benefit from the education, the drug companies are dependent on sales to the patients, and for this reason may well be ready to provide financial help. Certainly no one should be out of pocket; therefore, adequate funding is essential from the start. One further point is that it may be viable to charge each patient a nominal fee in order to cover expenses.

Suggested topics for discussion might be:

1. Disease process
2. Joint protection
3. Drug therapy
4. Social benefits

Printed hand-outs and visual aids enhance these meetings and ease the burden upon the speaker. (If visual aids are to be used, a check must be made beforehand to ensure that electric sockets are available.) As already mentioned, time is limited, and therefore hand-outs and visual aids will help patients to assimilate much information for which there may not be sufficient time at the meeting.

Publicity. A specific telephone number can be displayed in the outpatient department, public libraries and meeting places for old-age pensioners or any public organisation which attracts a cross-section of the community. Patients could telephone this number and be advised where and when the next session would be held, and they would be encouraged to make a definite booking. Prior knowledge of approximate numbers to expect at a meeting can be invaluable to both speaker and organiser. A volunteer could man the telephone. The number publicised could be either the volunteer's own private number or one in the hospital to which the volunteer has access. Provided that the relevant information as to the times to telephone is clearly displayed alongside the number there should be little difficulty.

Evaluation. It is most important to evaluate the success of the scheme. The most simple way of assessing the rate of progress is by using questionnaires, which may be given out at the start and end of each session. They should include questions based upon the subject which is to be covered that evening. They must be simple and uncomplicated; multiple choice questions are a good idea. By the end of the evening the second questionnaire should reveal whether or not the patients have understood and therefore increased their knowledge in respect of rheumatology. Of course someone will have to be responsible for evaluating the questionnaires in order to determine whether or not positive results have been achieved and the sessions are worthwhile.

Inpatient Education

Group Sessions

A large number of rheumatology patients will impose upon paramedical disciplines the need to specialise in rheumatology, and such specialists are essential for the evolution of a successful inpatient education programme.

Patients have always been educated on a one-to-one basis, and the introduction of group sessions does not mean that this must cease. Not only will individual patient education continue, but it is hoped that it will improve, with all disciplines becoming acutely aware of their role of educator as well as therapist, nurse etc. Patient education in the group setting will reinforce what is already being taught individually. It will also help to create opportunities for patients and staff to come together on an informal basis to learn and discuss, thereby enlightening and enriching the patient's lives. An inpatient education programme will require a great deal of organisation, perhaps more than either of the two forms of education already mentioned, and once again cooperation from all quarters is essential in order to achieve success.

The audience in this instance will be a captive one. However, it must always be borne in mind that the people who will attend the group sessions are ill. Therefore, they cannot be treated like students in college, and every consideration for their disabilities must be taken into account when planning the programme.

Assuming that there is general agreement within the hospital on the value of inpatient education, the next step will be to appoint someone who will become an education coordinator. He or she will draw together a representative member from each discipline, and it is upon this basis that the education team can be formed.

Programme Aspects for Consideration

Disease

The members of the education team must decide which diseases are to be covered. Should the classes be directed towards RA only, or a mixture of rheumatic diseases? Both of these methods have proved successful in the United States. The decision will depend upon the number of patients admitted to the ward or unit. A larger number of patients can be included if a mixture of diseases is covered.

Speakers

The speakers should be drawn from all disciplines, and should include nurses, physiotherapists, occupational therapists, pharmacists, dieticians, medical social workers, psychiatrists, not forgetting the patients themselves. The reader may have noticed the omission of rheumatologists. This is not because nurses wish to exclude them; indeed their approval and cooperation are imperative for a successful programme to be implemented. However their actual participation in the classes is not really necessary. They will be busy applying their unique skills elsewhere.

It should be remembered that the speakers may never have faced a class before. Therefore, everyone who appears willing will not automatically be competent. The coordinator will have to be firm in accepting only those proven to be suitable, and the suitability of speakers should be constantly evaluated.

Subjects to be Taught

Each specialty will naturally decide exactly what should be taught. It is important, however, that once the content has been decided upon, each paper must be submitted to the education team for general scrutiny and discussion. The reason for this approval procedure is to ensure that all the speakers are fully aware of what their colleagues are saying. This is very important, otherwise patients could be unwittingly fed incorrect facts. It is worth mentioning here that all speakers must feel free at any time to admit openly to patients when they cannot answer a specific question, and to follow this with a promise to investigate further on the questioner's behalf.

The following is a suggested list of subjects and appropriate speakers (not in any order of priority):

1. Disease process	Nurse, drawing upon the advice of the medical staff
2. Joint protection, including ADL	Occupational therapist
3. Coping with a flare	Nurse, occupational therapist, physiotherapist
4. Exercise	Physiotherapist
5. Pacing, planning, priorities	Occupational therapist, physiotherapist, or nurse
6. Drug therapy	Pharmacist, or nurse in conjunction with pharmacist
7. Dietetics	Dietician, or nurse in conjunction with dietician
8. Social benefits etc.	Medical social worker/nurse
9. Quackery	Nurse/pharmacist
10. Patient experience	Patient
11. Mental adjustment	Psychiatrist

Where two speakers are suggested, this is to distribute the burden over as wide an area as possible. For example, there may well be only one or two social workers in a hospital, but many more nurses. As many members as possible from each discipline should be trained to take responsibility for a class. The burden then can be shared, and, most importantly in these days of staff shortages, individuals will not be called upon more than is necessary.

Educational Aids

No single method will suit every member of a class. However, by leaving time for open discussion at the end of a session, the speaker will be able to deal with any point on which a patient is unclear.

Planned talks may be backed by planned literature, slides, video tapes, films, blackboards, posters and models. These visual aids may be prepared by the education team themselves, or else bought or hired. Models may be supplied by drug companies. Incidentally, patients must never be left alone watching a film or slides which may cause them distress. They will always require a reassuring person nearby. Patients should be reminded to bring their glasses and a working hearing aid, if required.

Timetable and Location of Classes

Unlike the outpatient sessions, the educators will have access to the patient much more readily, and therefore the need to cram as much as possible into as short a time as possible does not arise. One suggestion is to hold classes of an hour's duration each weekday over a 2-week period. These will be ongoing classes repeated over and over again, with holidays being taken into account. Preference should be given to holding the classes at the same time each day, for example 10 a.m. (Mornings are perhaps the best time, as patients will not feel so tired.) This routine will ensure that each discipline in the hospital, including the medical staff, will become accustomed to the classes and will make allowances for them in planning their individual requirements. Visitors will also become familiar with the routine and may benefit by accompanying the patient in some instances.

Providing everyone (and this includes the patient taking part) knows in advance where and when the classes are to be held, then either one specific room or even a variety of rooms can be selected. Often size and the number of electrical points are governing factors. If patients can be encouraged to use the ward toilet before a class, then a convenient toilet should not be a prerequisite.

Selection of Patients for Education

Not every patient admitted will automatically be given the opportunity to attend classes. Unsuitable patients may fall into one, or more, of the following categories:

1. Patients who are too old or too ill to be receptive. These patients are not to be entirely excluded. As their condition improves they should be re-assessed.
2. Patients suffering from severe depression. In these instances, certain of the classes can be offered, for example a class on psychiatric aspects or a

class on quackery. As the patient's condition improves, other classes can be added.

3. Patients who have already attended classes during a previous hospitalisation or who have received the full benefit of the outpatient education programme. Again these patients should not be entirely excluded. Instead they should be offered the opportunity to update their previous knowledge, taking part in all or some of the classes, whichever they choose.

4. Disruptive patients. Unfortunately, they do exist but they cannot be excluded. Professional staff must learn how to cope with them. They may well benefit from the classes to such an extent that they no longer remain disruptive.

5. Patients suffering from non-specific rheumatic complaints, e.g. frozen shoulder, cervical pain, low back pain. Although these patients may benefit from certain classes only (i.e. pacing, planning, priorities and drug therapies), it remains a possibility that those with unusual organic disease are most likely to benefit from the extra attention received in class participation.

Who should make the final decision on patient suitability? Obviously the medical staff will wish to be consulted. It is hoped that selection will develop into a joint decision between the doctor and the ward sister, with the primary nurse's opinion being given considerable weight. Whatever the decision the result must be entered upon the patient's treatment sheet, and naturally the patient must also be informed.

In a large rheumatology hospital or unit patients should be given a list of classes, with the ones they are to attend being marked. The list should also include the venue and the time of each class. Providing patients are ambulant, they should be given the responsibility of attending the classes themselves. They should be instructed to report their departure by placing their names or a star upon a board informing everyone as to their whereabouts. If they are not ambulant, the process becomes a little more difficult, as a porter or nurse has to be alerted as escort. Incidentally, it is no use the patient turning up 10 min after the class has started. Escorts must therefore be reliable, and must be aware of the fact that these classes are an essential part of the patients' overall treatment, and not something frivolous thought up by the hierarchy!

Evaluation

Since many disciplines are involved in group classes, each discipline would be advised to draw up questionnaires for each class held. Ideally, the questionnaires would be evaluated by the education team as a whole. Certainly, if the patients are not improving their knowledge as judged by the returned questionnaires, then this aspect will need looking into carefully and diplomatically. It should be made clear at the outset to those instructing classes that it will be necessary for the education coordinator and team members to sit in on their colleagues' classes from time to time to evaluate their performance and to take action accordingly. It must not be assumed that patients have learned just because they have been taught.

Self-medication in the Hospital Setting

Because drug therapy plays an enormous part in the overall treatment of rheumatic patients, an educational self-medication programme could prove to be an invaluable addition to total patient care. Admission to hospital provides the perfect opportunity for educating rheumatic patients about their drug therapy.

In the current situation, expressed in simple terms, patients are being admitted to hospital or seen in the outpatient department for the prime reason of 'new medication'. Patients will be told the name of the new drug, when to take it and how many tablets to take. If it is a second-line drug (e.g. penicillamine), they will also be told to have their blood and urine tested at regular intervals. They will be very fortunate indeed if they are given more information than this—they may be told even less by their general practitioner. As the section title 'Self Medication in the Hospital Setting' suggests, we are advocating a moderately revolutionary idea, at least as far as the United Kingdom is concerned, and it should not be rejected out of hand.

Method of Self-medication

On admission to hospital, the patient is 'written up' for his drugs in the usual way (bearing in mind that most rheumatic patients are admitted for not less than 3 weeks), and may continue with the existing drug therapy or start immediately on a new one. In either case the medication will be given to the patient via the routine 'medicine round'.

Nurse's Role in Self-medication

Over the following 3 or 4 days the primary nurse, under whose care the patient has been placed, should familiarise herself with the patient's drugs in the following way:

1. Discover generic name of the drug, as well as its trade name.
2. Examine the tablets, taking note of colour and shape.
3. Note the different doses in which the drug is supplied.
4. Record the time of day and the number of times each day when the drug should be given.

5. Note whether the drug should be taken before or after meals.
6. Note whether the drug should be taken with food or on an empty stomach.
7. Make particular note of any possible side-effects and consequently any special precautions which should be taken.
8. Note any contraindications.

On approximately the fourth day, at a time set aside for education, the nurse begins the self-medication programme. Her first task will be explanatory, reassuring the patient by explaining that they will be going over the programme each day together until both are quite satisfied that the information has been absorbed. As each stage is passed a planning sheet is marked, until the final stage, that of self-medication, can begin. The medicine bottles containing a week's supply of tablets are placed in the patient's locker where they can be reached easily by the patient. Patients should be advised at this stage to carry the tablets with them should they leave their bedside for treatment. (Most rheumatic patients will be wearing their day clothes and will therefore have pockets or, in the case of ladies, handbags.) The patient is then supplied with a 'medication sheet' upon which are noted the times the medicine must be taken. All that remains is for the patient to take the drugs at the prescribed times and tick the sheet to say that it has been done. The primary nurse, or her deputy, will unobtrusively check at odd moments to see that this procedure has been carried out.

An alternative method is to give only 2 days' supply at a time. Checking for compliance then becomes easier and drug abuse less likely. The drawback to this method is the additional workload placed upon the pharmacy department. If an individual patient's drug therapy consists of many drugs (polypharmacy), then the task becomes more complicated. It is clear, however, that this patient is in greater need of education, when one considers how many permutations are possible for making mistakes after the patient is eventually discharged home. MacDonald et al. (1977) found that by 12 weeks after discharge, half their patients were taking less than half their tablets, while a further quarter were seriously overdosing themselves! Less than one quarter were still taking their tablets properly.

Drug Information Sheets

In order to simplify the task of educating the patient, DISs must be provided. The benefits of these are outstanding to both the patient and the nurse. These sheets are drawn up by the pharmacy department, the medical staff, or a combination of both. There should be a DIS produced for every drug dispensed to rheumatic patients, including peripheral drugs which are likely to be dispensed, e.g. anticoagulants, antidepressants, diuretics etc. Included upon the sheets are the points already mentioned under 'Nurse's Role in Education', and therefore her role as an educator becomes much easier. All she has to do before starting to educate a patient is to extract the individual sheets which refer specifically to the drugs which have been prescribed. With the DIS available to both the nurse and the patient there is less opportunity for mistakes to occur. The patient can retain the sheets and can refer to them at any time while in hospital and eventually take them home on discharge.

As mentioned already, the responsibility for updating these DISs should lie with the pharmacy department. Information on drugs may be sought directly from pharmaceutical companies.

Foreseeable Problems

When self-medication is first mooted, major resistance may be experienced from four particular groups—physicians, nursing officers, administrators and pharmacists. All will have legitimate reasons for concern, and all will cite the possibility of suicidal patients on every ward. In other words, it is the legal implications which so greatly concern them. However, such fears can easily be allayed. Providing that overall approval has been granted by the hospital authority, then a self-medication programme can be instigated. Patients are already allowed to retain in their lockers contraceptive pills, glyceryl trinitrate, Ventolin inhalers etc. Therefore, a precedent has already been set. It is merely one further step to allow patients to retain all of their medication—once they have been educated.

The nursing and pharmacy staff will see an immediate increase in their workload. In the case of the nursing staff, however, their job satisfaction should also increase. By their acceptance of patient self-medication they will be acknowledging a far more responsible role in relation to patient drug therapy. No longer will they be simply doling out drugs from a bottle; instead they will now be aware of the pharmacology behind each tablet and injection.

The pharmacy staff will certainly experience an increased workload. Instead of tablets being dispensed from ward stock bottles, they will now be asked to make up individual bottles for each patient. They may also feel threatened, as the nurse will appear to be taking over the pharmacist's role as drug educator.

It is to be hoped that no one will see overdosed patients littering the wards. That is not to say that it is definitely not a risk, although evidence so far would suggest otherwise. The vast majority of rheumatic patients suffer severe pain and are in possession at home of large quantities of analgesics, and yet how many ever commit suicide?

For a self-medication scheme to be successful a close relationship must develop between the nursing and pharmacy staff. The nurse must feel free to call upon the pharmacy staff at any time for advice with regard to a given drug. It could well be the task of the pharmacy staff to educate the nurse pharmacologically, while the nurse, because she has 24-h contact with the patient on the ward, is in the ideal situation to educate the patient. Pharmacists may wish to reinforce the nurses teaching, calling in on the ward to assess the situation and to answer any unanswered questions if they wish to do so.

The situation is bound to arise of the patient who is impossible to educate. The largest percentage of such patients will consist of the elderly, although not all elderly patients will automatically fall into this category—quite the contrary in fact. However, for those who do, the necessity for education becomes even more imperative. If they cannot understand the basic information regarding dose and time, what are they going to do when they return home, especially if they are living alone? For elderly patients living with an able-bodied partner or relative, or even in sheltered accommodation, the problem is eased somewhat. In such circumstances, instead of educating the patients, it is possible to educate the relatives or wardens. They will be visiting in hospital over a period of 3 weeks or more, and their visits could be used for that purpose. For patients living entirely alone the situation becomes more difficult, but not insurmountable. The district nurse could be informed of the drug regimen via the patient's medical social worker or general practitioner. They in turn could call upon neighbours whom they know are willing to help keep an eye upon the patient. Certainly someone other than the general practitioner should be fully informed. It should be remembered that these patients are probably taking a multitude of tablets; thus, it is morally wrong to discharge these patients without some form of back-up service. The DISs can be sent home with the patient as reference material for the district nurse or neighbour.

One very important point is that education may be a means of reducing pharmacy costs. After all, a patient who is fully informed about the prescribed drug therapy may well comply more closely, with the result of a better response to a chosen drug and so less wastage. A response which is all too familiar is, 'It doesn't suit me doctor. Can I have something else?', when the bottle is still half full. As Bullen (1980) stated, 'An informed patient will be more likely to cooperate than one who does not understand the rationale of treatment. Such patients will be ready to accept a share of the responsibility for their health and will discuss with their medical practitioner any problems that arise during treatment.'

Evaluation of Patients' Achievements

As with inpatient and outpatient education, the method of self-medication must be evaluated from the start. It is necessary to ensure in some way that patients are actually retaining, if not all, then at least a large amount of what is being taught. Questionnaires should be handed to the patients before and after the education programme, and a follow-up questionnaire could be given out after 6 months.

When patients are seen at their follow-up appointments and it is found that they have complied week after week as instructed, this will be an excellent indication of success. If inpatient group sessions have been established in the hospital, then the education coordinator and team members can evaluate the questionnaires. If not, the ward sisters or pharmacy staff could do so. The ward sister could also help in evaluation by accompanying a nurse and observing her performance while she educates a patient in self-medication.

References

Bullen MU (1980) What patients with hypertension should know about their medication. Drugs 19: 373–379

Cassileth, BR, Zupkis RV, Sutton-Smith K and March V (1980) Information and participation preference among cancer patients. Ann Internal Med 92 (6): 832–836

MacDonald ET, MacDonald JB and Phoenix M (1977) Br Med J 2: 618–621

Smith CR (1977) Patient education in ambulatory care. Nurs Clin North Am 12 (4): 595–607

Watson DS (1979) Health education for hypertension patients. Aust Fam Physician 8: 315–320

Further Reading

Arthritis patient education 'how to' guide (1976–77) American Arthritis Foundation, Atlanta, Georgia

8

Clinical Assessments in Rheumatology

Introduction

Access to serial assessments of the patient's progress over a period of time will be of great value to the clinician in deciding which type of drug to administer or what surgical procedure to employ in order to arrest the advance of the arthritis or to improve function. These assessments will show whether the disease state is improving or deteriorating. Nurses are trained in the taking of temperature, pulse, blood pressure and respiration. These are of considerable value in monitoring the progress of certain acute medical conditions, but for the purposes of rheumatic diseases alternative tests specific to joint function and inflammation have been developed. It is suggested that a sister or staff nurse working on a rheumatology ward might be trained to take a weekly Ritchie Articular Index or grip strength assessment just as her counterpart on an acute medical ward might take 4-hourly pulse and blood pressure measurements. This would assist the consultant rheumatologist and his or her assistants in planning future strategy on drug therapy and would provide an objective assessment of whether the patient was improving. At a more sophisticated level, serial clinical assessments on patients participating in clinical drug trials are essential to enable the physician to determine whether the drug under evaluation is more effective than placebo or a comparator compound.

This chapter deals entirely with the science of clinical measurement as applicable to senior nurses and other paramedical workers.

Measurement of Vital Functions in Rheumatology

Temperature

Routine 4-hourly sublingual or axillary temperature measurements may be required in the monitoring of patients with septic arthritis. Some patients with rheumatoid arthritis, often elderly males, present with a severe systemic illness characterised by a high swinging fever that mimics Hodgkin's disease. In this and in its juvenile counterpart, juvenile chronic polyarthritis (originally called 'Still's disease') with its high swinging fever, daily or twice-daily temperature recording is of value to the physician (Fig. 8.1). With these possible exceptions, however, routine temperature recording does not play such an important role in the management of rheumatic diseases as it does in other branches of acute general medicine. It should be remembered that the prescribing of steroids may mask infection in patients with arthritis. The inflammatory response is reduced and a pyrexia does not appear.

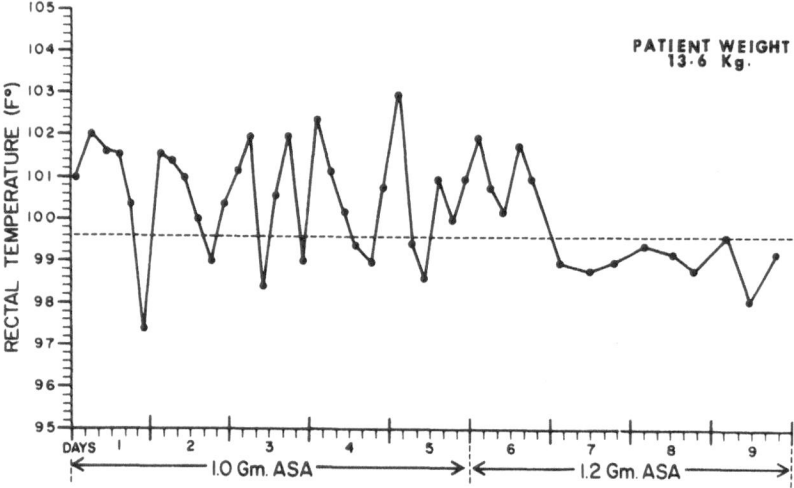

Fig. 8.1. Fluctuant temperature chart in a patient with Still's disease.

Pulse

A tachycardia can accompany any systemic arthritic involvement and may be associated with pain or overintensive physiotherapy. However, in general, routine monitoring of pulse rate is unlikely to help the physician much unless septic arthritis is suspected. Rheumatoid arthritis can involve the heart as nodules impinge upon the conducting tissue causing a bradycardia or even heart block. Heart involvement is equally likely to be caused by alternative pathologies. Seronegative spondarthritides, particularly ankylosing spondylitis and connective tissue disorders, (in particular SLE), can cause valvular lesions by endocardial involvement which in turn might produce a wide-volume pulse. This means that when blood pressure is taken there will be a big difference between the systolic and diastolic values. Blood pressure of 120/90 in a normal individual might become 150/70 in a patient with aortic incompetence.

Blood Pressure

Blood pressure may be abnormal in the septicaemic shock occasioned by septic arthritis and may be slightly raised in patients receiving corticosteriod or ACTH therapy. It may be raised in patients with renal involvement caused by rheumatic diseases, particularly that resulting from connective tissue disorders such as SLE. A raised blood pressure should alert the nurse to the routine testing of urine for protein. In clinical trials blood pressure may be recorded routinely if there is anxiety that a particular drug may cause hypotension or (less likely) hypertension as a side-effect. If this sometimes seems pedantic, it should be remembered that this may be information that is sought by the government licensing body rather than the physician. In general, routine monitoring of blood pressure adds little to the management of rheumatic diseases, although one interesting physical sign is the pain that can be caused to a patient with polymyalgia rheumatica or polymyositis as the blood pressure cuff is inflated around the forearm. (Polymyalgia rheumatica can also involve the pelvic girdle; the corresponding symptom is intense pain in the buttocks when the patient sits on a toilet seat or chair. The correct diagnosis of polymyalgia rheumatica was recently made by letter when a patient wrote to the Rheumatism Research Unit at Leeds claiming that her particular variant of arthritis was much relieved by the use of cushioned toilet seats!)

Respiration Rate

There may be restriction of thoracic excursion in ankylosing spondylitis, with a corresponding accentuation of diaphragmatic breathing; patients with rheumatoid arthritis occasionally develop pleural effusion sufficient to cause tachypnoea (a raised respiration rate). However, with these exceptions, measurement of respiration rate adds little to the management of rheumatic diseases.

Urine Testing

In contrast to the measurements already mentioned, urine testing is of considerable importance in rheumatology. The kidney can be involved in rheumatoid arthritis of long-standing duration, when amyloid is deposited, and in connective tissue disorders such as SLE or polyarteritis nodosa. For this reason a monthly or 3-monthly testing of urine for protein might be regarded as routine in these conditions.

In practice, the more common cause of proteinuria in rheumatic diseases is nephrotoxicity following the use of sodium aurothiomalate or D-penicillamine. Patients taking either of these drugs should be instructed on the regular use of Albustix (usually at weekly intervals), and patients should be referred to a physician if albuminuria occurs during treatment with either of these drugs. The renal involvement with gold, although probably less frequently seen than with penicillamine, is likely to be more severe, and our own practice in Leeds is to review gold therapy critically once Albustix has recorded 2+ for protein on two occasions. For patients receiving penicillamine we wait until the urine is 3+ on at least two occasions before arranging a 24-h urine assay for protein; many physicians advocate continuation of penicillamine therapy if it is helping the patients, providing the 24-h urinary protein does not exceed 2.0 g. If a trace of blood is found in addition to a trace of protein, this is more significant and should be referred to a physician, since the presence of blood denotes more serious renal structural damage than the leak of protein alone through the glomerular basement membrane. Most rheumatologists would discontinue the drug. Although there is a fairly large literature (mainly from Australia) suggesting that analgesic nephropathy is a serious complication of the use of analgesics and non-steroidal anti-inflammatory agents in chronic inflammatory diseases, our own experience suggests that the danger may be exaggerated. We do not advocate frequent testing of urine for protein and blood in patients receiving anti-inflammatory agents or analgesics alone.

Subjective Evaluation of Pain and Stiffness

The subjective evaluation of pain and stiffness is applicable to a variety of rheumatic diseases, including osteoarthrosis (monoarticular or polyarticular), seronegative spondarthritis, rheumatoid arthritis and variants, connective tissue disorders and polymyalgia rheumatica. It may also be relevant to the management of soft tissue rheumatism, a condition more frequently seen in general practice than in hospital clinics.

Visual Analogue Scales

Pain and stiffness are assessed by visual analogue scales. They consist of a horizontal (sometimes vertical) line 10 cm long, marked at one end with the words 'no pain at all' and at the other end with 'unbearable pain' (Fig. 8.2). Patients are invited to place a cross on the line in a position which, in their opinion, represents the *worst* pain that they have experienced over a given period, either that day if they are completing them daily, or over the

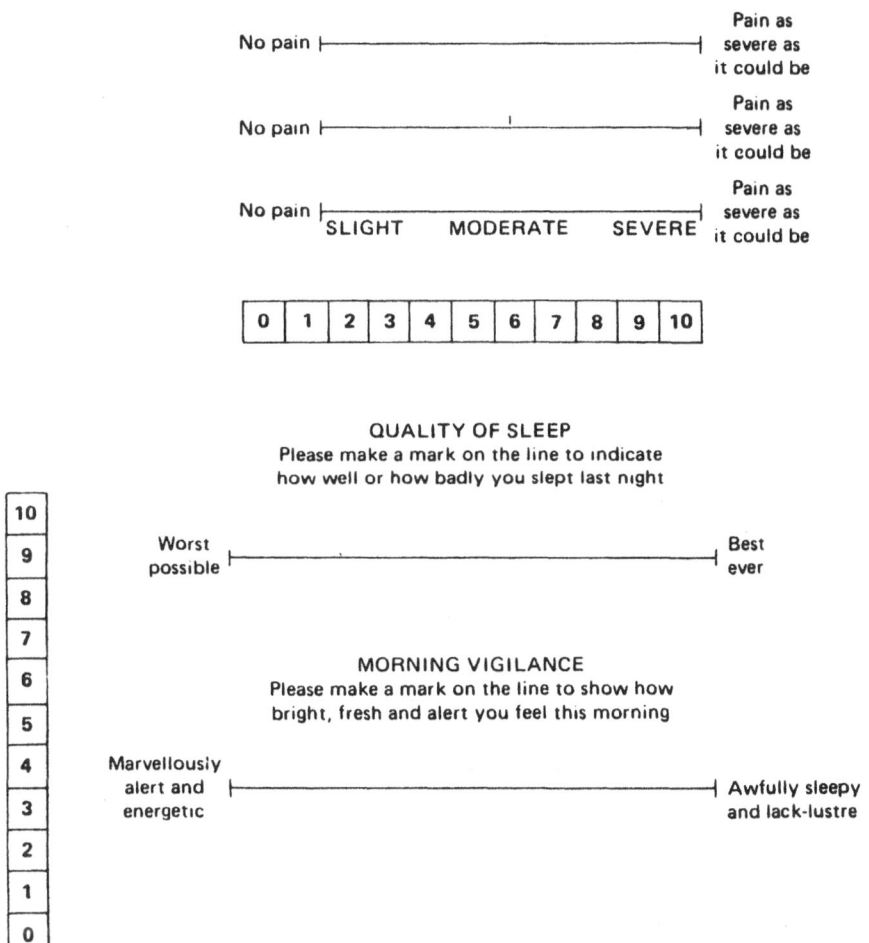

Fig. 8.2. Examples of visual analogue scales. (Bird and Wright 1982)

past week if the interval is greater. It is the worst pain the patient has suffered that the physician is interested in. The distance from the 'no pain' end to the cross is measured in centimetres. This first recording by the patient is the baseline, and future scores are then compared with it.

Visual analogue scales can be used for the assessment of aspects other than pain or stiffness, such as sleep after the use of hypnotics. In this case they might be used to determine the quality of sleep or the morning vigilance or 'hangover' effect resulting from the sleeping tablet.

There is controversy as to whether patients should be allowed access to their previous scores. The danger is that patients may be biased by their previous result; however, some researchers have claimed that this improves the use of visual analogue scales. We do not allow patients to have access to assessments made at weekly or monthly intervals. However, if a daily record is being compiled at home, then obviously the patient has access to previous scores.

Patients appear to relate more easily to the 1–5 (no pain–unbearable pain) type of scale rather than the unmarked 10 cm line. It is important that patients always view the visual analogue scale from above, since if they view it from the side, the point at which they mark it may be different.

Summated Change Score

A variant of the simple visual analogue scale described above is the summated change score. Here patients are presented with a vertical line 20 cm long marked midway at the 10 cm point by a small horizontal line (Fig. 8.3). At

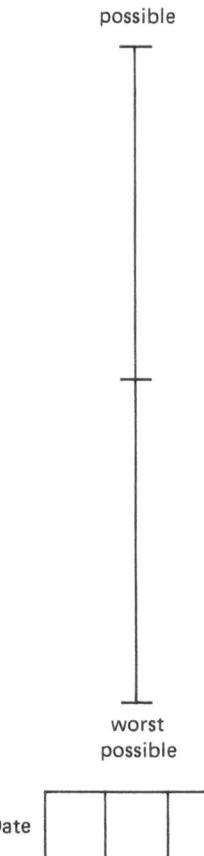

Fig. 8.3. Summated change score.

the top are the words 'best ever' and at the bottom are the words 'worst ever'. Patients are asked, 'Assuming you placed a cross in the centre at your last visit, do you now feel better, worse or the same?' The degree of improvement or deterioration is registered by the distance the cross is placed from the midpoint towards top or bottom of the scale. The answer, 'same as before' would register as a cross at the midpoint. The distance is measured, starting from the midpoint, and recorded.

Visual analogue scales and summated change scores may be subject to various further errors that are listed elsewhere (Bird and Wright 1982). Nevertheless, they have found acceptability in a difficult field where few suitable alternatives exist.

Daily Diary Cards

The most important subjective phenomenon associated with arthritis is pain, followed closely by stiffness. If we had to recommend one method of assessing daily pain and stiffness, we would certainly opt for the use of the daily diary card (DDC) (Fig. 8.4). DDCs are convenient and easy to use. They can be given to inpatients, or to outpatients who attend on a regular basis. Information presented in such a fashion:

1. Forms a basis for positive discussion with the patient
2. Allows the practitioner and patient to reach a joint decision on future treatment
3. Provides an invaluable record of progress, compiled by the patient, which saves clinic time

If DDCs are introduced for 1 or 2 weeks prior to starting new therapy, a baseline can be obtained. Over the following weeks and months a clear picture of the degree of the pain and stiffness emerges. The analgesic intake is an indication of the patient's pain threshold and an excellent guide of pain control, or the lack of it. Used in conjunction with objective assessments such as articular index and laboratory variables such as ESR, plasma viscosity, CRP and haemoglobin, a picture develops which demonstrates graphically the extent of disease activity combined with the efficiency of drug control.

One novel example of an additional use of the DDC is in the therapeutic test of prednisolone for patients suspected of having polymyalgia rheumatica. The patient takes home a supply of placebo tablets for 1 week, followed by a supply of prednisolone tablets for 1 week, and completes a DDC on each day of the 2-week period. Patients with polymyalgia rheumatica experience a dramatic improvement in pain and stiffness on the first or second day after starting the prednisolone tablets, and this can almost be used as a diagnostic test. Improvement in rheumatoid arthritis is said to be slower.

Name:

Study No:

Date	Pain				
	1	2	3	4	5
	1	2	3	4	5
	1	2	3	4	5
	1	2	3	4	5
	1	2	3	4	5
	1	2	3	4	5
	1	2	3	4	5

Duration of Morning Stiffness		No of paracetamol taken today
Hrs	Mins	

Date	Pain				
	1	2	3	4	5
	1	2	3	4	5
	1	2	3	4	5
	1	2	3	4	5
	1	2	3	4	5
	1	2	3	4	5
	1	2	3	4	5

Duration of Morning Stiffness		No of paracetamol taken today
Hrs	Mins	

HINTS

1. Please complete this form each evening just before going to bed.

2. PAIN – ring the appropriate number.

   1 = no pain
   2 = mild pain
   3 = moderate pain
   4 = severe pain
   5 = unbearable pain

3. MORNING STIFFNESS – fill in the duration in hours and minutes.

4. When you visit the out-patient clinic, take with you your completed record cards and tubes of tablets.

Fig. 8.4. Example of a DDC.

Objective Assessments in Inflammatory Polyarthritis

Objective assessments, none of them perfect, rely less on the patient's judgement and more on the independent observer's skill in eliciting the degree of inflammation present. These tests are of particular value in rheumatoid arthritis and in arthritides that involve the hands. There is a constant controversy in the medical literature as to whether it is safest to rely on what the patient feels (e.g. the subjective visual analogue scales described above) or on what an observer measures. In fact, both assessment methods may be equally important.

Grip Strength

Grip strength is a function with many factors and is not relevant to patients who lack hand involvement or who have such extreme rheumatoid arthritis that they have severe hand deformities. It relies on the integrity of the joints in the hand, the ability to hold the cuff, the integrity of the hand and forearm musculature and the integrity of the tendons. Neurological coordination is also required.

Grip strength as a means of assessment has been used for over two decades. Various instruments of measurement have been used over the years, and today a dynamo sphygmomanometer is used. The model illustrated (Fig. 8.5) is light, portable, fairly reliable and costs approximately £18. These machines are difficult to acquire and have a surprisingly short life when in constant use.

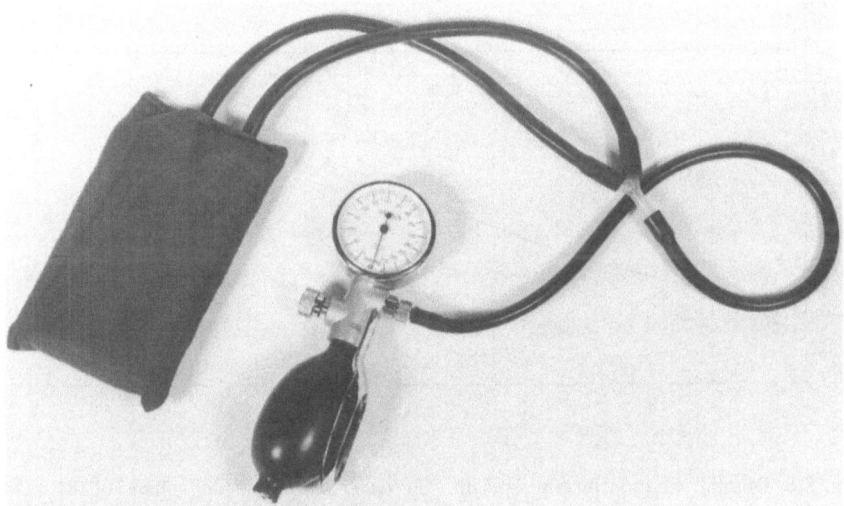

Fig. 8.5. Grip strength cuff.

Variations in grip strength can be used as an indication of disease activity. The painful swollen hand will perform poorly in comparison with one unencumbered by inflammation. Regular assessments of grip strength may be carried out weekly, 2-weekly or monthly, depending upon access to the patients. Once a baseline has been established, grip strength can be introduced prior to starting new treatment as a means of assessing ongoing disease activity. New treatment might involve drug therapy, physiotherapy or even occupational therapy. Grip strength can also be used as a guide to functional capacity, postoperatively or following development of hand deformity. It is important whenever possible to perform the test at approximately the same time each day (as with all other objective assessments for information). Figure 8.6 shows the diurnal variation that can occur in grip strength over a 24-h period.

The scale on the sphygmomanometer dial ranges from 20 to 300 mmHg. Before starting an assessment the indicator is set to 30 mmHg, a universally agreed starting point which provides the patient with a well-inflated bag on which to squeeze. Three readings are taken of each hand, alternating between left and right. The mean of the readings from each hand is recorded in an attempt to negate the learning effect, which differs between individuals (though others have argued that a single reading from each hand is equally effective). We prefer to allow the patient to use alternate hands, as the brief respite experienced between squeezing appears to cause less pain and

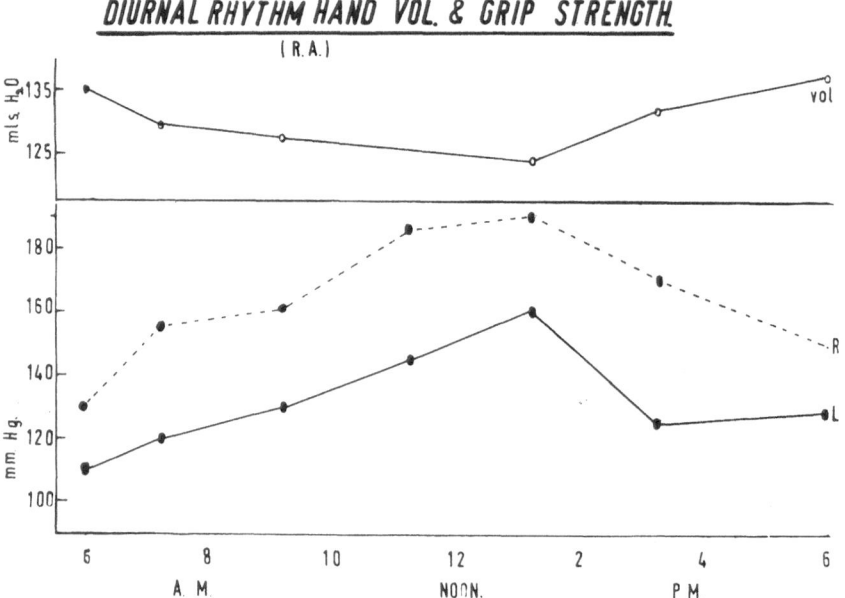

Fig. 8.6. Diurnal variation in grip strength. The *upper line* shows the volume of the hand, measured in millilitres of water displaced from a water bath. As the hand volume changes throughout the day, the grip strength (*lower two lines*) alters accordingly.

discomfort; others have taken three consecutive readings from each hand in turn. The same machine should be used for each patient as it is surprising how different machines of the same model can differ in performance.

A normal individual, male or female, devoid of hand involvement, can obtain a reading in excess of 300 mmHg without difficulty. A patient with active disease and early hand deformity may obtain a score with a mean value of between 30 and 120 mmHg. It is rare, even when the disease is brought under control, for a normal score of over 300 mmHg to be achieved. Nonetheless, serial improvement can be demonstrated once treatment begins to work, and positive results prove particularly satisfying to the patient. All patients with hand deformity need not be excluded from this form of assessment, providing they can squeeze the bag in whatever fashion they are capable of. A reading can be taken which provides a baseline to work from. A patient with ulnar deviation may indeed have difficulty squeezing the bag; however, providing they can still record a reading, this assessment can be used to follow their performance in a trial.

Digital Joint Circumference

Measurement of the proximal interphalangeal joint size was first suggested in 1951. The instrument used for taking this measurement has passed through various stages of development, starting with the jeweller's ring gauge and finally ending with the arthrocircometer, the most widely used instrument today (Fig. 8.7). Unfortunately, they are difficult to acquire and therefore costly. An inexpensive plastic version is readily available in which gauge

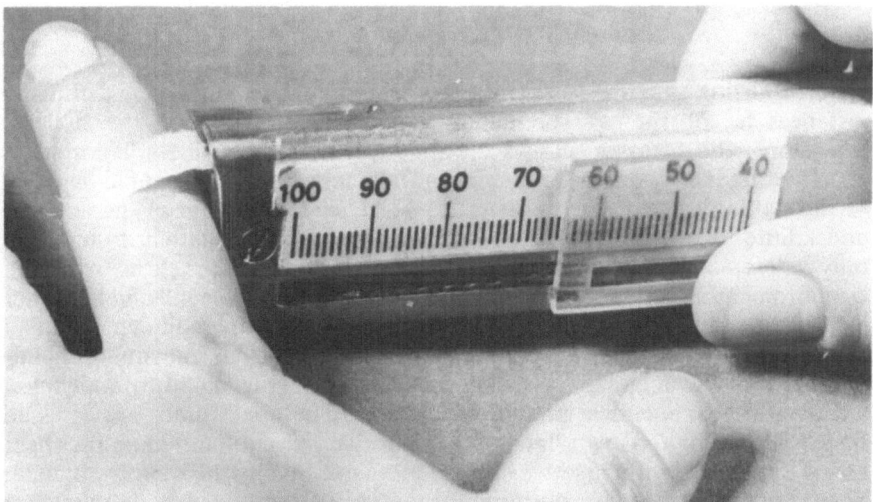

Fig. 8.7. Arthrocircometer for measuring joint circumference at the proximal interphalangeal joint.

marking is in the form of a transfer which wears off very quickly. The metal arthrocircometer shown in Fig. 8.7 is fitted with a flexible nylon loop attached to a spring. The loop circling the joint is pulled tight, and the circumference of the joint is read off the scale in millimetres. Comparison is then made with previous readings, the same instrument should always be used for individual patients. Clearly there is no quotable normal range since everyone possesses individually sized joints, and the joints themselves may have varying degrees of effusion.

Assessment of digital joints by this method is more suitable for those suffering from soft tissue swelling, particularly among patients exhibiting arthritis of the proximal and/or terminal interphalangeal joints. The latter is a feature more common in seronegative spondarthritides, to which this index is well suited. Certainly patients who have significant bony deformity would not benefit from this assessment, and therefore it is of limited value.

Ritchie Articular Index

The articular index (AI) was devised in 1964 by Dorothy M. Ritchie, an occupational therapist and her colleagues of the Centre for Rheumatic Diseases, University Department of Medicine, Royal Infirmary, Glasgow. It is based upon an earlier articular assessment used by the Co-operating Clinics Committee of the American Rheumatism Association.

The Ritchie clinical study was the result of a search for a single, reliable and clinically convenient measurement of inflammation and pain in joints in patients with rheumatoid arthritis. The actual study undertook the construction of a simple scoring system for joint tenderness (Ritchie et al. 1968).

Method

Before starting the assessment, the assessor should remember that in many instances he or she will be inflicting additional pain upon the patient. Therefore, the assessor should always explain to the patient beforehand exactly what is happening, although naturally no information should be given of the scoring system. The patient should be seated in front of the assessor and a little to the left or right. There is no need for the patient to undress, only to remove a heavy coat and shoes. The assessor starts with the temporomandibular joint, placing the first two fingers of each hand on either side of the patient's head immediately over the temporomandibular joint and squeezing simultaneously. Both joints score as one. Then, moving his hands gradually downwards, the assessor squeezes each joint in turn, applying a steady and near identical pressure each time. The upper limbs are assessed first, followed by the lower limbs. Each positive score is entered on the sheet as it is observed, with negative scores left blank. Finally the score is totalled. The first articular index performed on a patient produces a baseline for reference and comparison for that particular patient. With the exception of the cervical spine, hip joints, talocalcaneal and midtarsal joints, tenderness is elicited by applying firm pressure (squeezing) over the joint margin. In the case of the four sites mentioned above, tenderness is elicited by passive movement of the joint. The assessor observes and scores the patient's response throughout as follows:

1. If the patient feels no pain or tenderness   Score 0
2. If the patient feels pain and says so   Score 1
3. If the patient feels pain and winces   Score 2
4. If the patient feels pain, winces and withdraws   Score 3

The following joints are treated as a single unit: temporomandibular, cervical spine, sternoclavicular, acromioclavicular, the MCP and PIP joints of each hand and the midtarsal and metatarsal joints of each foot. For example, the maximum score for the PIP joints will be 3, not 15, and for the two acromioclavicular joints the maximum score is 3, not 6. The hips are difficult to assess unless the patient is lying down, in which case a simple passive abduction can be performed. In a busy outpatient clinic patients rarely have time to lie down, and therefore the assessor should ask if the patient experiences hip pain when lying in bed. If the reply is positive, the patient should be asked to score the pain as mild (score 1), moderate (score 2), or severe (score 3), for each hip.

Evaluation of Scores

The highest score possible would be 78, in which case every joint would have scored 3. Fortunately, this does not happen too often. The following points are made to help assist in the interpretation of certain scores:

1. An extremely high score in excess of 30 would indicate extreme disease activity and would call for a rapid reassessment of present drug therapy.
2. A score of over 15 (made up mainly of scores of 1) could indicate widespread but mild activity.
3. A score of 9 must not be considered insignificant. Although this may have been produced by only three joints, they may have been functionally important joints conferring considerable disability upon the patient. These particular joints might need joint protection (splinting), and an isolated high score at a single joint in a patient who is otherwise quiescent might alert the observer to the suspicion of local septic arthritis.
4. A diminishing score observed over days or weeks could indicate a successful response to treatment or spontaneous remission. Consideration should be given to discontinuing drug therapy to distinguish between these two (if that is felt ethical).
5. Conversely, a score which is steadily climbing might well suggest the need for a reappraisal of treatment or a much closer investigation into the patient's life style.

The total score is most important when extremely high, and, as mentioned, a reappraisal of treatment should be made. However, as the score drops, individual joint scores need closer attention. An isolated score of 3 might suggest either a slow response to treatment or a completely new flare of disease activity. The difference is important. The score should be verified by checking previous score sheets.

An AI needs to be repeated weekly, 2-weekly or monthly, depending on accessibility to patients. There is probably little point in doing it more often. Each score is compared with the previous score and, if necessary, referred back to the first score. Each assessment should be performed by the same person on each occasion, thus obviating inter-observer error. Each individual has a different concept of what constitutes a squeeze. Although it is possible to eliminate or reduce inter-observer error by regular blind synchronisation of observers, it is most certainly not as satisfactory as the same person performing the assessment each time. Even if the same person performs the assessment each time,there may be an intra-observer error. The assessor may squeeze the joints harder on some days than on others, and care should be taken to avoid this.

If the aim is to assess the severity of disease activity by relating it to the amount of pain felt, then the assessor would be advised to use the Ritchie articular index, as it is both simple and adequate. A scoring chart (Fig. 8.8) can be used which ensures that no joints are forgotten. Other articular indices exist, such as the Doyle index for osteoarthritis, and the scoring chart for this (Fig. 8.9) is even more complicated. The choice of index will be determined by the disease the patient has and the information the assessor hopes to gain from the results (though we prefer the Ritchie index for rheumatoid arthritis). In patients with secondary osteoarthritis that is confined to a small number of joints such as the hip or knee, there is little point in performing the full Doyle AI on each joint. It is simpler to squeeze the relevant joint prior to new treatment, be it drug therapy or physiotherapy, and to repeat this assessment on the same joint at regular intervals. This could give an indication of the success of treatment.

Rheumatoid arthritis is particularly difficult to assess as its manifestations are widespread and vary from day to day. The Ritchie AI attempts to quantify the patient's major problem for which he seeks relief, that is pain. Beecher (1959) has stated that 'pain is measured in terms of its relief'.

The Ritchie AI has been used worldwide since 1968 and has proved itself to be a practical and convenient method of assessing joint tenderness and pain.

Functional Assessments

The relatively objective assessments described above are most appropriate for measuring relatively short-term serial change in patients with polyarthritis (usually over not more than 1 year). However, it has been argued that in

Patient initials ☐☐☐

Articular Index Score

Observation Date
Day/Month/Year

Patient Study No.

Week No. ☐   ☐☐☐   ☐☐

Examiner ....

Temporomandibular	
Cervical Spine	
Sternoclavicular	
Acromioclavicular	
Shoulder	(Left)
	(Right)
Elbow	(Left)
	(Right)
Wrist	(Left)
	(Right)
M.C.P.	(Left)
	(Right)
P.I.P.	(Left)
	(Right)
Hip	(Left)
	(Right)
Knee	(Left)
	(Right)
Ankles	(Left)
	(Right)
Talocalcaneal	(Left)
	(Right)
Midtarsal	(Left)
	(Right)
M.T.P.	(Left)
	(Right)
TOTAL SCORE	

Fig. 8.8. Ritchie articular index scoring chart.

the last resort it is the patient's functional ability to perform simple everyday tasks that matters most. This in turn will reflect a combination of joint damage, inflammation, pain and stiffness.

A variety of 4- or 5-point scales are available for assessing functional activity, and a typical example is shown in Fig. 8.10. The assessment scores

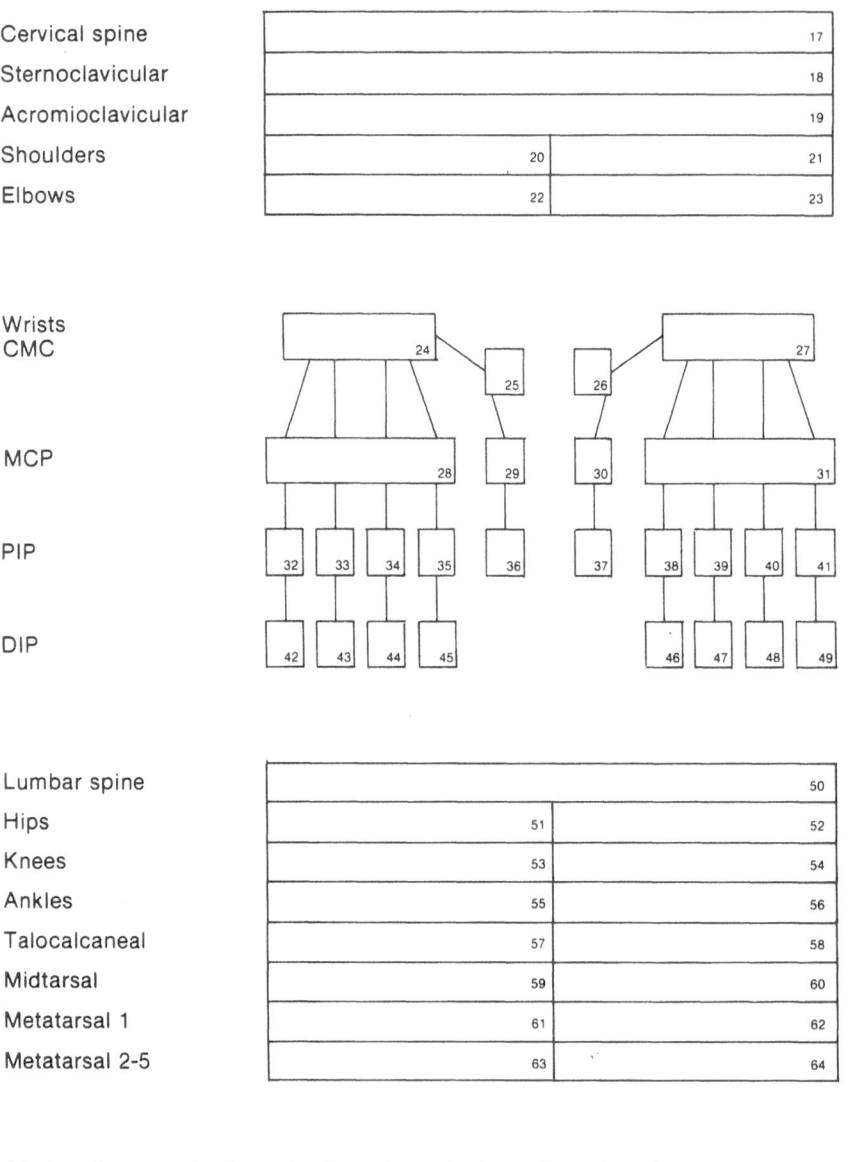

RIGHT   LEFT

Cervical spine		17
Sternoclavicular		18
Acromioclavicular		19
Shoulders	20	21
Elbows	22	23

Wrists CMC   24   25   26   27

MCP   28   29   30   31

PIP   32 33 34 35   36   37   38 39 40 41

DIP   42 43 44 45   46 47 48 49

Lumbar spine		50
Hips	51	52
Knees	53	54
Ankles	55	56
Talocalcaneal	57	58
Midtarsal	59	60
Metatarsal 1	61	62
Metatarsal 2-5	63	64

(Rating: 0 = no pain, 1 = pain, 2 = pain and wince, 3 = pain, wince and withdrawal)

Total score

65   67

Fig. 8.9. Doyle articular index for use in studies on osteoarthrosis.

Functional Grade (Tick as appropriate)

   1.   completely mobile

   2.   mobile with difficulty

   3.   mobile with stick

   4.   confined to house

   5.   bedfast

Fig. 8.10. Assessment scale for functional grade.

from 0 to 4 or 5 according to whether the patient is completely immobile and bed-fast at one extreme or fully functional and able to walk and carry on normal employment at the other extreme. This is a simple sort of functional assessment, but in our experience it adds little to short-term clinical trials.

Scales have been superseded by more complex assessments using tables of questions relating to different activities, which may total from 17 to 100. The patient is asked which of these 100 activities he or she can perform. Examples of simple tasks that might be included in such a questionnaire include the ability to walk 3 m or climb stairs. These would reflect function in the lower limbs. If the function in the hands was of most interest, the assessor would enquire about the patient's ability to tie a knot, strike a match, unscrew the cap of a drug container or to write his or her name. The test can be made more precise by timing the patient's ability to perform these tasks. The time taken in seconds to write the patient's name, for example, could be recorded using a stopwatch. Each test selected is likely to demonstrate change in a particular group of joints that are involved by the arthritis. The functional assessment result may improve as the patient gets bettter, but some of these tests are also influenced by learning, as the patient repeats the test on serial occasions while attending clinic.

Stanford Health Assessment Questionnaire

The Stanford Health Assessment Questionnaire, recently evaluated by Fries and his colleagues at Stanford University, California, concentrates on five dimensions: death, disability, discomfort, drug side-effects and economic impact. A total of 62 potential questions were reviewed and the best of these selected by a complex statistical analysis. The resultant questionnaire (Fig. 8.11) is relatively quick to complete and may be of particular value in the long-term (1 year or more) assessment of whether the drugs used for treating inflammatory polyarthritis really do influence the course of the diseases or not (Fries et al. 1982). The questionnaire has now been used with considerable effect in a large number of patients both with rheumatoid arthritis and with osteoarthritis.

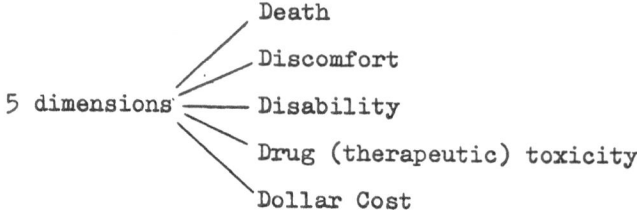

```
                        / Death
                      / Discomfort
 5 dimensions ———— Disability
                      \ Drug (therapeutic) toxicity
                        \ Dollar Cost
```

I. Death

II. Disability

    A. Physical

        1. Dressing
        2. Arising
        3. Eating
        4. Walking
        5. Hygiene
        6. Reach
        7. Grip
        8. Outside activity
        9. Sex

        Index

    B. Psychological

III. Discomfort

    A. Physical

        1. Severity
        2. Trend
        Index

    B. Psychological

    C. Dissatisfaction

IV. Drug (therapeutic) toxicity

    A. Medical

    B. Surgical

    C. Investigational

    Index

V. Dollar Costs

    A. Medical and surgical

        1. Medications
        2. Laboratory tests
        3. X-rays
        4. Physician visits
        5. Paramedical visits
        6. Devices
        7. Hospitalizations
        8. Surgeries

    B. Out-of-pocket

    C. Social

        1. Employment
        2. Domestic
        3. Transportation

    Total dollar cost

Fig. 8.11. The Stanford Health Assessment Questionnaire.

Monitoring of Side-effects

In part, the monitoring of side-effects is a subjective assessment, although some objectivity can be introduced, as in the photography of skin rashes and grading of histology of biopsied skin specimens. Unfortunately, eliciting side-effects may be liable to observer variation in interpretation. The enthusiasm with which side-effects are sought almost certainly accounts for the wide variation that can occur between centres in multicentre studies.

At Leeds, for studies on drugs that have been on the market some time, we use a simple standard question, 'Have the tablets upset you in any way? If so, was it mild, moderate or severe'? This is more satisfactory than a vague question such as, 'Did the tablets suit you?', which may be interpreted by the patient as seeking information both on side-effects and on clinical response. If patients are allowed to speculate on the way in which tablets upset them the interview can last for hours. We prefer to restrict patients to defining whether the side-effect was mild, moderate or severe.

For drugs recently introduced we prefer a standard check list of side-effects, and a typical example is shown in Fig. 8.12. This is shown to the patient at the start of a drug or therapeutic study so that baseline side-effects that may be a natural part of that patient's make-up can be recorded before the novel compound or drug is introduced. Side-effects elicited may be altered according to the drug under test. The patient is subsequently questioned at each clinic visit after receiving the new drug, and an overall profile of the side-effects of the compound is built up. It should be noted that patients tend to describe more side-effects at the start of a trial and fewer side-effects on successive clinic visits, possibly because they have a greater sense of security at successive visits.

Monitoring of Laboratory Changes

Routine checking of possible toxicology may be applicable to any new drug tried for any rheumatic disease. By contrast, the routine monitoring of laboratory indicators of inflammation will only be appropriate to systemic polyarthritides, particularly rheumatoid arthritis.

Routine Charting of Laboratory Side-effects

If new drugs are under evaluation it will be appropriate to perform regular haematological and biochemical screens on patients. In practice, haemoglobin, white blood cell count, platelet count and possibly differential white cell count from the haematology laboratory will suffice. It must be remembered that some of these tests may be abnormal in untreated rheumatic disease in any case (the normochromic normocytic anemia giving a low haemoglobin and the relative thrombocytosis or raised platelet count); therefore, it is important to have baseline data on each patient prior to embarking upon new therapy. We find the most satisfactory solution is to chart serial results on special sheets in the patient's notes, in addition to recording the routine laboratory returns. For hepatic function, bilirubin, SGOT or SGPT, alkaline phosphatase and total protein usually suffice, though gamma glutamyl transpeptidase may be requested as an extrasensitive test for early liver damage. Electrolytes, urea and particularly creatinine, together with routine urine testing, are the most reliable simple tests of renal function, though some

SIDE EFFECTS CHECK LIST

Please score: 1 = mild
                     2 = moderate
                     3 = severe

Tick as appropriate   DATE:

	day	month	year

	1	2	3
Headache			
Blurred vision			
Drowsiness			
Visual disturbance			
Tinnitus			
Dizziness			
Insomnia			
Tachycardia			
Sweating			
Nausea			
Vomiting			
Dry Mouth			
Diarrhoea			
Indigestion			
Constipation			
Micturition difficulty			
Skin rash			
Pruritis			
Other			

Fig. 8.12. Typical example of side-effects check list.

workers prefer a *N*-acetyl-glucosamine (NAG)/creatinine ratio as a very sensitive indicator of early renal damage. Again, because abnormalities may be present as part of the disease process (for example a raised alkaline phosphatase in rheumatoid arthritis), baseline values are essential. The physician's attention should be drawn to any abnormal values, whereupon the normal procedure is to repeat the test giving abnormal results. In the field of possible drug toxicity, matters can never be left to chance, and it is vital to draw the attention of the physician to the suspected abnormality at the earliest possible opportunity. (A list of the normal range of common haematological and biochemical laboratory values is included as Appendix A; see p. 289.)

Biochemical and Immunological Assessments of Disease Activity

The importance of biochemical and immunological assessments lies in the regular collection of all results for long-term review, rather than the regular and urgent seeking out of results of every blood test taken, as in the case of toxicology. The evaluations used will depend upon the disease and the study and the availability of tests in the particular laboratory involved. ESR and/or plasma viscosity are the most common haematological assessments; C-reactive protein, serum sulphydryl and possibly histidine are all biochemical assessments that may be performed. If the laboratory is immunologically orientated, particularly if the disease is SLE rather than rheumatoid arthritis, C_3, C_4 and possibly total circulating immune complexes, are likely to be available. Appendix A gives examples of the normal range for these more sophisticated laboratory assessments of inflammation, together with the extent to which they might be abnormal in active disease.

Radiological Assessment

Many physicians feel that in the last resort it is the serial radiological change (or rather lack of it) that determines whether a particular treatment has been successful in a particular rheumatic disease. With conventional radiological techniques, the time required for serial change to become apparent is relatively long. In the case of osteoarthrosis, radiographs should probably only be reviewed if they are taken at least 1 year apart, although in the unusual cases of ischaemic necrosis or neuropathic osteoarthrosis, change may be seen at an interval less than this. In rheumatoid arthritis the first easily observable radiological changes do not occur until 2–3 months after the onset of symptoms; as a rule of thumb radiographs should be read at least 6 months apart, and preferably at even longer intervals. In the majority of rheumatology units the assessment of radiographs will be done by a physician, often a radiologist; however, given adequate training (which is beyond the scope of this book), there is no reason why a nurse should not learn to assess serial radiological change.

Miscellaneous Clinical Assessments

The assessments hitherto described are the common ones used in rheumatic diseases. However, additional assessments may be applicable to certain research projects and are described briefly here.

Assessments of Joint size

Although the finger arthrocircometer probably represents the most reliable assessment of joint size, investigators may make serial assessments of the girth of other joints, the knee being an obvious example. Use of simple tape measure is satisfactory, and the secret lies in ensuring that the girth is always recorded at exactly the same point. If measurements are made over a short period of time a mark can be made on the skin with a marking pencil. If measurements are made over a longer period of time, the tape must always be sited at the same position in relation to a fixed landmark, possibly a naevus on the skin or else a fixed bony point such as the upper margin of the patella, or a set distance below the superior anterior iliac spine if the patella moves in relation to the size of the effusion, as sometimes happens. The need to measure a muscular girth sometimes arises, as in evaluation of a ruptured Baker's cyst or of quadriceps wasting before and after exercise therapy. Here attention must be paid to whether the patient is relaxed or has the muscles tensed at the time of measuring, and again a tape should be sited in relation to a fixed bony landmark on each occasion when a measurement is made.

Assessments in Ankylosing Spondylitis

Ankylosing spondylitis involves the spine and sacroiliac joints, and therefore the joint assessments described earlier are not usually applicable. Nurses are likely to become adept at measuring chest expansion using a tape measure levelled at the height of the nipples; it is important to state whether the measurement is performed in expiration or inspiration. Vital capacity measurements using a vitalograph, which records the volume of air exhaled in a single forced exhalation, provide an alternative assessment of chest expansion.

Assessments such as visual analogue scales for pain and stiffness can be used with effect in ankylosing spondylitis, but the Ritchie AI is not usually of value unless the patient has extensive peripheral joint involvement. It is more important to concentrate on assessments of the spine. Ankylosing spondylitis starts in the sacroiliac joints and works up through the thoracolumbar spine until finally the cervical spine is also involved. An initial assessment is therefore likely to be made of both sacroiliac joints. These are palpated from the back, with the patient standing in an erect position, and the resultant score is recorded on a 0–3 basis rather like the Ritchie AI.

The easiest way of assessing the lumber spine is to use Schober's test, which is illustrated in Fig. 8.13. Two marks are made with a ballpoint pen on the skin on either side of the point where a line joining the two dimples of Venus crosses the lumbar spine. The patient is then invited to bend forward as though trying to touch the toes, and the resultant distraction of the two marks as they move apart when the patient bends forward is measured in centimetres. This assessment has been shown to correlate well with radiological movement of the lumbar spine.

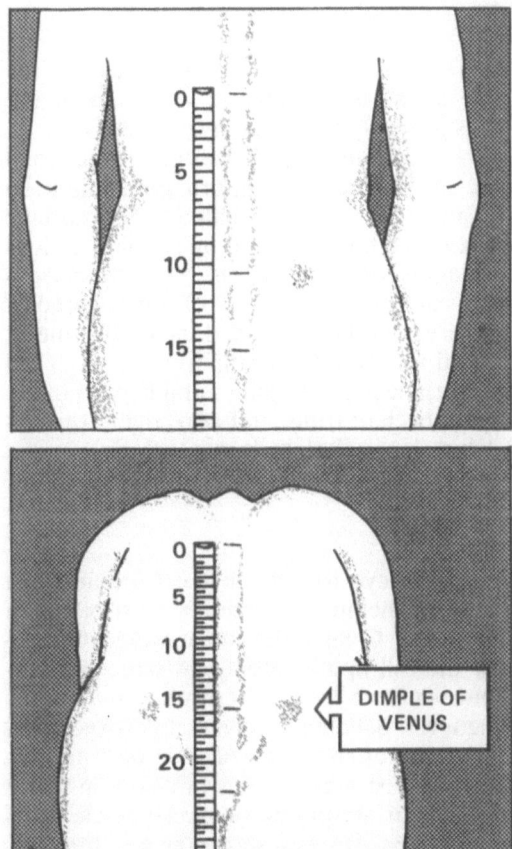

Fig. 8.13. Measurement of anterior spinal flexion by a modification of Schober's method. The *upper* diagram shows the essential landmarks. The middle mark lies at the point where a line through the dimples of Venus crosses the spine. The upper and lower marks are situated 10 and 5 cm respectively above and below the middle mark. The *lower* diagram shows measurement of the distraction between the upper and lower marks on anterior spinal flexion.

Lateral flexion of the lumbar spine, a movement lost early in active ankylosing spondylitis, is measured with the patient standing upright and the feet just slightly apart. The patient is asked to slide one hand down the lateral side of the thigh, first on the left side and then on the right. The distance the hand moves towards the knee is measured in centimetres with a tape-measure on serial occasions as the patient undergoes therapy. An alternative method for measuring movements of the lumbar spine is to use the angle goniometer, which is described in more detail later in this chapter.

Involvement of the thoracic spine is best assessed by measuring chest expansion at the level of the nipples as the patient inhales deeply. Assessment of the cervical spine involvement is best accomplished using the Loebl hydrogoniometer, also described later in this chapter.

Assessment in Psoriatic Arthritis

In general, most of the joint assessments described above will suffice, but the nurse may be called upon to give serial assessments of the state of the psoriasis in psoriatic arthritis. This is probably best done by concentrating on a single named plaque, one for each patient, and measuring its size and commenting on its appearance at each clinic visit. Information might be sought on the thickness, scaling and erythema of an individual's psoriatic plaque. Alternatively, the total area of the body covered by psoriatic lesions may be assessed using a simple diagram. If a treatment were to cause a complete remission of the skin lesions of psoriasis, the area of skin covered by the lesions would be reduced; this area can be quantified using the rule of nines, in which one point is allocated for any of nine different areas of the body that might be involved in the psoriatic process. Nine suitable parts of the body are head (scalp), anterior trunk, back of trunk, left arm, right arm, left upper leg, right upper leg, left lower leg and right lower leg.

Eye Testing

The responsibility for avoiding the rare eye toxicity that can occur when hydroxychloroquine is used for treating rheumatoid arthritis must rest with the rheumatologist and ophthalmologist. Clearly the nurse would not be expected to take responsibility for the full ophthalmological screening performed by an ophthalmologist, but we have found the routine use of the Ishihara colour-blindness test whenever patients receiving hydroxychloroquine attend a rheumatology clinic to be of some reassurance both to ourselves and to the patients. The Ishihara test uses a series of charts in which numbers formed out of dots of one colour are placed on circles made up of dots of a second colour. This may be regarded as a screening test for early colour-blindness, which is one of the first possible problems arising in hydroxychloroquine toxicity. The ability of those patients receiving hydroxychloroquine to read the numbers accurately is recorded on each clinic visit. However, this test is not a substitute for adequate ophthalmological examination.

Measurement of Joint Movement

Clinically the range of movement of a joint is measured for several reasons:

1. To help evaluate the degree of mobility which a patient possesses
2. To monitor any changes in this function
3. To help establish if the range of motion at the joint is normal
4. To help diagnose what is causing any joint dysfunction

Normal Range of Joint Movement

It must be remembered that there is a marked difference between active and passive movement, the range of passive movement always being greater. Attention should be paid to whether the subjects are 'warmed up' or cold. This is certainly relevant in athletes, in whom the range of movement at certain joints may be almost doubled with appropriate training for stretching. Since there is a diurnal variation in the range of joint movements, assessments in clinical trials should always be made at approximately the same time of day. In general, females have a wider range of movement at any given joint than males, and joint movement also alters with age. It is maximal in the second decade and decreases through adult life as the joints become less supple with age. Attention should also be paid to whether the measurements are made on the dominant side or non-dominant side, particularly in the arms. Movements in the dominant hand tend to have a smaller range than in the non-dominant hand, possibly because of the extra muscle tone on the dominant side.

It should also be remembered that the joints in the body move in groups rather than in isolation. Restriction of movement between two consecutive vertebrae in the lumbar spine is likely to be compensated for by an increased range of movement at other vertebrae in the lumbar spine, such that the final functional range of spinal movement remains unaltered, at least in the early stages of localised disease.

Figure 8.14 emphasises that it is hard to define a normal range for a variety of factors, but lists the standard guidelines for the range of joint movement at common joints in the normal individual.

A recent monograph is available (Wright 1982) which provides more details on the range of movement at each joint. This supplements the earlier book published by the American Academy of Orthopedic Surgeons (1965), which gives, in simpler form, the methods for measuring and recording the range of joint motion at all the joints in the body.

ESTIMATES OF
AVERAGE RANGES OF JOINT MOTION

The average ranges of joint motion can not be accurately determined, due to the wide variation in the degrees of motion amongst individuals of varying physical build and age groups. The following estimates are to serve merely as a guide, and not as a standard. The patient's opposite extremity is perhaps the best "normal" standard. In those instances when the opposite extremity has been injured, or is not present, these figures may prove helpful. Four sources are used for references. An average of these estimates is given. The sources are as follows:

Column (1)

The Committee on Medical Rating of Physical Impairment, Journal American Medical Association, (JAMA, 15 Feb. 1958, pp 1-112).

Column (2)

The Committee of the California Medical Association and Industrial Accident Commission of the State of California (Evaluation of industrial disability. Oxford University Press, 1960).

Column (3)

A System of Joint Measurements, William A. Clarke, Mayo Clinic (J Orthop Surg, vol. 2, no. 12, Dec. 1920).

Column (4)

The Committee on Joint Motion, American Academy of Orthopaedic Surgeons.

AVERAGE RANGES OF JOINT MOTION

SOURCES

JOINT	(1)	(2)	(3)	(4)	AVERAGES
ELBOW =					
FLEXION	150	135	150	150	146
HYPEREXTENSION	0	0	0	0	0

Fig. 8.14. Range of movement of joints. [American Academy of Orthopedic Surgeons 1965: *ref 12*, A guide to the evaluation of permanent impairment of the extremities and back (1958) JAMA special edn, pp. 1–112; *ref. 5*, Evaluation of industrial disability (1960) Oxford University Press, Oxford; *ref 3*, Clarke WA (1920) A system of joint measurements. J Orthop Surg 2(12)]

Fig. 8.14. (*continued*)

FOREARM =

PRONATION	80	75	50	80	71
SUPINATION	80	85	90	80	84

WRIST =

EXTENSION	60	65	90	70	71
FLEXION	70	70		80	73
ULNAR DEV.	30	40	30	30	33
RADIAL DEV.	20	20	15	20	19

THUMB =

ABDUCTION		55	50	70	58
FLEXION					
I-P Jt.	80	75	90	80	81
M — P	60	50	50	50	53
M — C				15	15
EXTENSION					
Distal Jt.		20	10	20	17
M — P		5	10	0	8
M — C				20	20

FINGERS =

FLEXION					
Distal Jt.	70	70	90	90	80
Middle Jt.	100	100		100	100
Proximal Jt.	90	90		90	90

KNEE =

FLEXION	120	135	145	135	134
HYPEREXTENSION			10	10	10

ANKLE =

FLEXION (plantar flexion)	40	50	50	50	48
EXTENSION (dorsiflexion)	20	15	15	20	18

HIND FOOT (subtalar) =

INVERSION				5	5
EVERSION				5	5

FORE FOOT =

INVERSION	30	35		35	33
EVERSION	20	20		15	18

Fig. 8.14. (*continued*)

AVERAGE RANGES OF JOINT MOTION

SOURCES

JOINT	(1)	(2)	(3)	(4)	AVERAGES
TOES =					
GREAT TOE					
I-P Jt.					
Flexion	30			90	60
Extension	0			0	0
Proximal Jt.					
Flexion	30	35		45	37
Extension	50	70		70	63
2nd TO 5th TOES =					
FLEXION					
Distal Jt.	50			60	55
Middle Jt.	40			35	38
Proximal Jt.	30			40	35
Extension	40			40	40
FINGERS =					
EXTENSION					
Distal Jt.				0	0
Middle Jt.				0	0
Proximal Jt.			45	45	45
SHOULDER =					
FORWARD					
FLEXION	150	170	130	180	158
HORIZONTAL					
FLEXION				135	135
BACKWARD					
EXTENSION	40	30	80	60	53
ABDUCTION	150	170	180	180	170
ADDUCTION	30		45	75	50
ROTATION					
Arm at Side					
Int. Rot.	40	60	90	80	68
Ext. Rot.	90	80	40	60	68
Arm in Abduction (90°)					
Int. Rot.				70	70
Ext. Rot.				90	90
HIP =					
FLEXION	100	110	120	120	113
EXTENSION	30	30	20	30	28
ABDUCTION	40	50	55	45	48
ADDUCTION	20	30	45	30	31

Fig. 8.14. (*continued*)

AVERAGE RANGES OF JOINT MOTION

SOURCES

JOINT	(1)	(2)	(3)	(4)	AVERAGES
ROTATION					
In Flexion =					
Int. Rot.				45	45
Ext. Rot.				45	45
In Extension =					
Int. Rot.	40	35	20	45	35
Ext. Rot.	50	50	45	45	48
ABDUCTION					
In 90° of flexion		45 to 60			
		(depending on age)			
SPINE =					
CERVICAL					
FLEXION	30			45	38
EXTENSION	30			45	38
LAT. BENDING	40			45	43
ROTATION	30			60	45
THORACIC AND LUMBAR					
FLEXION	90			{80 4″	{85 4″
EXTENSION	30			20-30	30
LAT. BENDING	20			35	28
ROTATION	30			45	38

Instruments for Measuring Joint Movement

Instruments that measure the range of joint movement are called gonio-meters. The various models which are available on the market fall into two main designs:

1. The hydrogoniometer, designed by Loebl and also known as the spirit inclinometer, is shown in its simplest form in Fig. 8.15b. If placed in the correct position it can be used to measure the range of movement at any joint.
2. The Zimmer angle goniometer, also known as the standard or adapted goniometer, is illustrated in Fig. 8.15a. This can only be used for the measurement of the range of movement at hinge joints such as the knee and elbow.

Ideally a goniometer should be inexpensive, portable, easy to read, reasonably accurate and require little expertise to operate. Joints suited to assessment using goniometry are the cervical spine, shoulder, elbow, wrist, lumbar spine, hip and knee. Each of these will now be considered in turn.

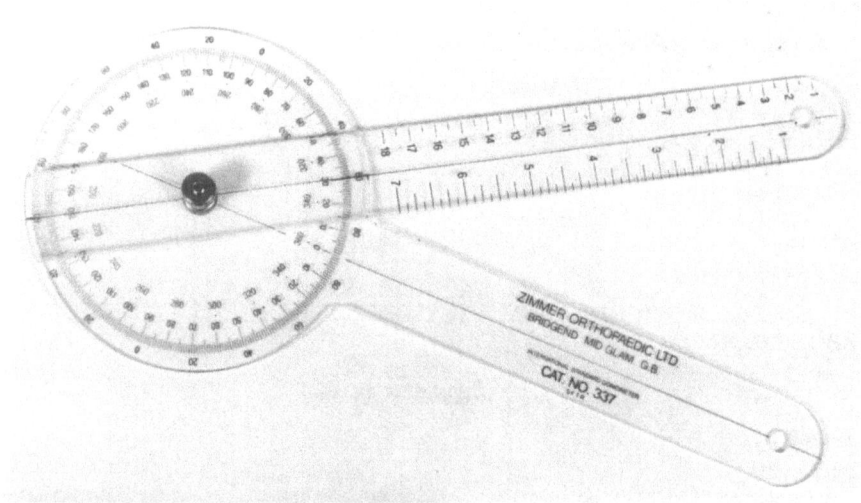

a

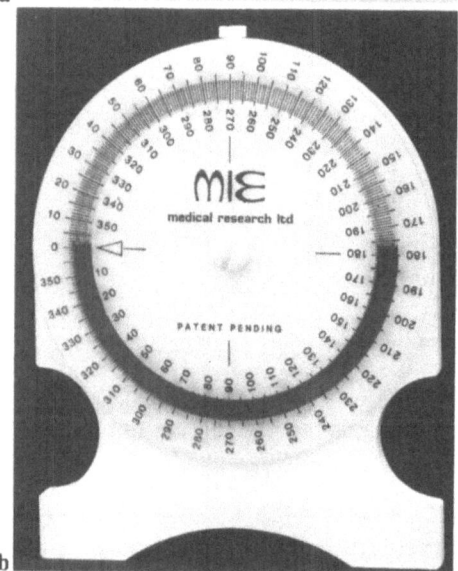

b

Fig. 8.15. a An angle ('Hinge') goniometer. b A hydrogoniometer.

Cervical Spine

More movement occurs, in all directions, within the cervical spine than in the whole of the remainder of the spinal column. It can be divided into two distinct segments: (1) the superior or suboccipital segment and (2) the inferior segment.

1. The superior segment consists of the occiput, atlas and axis and has three degrees of freedom. These are flexion/extension, rotation and lateral flexion to a minor degree (20%).
2. The inferior segment, which extends from the inferior surface of the axis through C3 and C7 to the superior surface of Tl has only two degrees of freedom—flexion/extension and lateral flexion.

Thus in disease the range and the way in which movement is limited can give some guide to the area of the cervical spine affected.

By using the Loebl hydrogoniometer, flexion/extension, rotation and lateral flexion can all be measured. The hydrogoniometer is portable, simple to use and atraumatic to the patient. It costs approximately £40, but unfortunately has a very short life, however carefully it is used. For measuring flexion/extension the instrument is placed vertically over the sagittal plane on the crown of the head, with the patient in the vertical (sitting) position. With the patient's head in an upright position the instrument is zeroed by rotating the dial, and the patient is then invited to flex and extend the head as far as possible. For lateral flexion the patient remains in the same position, but the instrument is placed vertically and on the coronal plane on the crown of the head. The instrument is zeroed, and the patient is invited to attempt to touch the shoulder with the ears, first in one direction then in the other. For measurement of rotation the patient lies flat and the goniometer is placed on the forehead horizontally. Rotation to the left and right can then be measured.

Shoulder

The shoulder is the most mobile joint in the body and is capable of movement in every direction—flexion, extension, adduction, abduction, circumduction and rotation. However, complete functional evaluation is not easy, and the reader should refer to Wright (1982) for a detailed consideration of the way in which the different muscle groups contribute to the various movements made at this joint.

Movements are best measured with the Loebl hydrogoniometer starting from a standard reference position in which the patient's arm is hanging down by the side of the body with the palm of the hand facing inwards and the thumb pointing forwards. The range of movement for each of the movements can then be determined (Fig. 8.16), as the patient's arm is moved actively and passively through the various arcs of movement. In flexion the arm is raised in front of the body and in extension the arm is raised backwards behind the body. It is moved out from the body for abduction and in across the trunk for adduction. With the elbow then flexed to 90°, internal rotation (forearm moving across the front of the body) and external rotation (forearm levered out away from the body) can be measured.

Finally, use may be made of the 'triple point'. This is situated on the back at the scapular level and can be reached by the opposite hand in three different ways: over the shoulder, behind the nape of the neck and up the back. It is

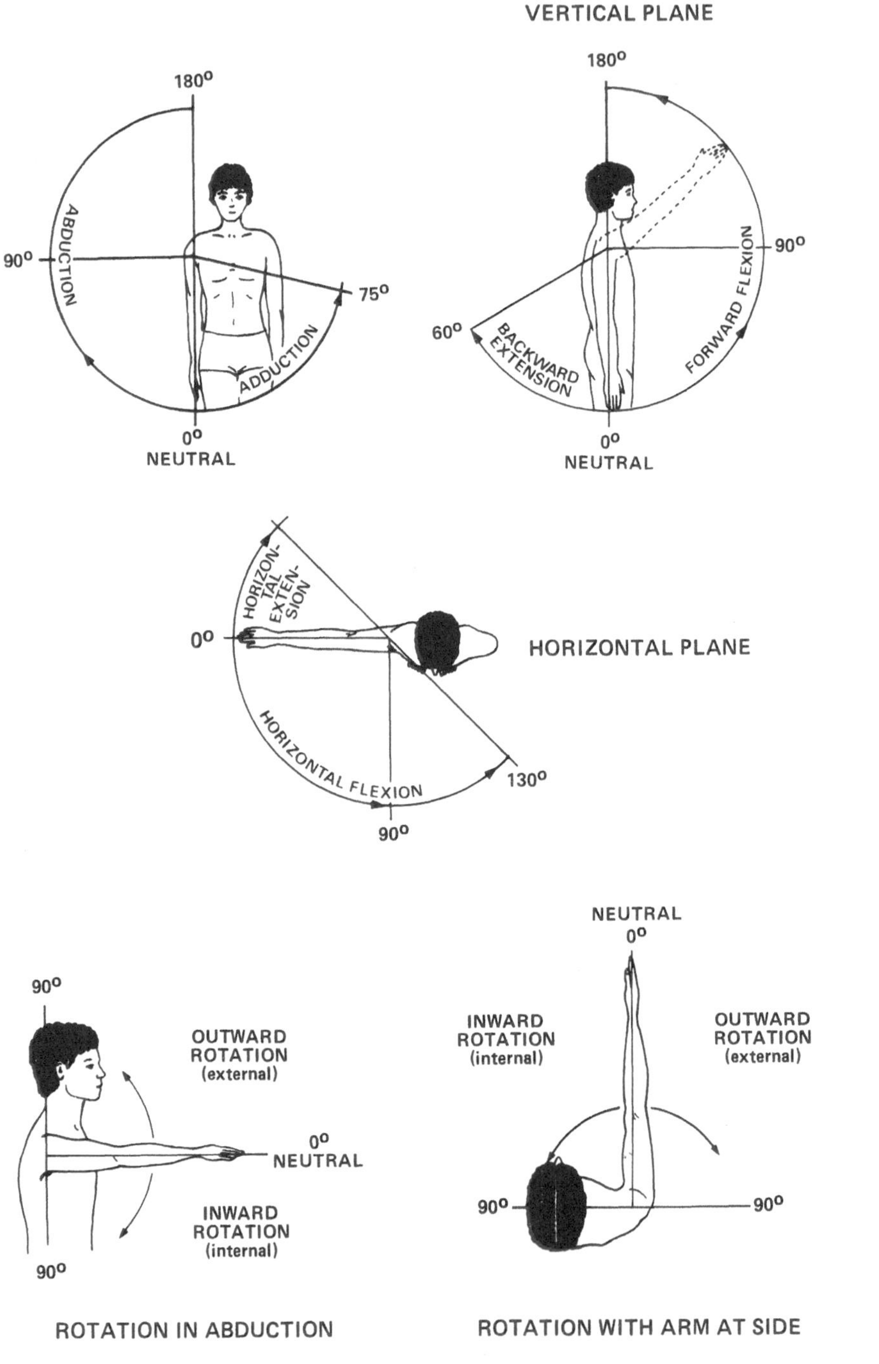

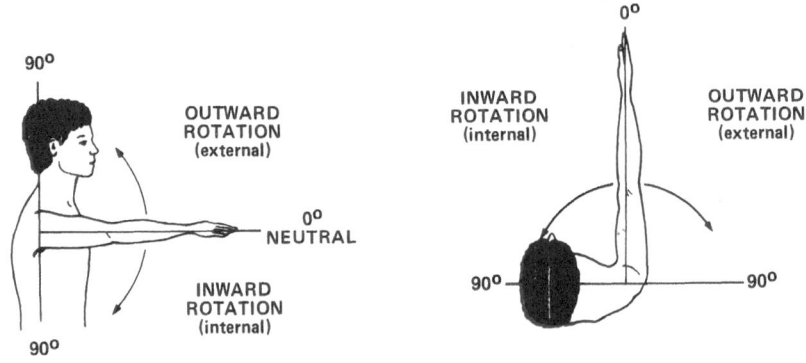

Fig. 8.16. Measurement of range of movement at the shoulder. (American Academy of Orthopedic Surgeons 1965)

helpful to know that a patient who can reach his or her 'triple point' by each of these three methods must have a full and healthy range of shoulder movement.

Elbow

Measurement of the range of elbow movement is best performed with a Zimmer goniometer. The goniometer arm should be as long as the limb segment to be measured, otherwise there will be inaccuracy because of the need for visual extrapolation from the ends of the goniometer arms to the landmarks at the wrists and shoulders. Patients should be sitting or standing, but the arms should be relaxed. The two arms of the goniometer are lined up with the upper arm and the lower arm respectively and the range of movements read off. In a recent survey (Amis and Miller 1982) of 208 rheumatic patients an average flexion mobility of 20°–137° was shown (mean range 117°). It was suggested that the clinical impression of the stiff elbow in rheumatoid arthritis may be overexaggerated. As mobility decreased, the elbow tended to stiffen towards a position of 90° flexion.

Wrist

An angle goniometer should be used for measuring the movement of the wrist. The conventional Zimmer angle goniometer has arms that are too long, but it may be possible to saw off one of these. The range of movement at the wrist joint is flexion/extension and adduction/abduction. In fact the 'wrist' is a composite joint, with movement occurring at the articulation between the radius and ulna with the carpus and also at the midcarpal articulations.

With the patient sitting and relaxed, the long arm of the goniometer is lined up along the radius/ulna. The short arm of the goniometer is lined up along the middle finger, the goniometer being placed on the back of the wrist, and abduction and adduction are measured. For flexion and extension the goniometer is placed at the side of the wrist joint, and the patient's hand is moved up and down.

Lumbar Spine

The lumbar spine is a composite set of vertebrae that move in conjunction with each other. In addition, many of the functional movements that may be attributed to the lumbar spine depend to a considerable degree on the flexibility of the hip joints. The test of bending forward to place the hands on the toes is as much a test of hip function as of lumbar spine function. With immobile lumbar spine but supple hips this movement can still be achieved.

One method for measuring the range of movement at the lumbar spine is Schober's test, which has already been described in the section on ankylosing spondylitis. The alternative method is to use the Loebl hydrogoniometer. The arcs of movement of the lumbar spine are flexion/extension, lateral flexion and rotation with the pelvis anchored. For flexion and extension the base of the Loebl hydrogoniometer is placed along the line of the vertebrae at the lumbar spine, the circular dial is zeroed and the angles of flexion and extension are read off. For lateral flexion the patient is invited to stretch one hand down the side of the leg towards the knee. The Loebl goniometer is held flat against the back over the lumbar spine and the angle of deflection to each side is measured. Rotation in the lumbar spine is notoriously difficult to measure and is probably best ignored for routine clinical purposes.

Hip Joint

The hip joint is also capable of a vast range of movements and no simple method of measurement is completely suitable. Both the Loebl hydrogoniometer and the Zimmer angle goniometer can be used but are prone to intra- and inter-operator error. However, for routine clinical use these instruments will be favoured by most clinicians. More complex methods for assessing hip mobility are:

1. An electromechanical goniometer, which is far more accurate than those already mentioned but which requires expertise both in operation and analysis of results
2. An optical system to determine movement. The polarised light goniometer measures limb angles by means of light-sensing devices, but is costly. However, this is probably cheaper than the cine camera technique, which involves placing markers on the patient's body and exposing the patient under suitable lighting conditions.

The standard movements that are normally measured at the hip joint are demonstrated in Fig. 8.17. It must be remembered that movement in the lumbar spine can easily contribute to hip movement. Ideally patients should be lying on a bed with an assistant anchoring their pelvis with both hands while the observer moves and measures the hip joints. For measurement of flexion the hydrogoniometer is placed vertically just above the knee joint, and a first reading is taken. The patient is then invited to flex the hip. The hydrogoniometer is replaced in exactly the same position (possibly marked with a marking pencil), and a second reading is obtained.

For measurement of extension the patient should be lying face down as far as is possible. The hydrogoniometer reading is taken with the device placed upright on the back of the thigh just above the knee, and the leg is then extended by the observer. A second reading is taken at the same site once the leg is in the air. For measurement of abduction and adduction, the Zimmer goniometer is probably the most satisfactory device with the patient lying face up on the couch again with the pelvis anchored. The straight leg is moved out from the midline and the resultant angle of abduction measured. The leg is then moved back across the midline and the resultant angle of adduction measured from the 'legs straight' position. The hip can then be bent to 90°

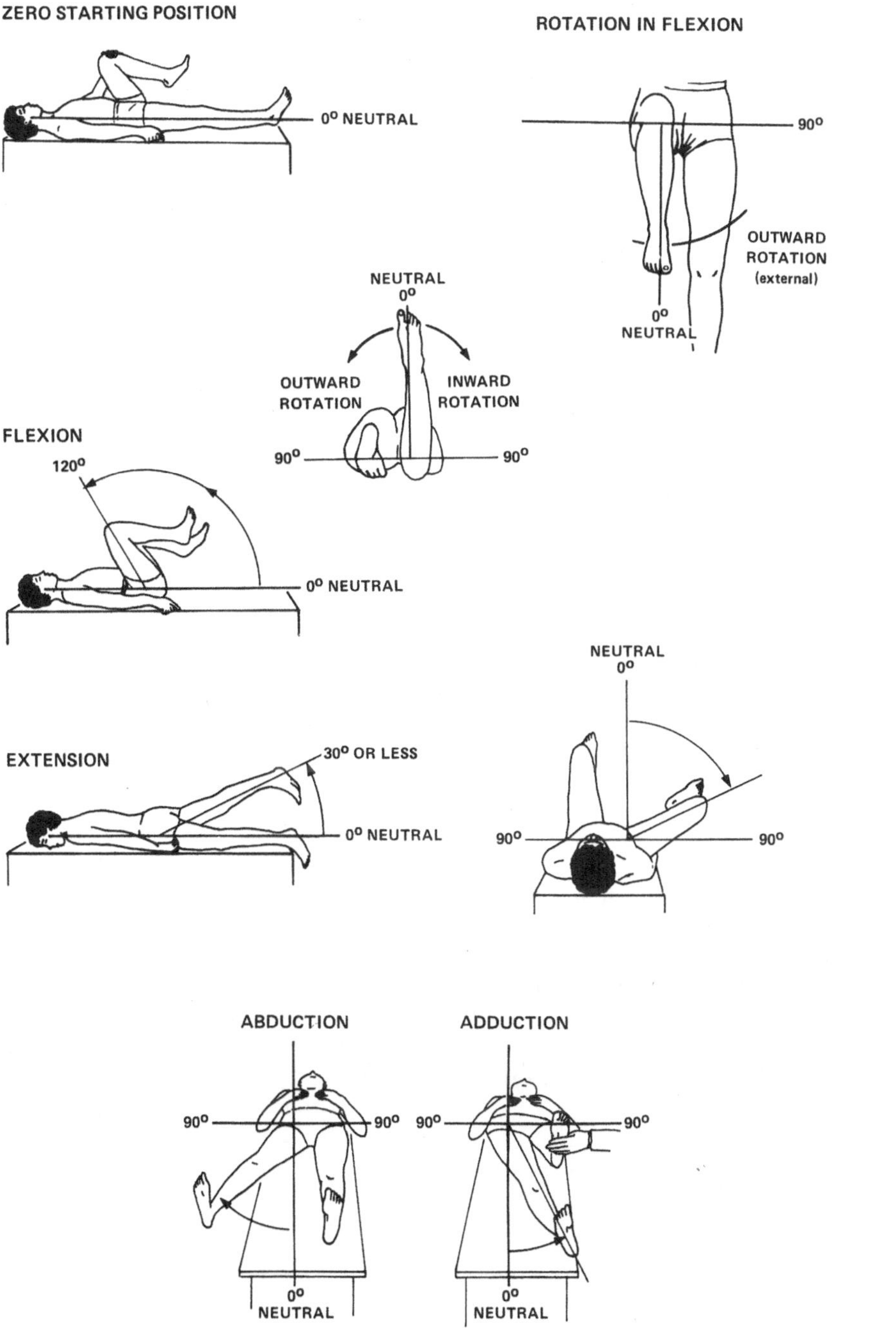

ZERO STARTING POSITION

ROTATION IN FLEXION

0° NEUTRAL

90°

OUTWARD
ROTATION
(external)

0°
NEUTRAL

NEUTRAL
0°

OUTWARD   INWARD
ROTATION   ROTATION

FLEXION

120°

90° ───── ───── 90°

0° NEUTRAL

EXTENSION

NEUTRAL
0°

30° OR LESS

0° NEUTRAL

90° ───── ───── 90°

ABDUCTION   ADDUCTION

90° ───── ───── 90°   90° ───── ───── 90°

0°
NEUTRAL

0°
NEUTRAL

Fig. 8.17. Measurement of range of movement at the hip. (American Academy of Orthopedic Surgeons 1965)

with the patient lying face up on the couch; the lower leg can now be used as a marker to determine internal rotation in flexion and external rotation in flexion, both of these being measured from a neutral position in which the lower leg is pointing towards the other foot.

Knee Joint

Although at first sight the knee appears to be a simple hinge joint, it is capable of some rotational movement. In practice, however, this is restricted, and flexion and extension are the only movements assessed routinely. The Zimmer angle goniometer is used and is placed on one side of the knee joint with the centre of the goniometer aligned to the axis of rotation of the knee joint. Some individuals can hyperextend their knee and this may be recorded as $-10°$ or $-15°$. Zero baseline is taken as the position in which the knee is straight; the angle of flexion can then be measured, the upper arm of the goniometer being levelled against the side of the thigh and the lower arm of the goniometer being levelled against the side of the lower leg.

Ankle Joint

An angle goniometer is used to measure flexion/extension (plantar flexion and dorsal flexion) and abduction/adduction of the ankle joint. In each case the axis of the angle goniometer is lined up with the axis of movement of the joint to be examined and the resultant deflection measured from a zero point.

Hands and Feet

It may also be useful to measure the range of movement at the inter-phalangeal joints in the hands and at the joints within the foot (though measurements of range of movement within the foot joints is of little use practically). For measurement of the range of movement at interphalangeal joints in the hands, a small angle goniometer is used. Various devices can be purchased, each with arms about 5 cm in length. These allow ulnar and radial deviation of the hand and flexion/extension at each of the interphalangeal joints to be quantified.

Sophisticated Objective Assessments of Joint Function

Isotope Uptake

The administration of isotope is likely to be performed by a physician in conjunction with a medical physicist, since this is an invasive technique. Isotopes may be used diagnostically or, if given on several occasions, in the serial assessment of joint inflammation. This isotope may be injected intravenously and the uptake counted over involved joints. Alternatively the isotope is injected into the involved joint and its speed of excretion from that joint measured by an isotopic method. The medical physics department is likely to provide the results for entry on the patient's data sheet.

Thermography

Thermography is a non-invasive assessment technique and can be repeated an unlimited number of times on patients. The same joint or area of a joint is scanned on each occasion using a heat-sensitive camera and the resultant thermographic index calculated on a computer. This will produce a print out for inclusion in the patient's notes.

Objective Assessments of Stiffness

The Leeds group have pioneered the use of a finger hyperextensometer (mainly for studies on hyperlaxity) and a finger arthrograph, which may be more relevant in determining the relief of stiffness by anti-inflammatory drugs. Both machines can be regarded as experimental at present, but the finger hyperextensometer may come into more general use for epidemiological studies on the range of movement at the metacarpophalangeal joint of the finger. Both machines can be operated by a suitably trained person, since they are non-invasive and do not require detailed mechanical or electrical knowledge on the part of the operator.

Arthroscopy

There are ethical problems in the serial use of arthroscopy in clinical trials, and the evidence is that the results are not particularly valuable in any case. The procedure of arthroscopy has already been described in Chapter 2 (see p. 48) and the nursing care of arthroscopy patients in Chapter 4 (see p. 126).

References

American Academy of Orthopedic Surgeons (1965) Joint motion. Method of measuring and recording. [Reprinted (1966) Churchill Livingstone, Edinburgh]

Amis AA and Miller JA (1982) The elbow. Clin Rheum Dis 8: 571–593

Beecher HK (1959) Measurement of subjective responses. Quantitative effects of drugs. New York. (Cited by Ritchie et al. 1968)

Bird HA and Wright V (1982) Assessments in the rheumatic diseases. In: Applied drug therapy of the rheumatic diseases. Wright, Bristol, pp 40–61

Fries JF, Spitz BW and Young DI (1982) The dimensions of health outcomes: the health assessment questionnaire, disability and pain scales. J Rheumatol 9: 789–793

Ritchie DM, Boyle JA, McInnes JM et al. (1968) Clinical studies with an articular index for the assessment of joint tenderness in patients with rheumatoid arthritis. Q J Med 37: 393–406

Wright V (ed) (1982) Measurement of joint movement. Clin Rheum Dis 8(3): 521–722

9
Psychological Aspects

Introduction

Much attention is paid to the medical and physical aspects of rheumatic disease; however, when treating a painful, potentially deforming and unpredictable chronic disease such as rheumatoid arthritis it is important to take into consideration the effect that it has on every aspect of the patient's life. A chronic disabling disease will undoubtedly have emotional as well as physical effects. Without help and understanding the patient's personal and social relationships can become strained or non-existent. Some patients may become hostile towards the health professionals, and others cease to comply with their treatment, making the management of their disease doubly difficult. To enable patients to adjust to their situation they need some understanding of the psychological consequences of their disease, which will allow them to take full advantage of the health care available to them.

Reactions of Patients to their Disease

Patients suffering from rheumatoid arthritis share certain fundamental responses with patients suffering from other chronic diseases. These are listed by Sinescu (1963) as fear or anxiety, dependency, anger and loss of gratification. However, it must be accepted that each patient is an individual, and the psychological response of each patient to the disease will vary accordingly.

Initially many patients go through a period of grieving for their loss of life style or self-image. This can involve stages of:

1. Shock, denial, disbelief
2. Anger
3. Bargaining
4. Depression
5. Eventual acceptance.

Each patient's grieving process is unique; not all patients can go through all these stages in sequence. Patients sometimes bypass a stage or swing back and forth between stages or even experience an overlap of stages. It is important that patients are allowed their grief and that they are given time to work through the grieving process in their own way. Less normal are exaggerated responses such as severe depression, hyperanxiety and continual denial of their disease. These abnormal responses can interfere with the patient's treatment. Patients who are denying their disease will not feel inclined to accept treatment for it or from health professionals to whom they feel hostility. When treating a hostile patient it should be accepted that he needs to be allowed to express his feelings. It is vital not to react negatively by meeting hostility with hostility as this can stop the patient trying to communicate.

The capacity to accept the disease varies from patient to patient, and whilst one patient who is severely deformed may lead a full and satisfying life, another patient with only mild physical disability may be 'emotionally crippled' and unable to function on both a personal and social level. Nor does the psychological adjustment of patients necessarily reflect the changes in their physical situation; patients showing physical improvement do not automatically show a corresponding psychological improvement.

Life for everyone is full of uncertainties with which each individual must come to terms by continually weighing the options and then making choices. For a patient suffering from a chronic disabling disease, however, the options slowly diminish, and so the choices become increasingly limited, making life difficult and frustrating. When there is added to this the unpredictability and uncertainty of rheumatoid arthritis with its periods of flares and quiescence, it is not surprising that at times the burden must feel intolerable (Weiner 1974).

Problems Arising from Physical Disability

The physical manifestations of chronic rheumatic disease are complex and manifold, and each will have its own impact on the patient's personality. An individual patient's vulnerability to a particular manifestation will in part depend upon personality and in part on how important that particular loss is in relation to life style and self-image.

Chronic Pain

Chronic pain can create great difficulties for the patient, and each will cope with it in a different way. The experience of pain is complex and varies not only for different patients but also for the same patient in different circumstances. For example, pain experienced in the early hours of the morning whilst the patient is trying to sleep can be far worse than the same pain experienced while the patient is engaged in an enjoyable activity. Distraction is therefore a good strategy for pain relief and if combined with relaxation can bring great relief (Slucki 1975). It is important for patients to keep mentally active, and the search for new interests, which do not damage the joints, will act as both stimulation and distraction.

The complaints of pain which patients express may bear little relationship to the severity and constancy of the pain which they experience. For instance, a patient with mild, sporadic pain may be more vocal than one whose pain is chronic and severe. Some patients deal with their pain by raising their pain threshold, and it is not unknown for an arthritic patient to allow a fractured limb to go unrecognised for weeks by simply assuming that the increased pain is associated with their arthritis.

Many patients have a fear of taking drugs. They are afraid that they will suffer serious side-effects or that they will become addicted by taking too many tablets over a long period. This anxiety can create a vicious circle. The patient is anxious about taking drugs and so will take less than is needed to bring about adequate analgesic effect. This will lead to inadequate pain control, which in turn will lead to further anxiety and emotional stress. The circle can be broken if the patient is taught the significance of the pain and is well informed about the medication. A recent study carried out on surgical patients showed that patients who were educated before their surgery required less postoperative analgesia than those who were given no preoperative education (Haywood 1975). If this is so with surgical patients experiencing acute pain, it is reasonable to expect that patients experiencing chronic pain, if educated in a similar manner, will react in a similar way.

Hostility, anger and bitterness are defence mechanisms that some patients use to help them to overcome their pain. Life can become very difficult for the immediate relatives and close friends of such patients as the feelings of anger are liable to be expressed towards those who are nearest and dearest. People closely connected with rheumatic patients need counselling and adequate information to help them to be understanding and tolerant and able to cope in these difficult circumstances.

When a good relationship exists between health professional and patient, the placebo effect should not be underestimated. If a medication or a treatment is highly endorsed by either a physician or paramedical worker whom the patient holds in high esteem, it can have a powerful positive effect on the outcome of treatment.

Patients experiencing chronic pain need to be treated with sensitivity and understanding. They need to be 'allowed to have their pain'. The following quotation from the diary of a patient who was interviewed in an American study expresses this well: 'Pain is essentially private. Sometimes you wish for someone to understand and to be patient with your pain. To allow you to have it! I do not mean sympathy or pity.'

Loss of Functional Ability

Maintaining psychological equilibrium in the face of an ever-changing situation is, to say the least, difficult, but patients with rheumatoid arthritis must achieve this if they are to live a full and satisfying life. Their functional abilities are slowly but constantly changing, bringing new problems and challenges.

As patients become more disabled they worry that they will be unable to hold down their jobs and so be unable to support themselves or their families. To a certain extent this problem can be anticipated by the physician, who can refer the patient to the disablement resettlement officer for assessment and re-training. By this means most patients are able to be re-employed without loss of dignity or self-esteem. Unfortunately, not all patients can be re-trained, and a role change thus becomes inevitable. This can be an extremely difficult situation for the patient and their family to accept, as a successful adjustment will require a change in the attitude of all concerned. It is not only those who are employed outside the home who experience stress as advancing disablement makes change inevitable. A housewife who has kept house for many years may feel that her role is being eroded by her children or relatives when they try to help. She may even refuse help, striving to keep things as they are.

For those patients in whose lives athletic sports played an important role, adjustment to a lowered physical ability can be particularly difficult. They often try to carry on an activity far too long, putting additional stress on joints which are not capable of withstanding it. Patients must be able to differentiate between exercise and activity. Exercise is important in the treatment of rheumatic disease, whereas some activities are optional and need to be placed in order of priority in a patient's life.

As patients become less mobile their personal and social lives become more difficult. Because they tend to be confined to their homes, social stimulation is lost to them, and friendships can become strained as invitations are broken or accepted less frequently. Even close family members can become exasperated with what they regard as erratic behaviour. Patients can feel ill one day and well the next, and if this leads to the patient being unable to do something that their partner believes they do not want to do, they can infer that the patient is 'putting it on'. The importance of teaching and counselling relatives cannot be over-stressed, as this can help bring about the understanding that is necessary for the existence of a stable relationship.

Perhaps the outcome that patients fear most is that they will become crippled and destined to a wheelchair existence. They fear that they will become a burden to their families and dependent on others for existence, relinquishing some of the control they have over their own lives into the hands of someone else. For a small proportion of sufferers, between 5% and 10%, these fears turn into reality, and this section of the rheumatoid population will need great help both physically and psychologically. For the majority of patients, however, this fear stems from ignorance of their disease and its treatment. Patient education based upon sound knowledge, given in an authoritative and professional manner and in a way that the patient understands, will do much to alleviate this problem.

Deformity

The reaction of patients to physical deformity will in part depend upon the importance which they place upon their physical appearance and body image. For instance, a woman who is proud of her beautiful hands may be very emotionally distressed if they become ugly and deformed. Although a number of these patients can be helped by hand surgery, which in some cases can return the hand to a near-normal appearance, by far the most satisfactory treatment is achieved by the physician who anticipates such dilemmas and prescribes preventive therapy, such as splinting at an early stage of the disease process.

Similarly, patients with foot problems may refuse the comfort of surgical shoes in preference for their more fashionable but more painful normal shoes. Surgery may again be useful to some patients, but for those who cannot be helped in this way careful counselling can be of immense value. Patients should be told of the great benefits that surgical shoes can bring and the harm of cramming deformed feet into ill-fitting shoes. Once a female patient realises that surgical shoes are not all monstrous, heavy and black and that it is not essential that they are worn on that special occasion when she wants to look exceptionally pretty, they can seem more acceptable. Women suffering from knee involvement and the resultant muscle wasting in their legs may be in a happier position, as the wearing of trousers has become highly acceptable, irrespective of age.

Deformity can create social barriers between patients and normal or non-deformed persons. Society does not like to be reminded of sickness, and persons with deformed limbs using crutches or aids are an uncomfortable reminder.

The loss of body image can bring about psychosexual problems. A woman to whom physical appearance is important can feel unattractive to her partner; a man may feel 'less of a man', and this can lead to impotence. These problems should be anticipated. The topic of sexuality can be introduced by the health professional, thus giving a lead to the patient who wishes to pursue the topic. Psychosexual counselling may be outside the scope of the health professional, and if this is the case the patient should be referred to a specialist counsellor. However, many of the problems which do arise are purely practical, such as positioning, or worries over medical matters such as pregnancy and heredity. Many patients worry about how their partners may react if sexual intercourse becomes more difficult and painful. The couple must be encouraged to talk openly and frankly together about their true feelings.

How Patients Cope

Patients use various strategies to cope with their disease.

Hope

Patients hold on to hopes of remission or of relief from constant pain. This is illustrated well in our clinics at Leeds, where patients are prepared to wait for many weeks and travel long distances on numerous occasions to take part in a trial of a new and untried drug, in the hope that it as may be 'the one that works'. Some patients turn to alternative medicine or 'folk-lore', and cures are frequently secured from friends or other patients. Others try to pinpoint the cause of their disease, such as a diet or a knock or a fall, this being something that they can understand and have control over.

Covering Up

Covering up has been described as 'the rejection by the patient of the handicap as his total identity. In effect it is the rejection of the social significance of the handicap and not the handicap per se'. In other words, covering up is not a denial of the disease itself, but rather a social strategy, and it is often used by patients when friends or family ask how they are. They say, 'I feel fine', when it is obvious they do not. This covering up can also happen when patients do not want to bother medical and nursing staff who appear to be busy, and it is therefore important to observe the non-verbal language of patients, such as wincing and facial expressions, when communicating with them.

The use of aids and appliances can be seen as a disadvantage by the patient who uses covering up as a social strategy, yet refusal to use them can cause problems in unexpected ways. Recently a patient attending one of our clinics disclosed that she had been refused a financial allowance. When closely questioned she admitted that she had refused to use her wheelchair (on which she was almost wholly dependent) to enter the department when she was to be assessed. With superhuman effort she had walked into the office with the aid of crutches and had subsequently been refused financial support on the grounds that she was able to walk!

Lowering of Expectations and Activities

As patients become less mobile and more deformed many learn to revise their expectations of themselves. They begin to set achievable goals and once they have reached those goals they feel a real sense of accomplishment and also preserve their self-image.

Pacing

Many patients appraise themselves by the activities that they can carry out. Rheumatic patients learn to pace themselves so that they are able to carry out activities which are important to them if interspaced by frequent rests. It has been shown that patients who improve their performance in ADL activities show a concomitant improvement in their social adjustment (Vignos et al. 1972)

Conclusion

Patients with chronic, painful diseases which affect them emotionally as well as physically will need the security of continuity of care. They also need time to come to terms with the disease and time to adjust to the emotional manifestations which inevitably present. The health professionals must convey to the patient and their families a sympathetic and understanding attitude that will enable a trusting relationship to develop.

Many patients are fearful of their disease and the effects it will have on the lives of themselves and their families. Some of these fears are well founded, but many are based on ignorance and folk-lore. It has been shown that patients react in a positive way when their disease and its prognosis is explained to them by an authoritative health professional. Patient education is an invaluable adjunct to physical treatment and helps patients to understand the rationale behind the management of their disease and so leads to greater compliance with their treatment. Similarly, if patients and their families are taught about their mental as well as their physical wellbeing, this knowledge will help to bring about the physical and psychological equilibrium which is necessary for leading a full and satisfying life.

References

Haywood J (1975) Information: prescription against pain. Royal College of Nurses, London
Sinescu RA (1963) The development of emotional complications in the patient with cancer. J Chron Dis 16: 813
Slucki H (1975) Reported in Rachman S (ed) Contributions to medical psychology, vol I. Pergamon, Oxford, p 2
Vignos, PJ Jr, Thompson HM, Katz S, Moskowitz RW, Fink S and Svec KH (1972) Comprehensive care and psycho-social factors in rehabilitation in chronic R.A.: a controlled study. J Chron Dis 25: 388
Weiner CL (1974) The burden of R.A.: tolerating the uncertainty. Social Sci Med 9: 97–104

10

Organisation and Development of Combined Care in the Outpatient Clinic

Introduction

Combined patient care, shared by physicians and rheumatology nurses, has been evolving in the outpatient clinics at the General Infirmary at Leeds for several years. This chapter reviews its history, its current status and its possible future development. The chapter is divided into two parts. The first, written by a physician, gives the physician's point of view on the way the combined service has developed. The second, written by the nursing sisters, evaluates the division of responsibility from the nurse's point of view and considers the way the combined patient care system may act as a starting point for the development of rheumatology nurse practitioners in the United Kingdom, in response to the needs of patients.

Combined Care in the Outpatient Clinic— the Physician's View

The Nurse as a Research Assistant

The role of the clinical metrologist has developed at Leeds over a period of about 10 years. The initial step was to employ state-registered nurses as research assistants. Such work, normally carried out within social working hours and usually limited to only a few hours a week provided satisfactory part-time employment to nursing sisters who did not want to be involved in a full-time job.

Clearly nurses can be of enormous use to the physician. They are well qualified to talk to patients, and this communication is appreciated by patients. Typical projects that might be tackled by a part-time research nurse include the completing of patient questionnaires on matters as diverse as information about medication and information about aids and appliances, the tabulation of data and the performing of routine clinical tasks such as the measurement of blood pressure, weight, height and temperature. Many consultants already use their clinic nurses to take blood pressure and complete investigation forms, and the use of nurses as research assistants simply represents an extension of this traditional role. Nevertheless, from the nursing point of view, one can see that such a job, although performed in social hours, lacks professional satisfaction. Moreover, the move by the Royal College of Nurses to instigate nursing research has led to the training of nurses in research methodology and statistical aspects of clinical trials so that they can conduct pure nursing research rather than act as handmaidens to physicians.

The use of a nurse as a research assistant may well be appropriate to physicians who have only a small research commitment, and the appointment is certainly likely to be more cost effective than the use of a succession of junior hospital doctors. Moreover, a nursing research assistant is less likely to move at 6-monthly intervals than a junior hospital doctor and, with luck, will not require re-training at regular intervals.

Advent of Clinical Metrologists

The transition of nursing research assistants into clinical metrologists was partly dictated by the inception of a Clinical Pharmacology Unit within the Rheumatism Research Unit at the University of Leeds. It is interesting to recall that initially the establishment in this Clinical Pharmacology Unit for the conduct of clinical trials into drugs that might relieve arthritis was envisaged as one consultant physician and one or two medical officers employed as clinical assistants or equivalent. However, the general practitioners who were employed as clinical assistants for one or two sessions each week were unable to cope with the large volume of trial work 'that accumulated and had to give priority to the needs of their practices. As a result, a decision, experimental at that stage, was made to employ two senior nursing sisters as clinical metrologists instead of the junior hospital doctors originally envisaged. It was hoped that the nursing incumbents would be available for longer hours than general practitioners and, after appropriate training, might be available for the performance of their duties for a longer time span than the normal short stay of a hospital doctor. As the Clinical Pharmacology Unit has expanded and the number of clinical trials has increased, successive metrologists working in the Unit have normally been keen to increase their working hours, when given the opportunity.

The way in which the clinical metrologist works has been described elsewhere (Bird et al. 1980; Bird et al. 1981) and will be discussed only briefly here. The state registered nurses employed as clinical metrologists are likely to work a 4-day week, though hours can often be increased or reduced by arrangement. Apart from the fixed clinic times, the hours may be relatively flexible, and our metrologists have been able to combine bringing up a family with working at their job. Indeed, the physician may prefer the metrologists to work on a 'flexi-hour' system rather like the nursing shift system since this provides a greater range of cover for inpatient pharmacokinetic profiles, which may start as early as 7.30 a.m. and finish as late as 9.00 p.m.

By virtue of our geographical area, the duties are divided between the General Infirmary at Leeds and the Royal Bath Hospital in Harrogate, and therefore metrologists have to work at both places. The General Infirmary at Leeds has a busy rheumatology clinic from 9.00 a.m. to 1.00 p.m. on a Monday morning and from 1.00 p.m. to 5.00 p.m. on a Friday afternoon. There are only a handful of rheumatology beds in Leeds, and patients from a catchment area as large as almost 2 million people are referred to this single clinic, which, although large, is one of the few rheumatology clinics in Yorkshire. By contrast, for historical reasons the Royal Bath Hospital in Harrogate has 120 inpatient beds devoted to the treatment of rheumatic diseases. This is only 15 miles away from Leeds and all patients from the West Yorkshire industrial conurbation who require inpatient care are automatically admitted to the hospital in Harrogate.

The metrologists work throughout the whole of both these long clinic sessions. At the clinic, each metrologist has her own room, which is likely to be adjacent to one of the rooms used by a consultant rheumatologist or a senior registrar. The metrologists work their way through a booked list of patients. This list is available beforehand so that the appropriate paperwork for patients attending a particular clinic can be assembled in advance. On a typical clinic day, when the consultant is seeing four or five new patients, each with 20-min appointments, and up to 20 or 25 old patients, each with 5-min appointments, the metrologist will each be seeing 10–12 patients, each patient having a 15-min metrology appointment. Patients are referred to the metrologist by the clinicians, often because they are suitable for inclusion in clinical trials, and the clinician will be responsible for obtaining informed consent from the patient and explaining the general details of the trial under question. However, once the patient has agreed to participate, from that point onwards, all appointments will be with the metrologist. The metrologist will explain the trial protocol in further detail and make certain that the patient understands everything needed to be known and to be done. The metrologist then prescribes the trial medicine, working according to the trial protocol, requests the appropriate blood tests, as required by the protocol, and checks the results. Metrologists are responsible for drawing the attention of the clinician to any seriously abnormal values. Since the clinician is always in the room next door, providing medical cover to the metrologists, any problems that arise when the patient attends the metrology clinic can be immediately referred to the physician. With this proviso, however, the patient will remain entirely under metrology care until the end of the trial. If the trial is of 6-months' duration—for example the investigation of a second-line agent—the patient will not see a clinician between the start and end of the study unless the patient particularly requests to do so.

Metrologists are assisted in their work by other members of staff employed by the University through the Rheumatism Research Unit. The Rheumatism Research Unit contributes to the salary of a trials pharmacist at Leeds General Infirmary, who liaises closely with the metrologists in the providing of drug supplies. The metrologists also have the services of a metrologists' clerk who works 2 days a week filing results and sets of notes. Finally, there is a part-time phlebotomist employed to be present at the times of the clinics so that blood samples can be taken in conjunction with clinical trials.

On their other working days the metrologists are employed in Harrogate. Here the Clinical Pharmacology Unit has its laboratory, and within the Unit the metrologists have their desk space, filing cabinets and bookshelves. From this base in Harrogate they supervise the conduct of inpatient clinical trials, for example pharmacokinetic profiles on non-steroidal anti-inflammatory agents, particularly in elderly rheumatic patients, and faecal blood loss studies, which are often more easily supervised on inpatients than on outpatients. At one time, much of the day was taken up with tabulation of patient data record forms, particularly with the advent of the extensive patient monitoring that is now required by the American Food and Drug Administration. This job has been somewhat eased by the employment of a metrologists' clerk.

Metrologists are expected to be proficient in all the measurement techniques already described (see Chap. 8), and appropriate training is provided by existing metrologists and the clinicians. Much of this training takes the form of an apprenticeship, but a reading list of appropriate rheumatology textbooks is provided, and the metrologists are encouraged to attend the lectures on rheumatology provided for medical students in the University of Leeds as part of their education.

Development of Combined Patient Care from Clinical Metrology

We may be fortunate in the Leeds area in that we have almost 25 applicants for each University Clinical Metrology post. This enables us to select well-motivated, intelligent and highly qualified nursing sisters for our posts. It was perhaps inevitable that after the period of apprenticeship and a couple of years spent learning the intricacies of clinical trials, the job would come to lack some of its initial appeal. To some extent it was possible to offset the relative tedium of performing clinical trials by expanding clinical metrology to its utmost point. Thus clinical metrologists were invited to be present at the planning stage of clinical trials and became experts on advising drug companies on the most appropriate assessments to use and the best method of tabulating them, and the best way to design the data recording booklets that are used in clinical trials. A wide range of trials was also provided so that metrologists became skilled in the routine conduct of trials in outpatients, in intravenous cannulation for pharmacokinetic assessments and in trials of non-rheumatic drugs such as hypnotics, anxiolytics and even antibiotics, with the appropriate assessments of precautions that were involved in assessing these compounds. Thus some variety was provided as a change from rheumatological trials on anti-inflammatory agents. With the advent of more trials on 'second-line' agents, it became possible for the metrologists to see the patients over a 6-month period as we judged whether they responded to penicillamine or comparable compounds. This allowed closer contact between metrologists and patients over a longer period of time, which was to the mutual advantage of both.

Nevertheless there is a limit to the interest that can be sustained by trials, and we have therefore sought to make the job itself more varied. This endeavour was helped by the provision of honorary nursing sister contracts by the local area health authorities of the NHS and also by the availability of university travelling bursaries that enable the metrologists to visit centres of rheumatological nursing excellence, particularly in the United States. As a result, the metrologists assumed more responsibility for total patient care. Many aspects of this, such as patient education and the explanation of appropriate physiotherapy and occupational therapy services, are easily neglected in an area such as West Yorkshire, which has one of the lowest numbers of rheumatologists per head of population in the country. The physician's dilemma is whether to restrict access to the clinics, thus preventing some patients with arthritis from getting specialist care, or whether to admit all-comers but restrict the time of their access to the physicians. Although neither of these is an enviable choice, we opted for the latter and encouraged patients attending clinic not only to see a physician but also to see a nurse counsellor for patient education and advice on aids and appliances. This system leaves the rehabilitation physicians with a freer hand to work on the more complex rehabilitation problems. It also allows the physicians more time to concentrate on differential diagnosis and the overall coordination of therapy, including drug therapy, for both of which functions they have received particular training. This evolution of combined patient care is described in more detail elsewhere (Bird 1983). It remains a possibility that our own clinical nurse metrologists will develop to become the first hospital nurse practitioners in the United Kingdom. Nurse practitioners or equivalent are used extensively in the United States in the provision of health care programmes for patients with chronic medical complaints such as arthritis, and it is likely that the British system could be improved in this respect by comparable provision of such health professionals.

Whether nurse practitioners will become an accepted career grade in the NHS and appropriate funding be provided for them, or whether they will be seen to be poaching on territory normally confined to doctors with their more extensive medical qualifications, remains to be seen. At present our own 'nurse practitioners' have to be recruited and funded as 'clinical metrologists', since with the current financial stringencies in the NHS, we are unlikely to find immediate funding elsewhere.

Establishment of a Clinical Metrology Post

Physicians reading this book will find this section of value; nurses who aspire to clinical metrology may persuade their physician colleagues to act along similar lines.

At present, clinical metrologists are likely to be paid from the 'soft funds' provided by the pharmaceutical industry for the conduct of clinical trials. Standard practice is for the pharmaceutical company to agree a contracted price for the conduct of each and every clinical trial. This will be done with the physician responsible for the trial, and the price asked by the physician will reflect the need for laboratory assessments, medical time, metrology time and secretarial time and facilities.

Clearly the number of metrology hours required will depend upon the number of trials to be conducted and this in turn will dictate the finances required. The clinician should consider undertaking a sufficient number of trials to employ two metrologists. Once trained, metrologists are extremely cost effective, and the advantages of having two metrologists are considerable, for example one can do clinical assessments when the other is sick or on holiday. Two metrologists also allow the flexibility needed for a wide variety of clinical trial designs, including true double-blind work; one metrologist can be used to evaluate the patients' clinical progress and the other metrologist to check the side-effects.

Ideally the physician should work out the number of trials he will be able to undertake, should cost them and should then work out the number of metrologists he will be able to afford, the hours they will work and the sort of contract they will have. Where possible the clinician should seek either a long-term study or, perhaps preferably, a package deal with a large pharmaceutical company such that he will perform several studies over the course of a 2-year period. This means that the metrologists can initially be given 2-year contracts rather than being employed on an item of service basis according to the trial work that comes in. Our own metrologists are paid on the Whitley salary scales, and this linking of the clinical metrologist's salary to the nationally agreed and negotiated professional salary scales avoids the possible embarrassment to the physician of seeming to decide the salary on an ad hoc basis. It implies some obligation for the pharmaceutical company to observe the nationally negotiated salary scales.

In Leeds we are fortunate to be able to employ the metrologists through the University administration. Although they are paid in accordance with the NHS recommended scales, the metrologists have access to all University facilities as academic-related staff, including the University library and central education services. Just as University lecturers and senior lecturers are awarded appropriate NHS honorary contracts, so our University-employed metrologists have been awarded the equivalent NHS nursing contracts. This in turn implies that they are available for education purposes within the NHS nursing schools. Our own metrologists are also encouraged to be active members of the Rheumatology Nursing Forum of the Royal College of Nurses. Nurses who are members of the Royal College are provided with appropriate professional insurance.

A specimen job description for one of our own Clinical Metrology posts is included as Appendix B at the end of the book. (This reflects our own local requirements and may not be applicable to the requirements of other research or service rheumatology units.) The actual starting salary may be determined by the University in the light of previous posts held in the NHS and the age and experience of the appointee.

Selection of Applicants

We are often asked whether other paramedical professionals should be considered for Clinical Metrology appointments. We are exceptionally lucky in the Rheumatism Research Unit in Leeds in that we also have access to a research physiotherapist, a research occupational therapist and a research speech therapist. Any project that would seem to be particularly applicable to the skills of one of these workers would be delegated to them. Partly because of this, we have always preferred state registered nurses as metrologists; however, in units with more limited personnel, local preferences may dictate a different choice. A unit concentrating on studies in spinal movement in ankylosing spondylitis, for example, might prefer a physiotherapist rather than a nurse as a metrologist.

If the predominant research interest is clinical pharmacology or clinical trials, however, there seem to be excellent reasons for preferring nurses, and we have always stipulated this in our advertisements for metrologists on the clinical pharmacology side. Nurses are often trained to take blood samples, particularly if they have worked as district nursing sisters, and this skill is not always acquired easily by physiotherapists and occupational therapists. Many trials may involve intramuscular injection, and again nurses are trained and qualified to give these. If intravenous cannulation techniques are required for pharmacokinetic procedures, the physician will be relieved that his nurse metrologist has a thorough grounding in sterile techniques and aseptic care of cannulae sites. Members of the Royal College of Nurses will be covered by the insurance schemes of the College in respect of professional duties of this sort. Finally, certain clinical trials may involve unusual hours, and a nursing education, based as it is on the shift system to provide 24-h patient care, equips the appointee well for the strenuous demands. Although physicians, nurses, occupational therapists and physiotherapists all give high standards of patient care, it is only the first two groups that are expected to provide routine service over bank holidays and to work on Christmas Day.

Since our metrologists are employed by the University, we have felt it appropriate to follow the guidelines laid down by the University in making appointments. This means that it is not mandatory to have the presence of senior nursing administrators on the appointing panel. Although we have been most grateful for the honorary NHS contracts provided by the senior nursing administrators once the University had made the appointment, we have felt that the freedom to appoint directly within the University has allowed us to make less conventional choices (with definite benefit to the Research Unit) than might otherwise have been made if we had had to contend with the formal NHS appointing machinery.

An analysis of 20 candidates who applied formally for a recent metrology post in Leeds showed that 16 of these visited the Unit, partly because they were expected to and partly because the unusual nature of the job prompted them to come and find out more about it. All applicants were female, and 18 of the 20 were married. The age range was 30–52 years, 13 applicants being between 35 and 45 years. Many patients are anxious if the clinical trial in which they are participating appears to be conducted by a nurse just recently out of training school. Of the 18 married women 16 had children, and 19 of the 20 lived locally. Although we had advertised in the national nursing press and in local papers, 18 of the 20 had seen the advertisement in local papers, possibly the most fertile source of part-time jobs.

The majority of nurses applying stated similar reasons for wanting the job. The part-time nature of the appointment and flexibility of hours were important, but most importance was attached to the extra responsibility and increased job satisfaction likely to be derived from the post, which compensated, in the case of some applicants, for the drop in salary from the senior Whitley nursing scale. Those applicants who did not want to become nursing tutors or nursing administrators saw the post as a means of achieving increased responsibility and close patient contact without being tied down by bureaucracy in their conditions of duty. Many applicants commented that under existing health service administration there was little scope for personal initiative. To our surprise, only three candidates mentioned an interest in research, an aspect that had deliberately been given prominence in the job description. This may be because nurses are not given the opportunity to become familiar with the excitement of doing original research as part of their basic training.

We encourage applicants to visit the Unit since the job is relatively unusual compared to routine nursing duties. The appointee is ultimately selected by the Head of Department in conjunction with the physicians under whom the metrologist will be working, although the existing clinical metrologists are asked to meet all applicants and serve in an advisory capacity, their views carrying considerable weight. It may be that this appointing machinery, which is less conventional than the standard NHS appointing machinery for nurses, enables us to consider applicants who are a little outside the conventional NHS career ladder.

All of the 20 candidates who made application had wide experience within hospitals. Nevertheless, it should not go unnoticed that although three applicants were selected for interview on the basis of their ability, confidence and initiative, all three had worked for relatively long periods of time outside the NHS nursing service. One had trained for 3 years as a laboratory technician and was thus doubly qualified, one had extensive experience in industrial, private and district nursing and one had worked for 8 years as a residential social worker (with particular responsibility for nursing aspects) in a special school for maladjusted but intelligent adolescent females with inadequate family backgrounds.

Inevitably, a career structure for clinical metrologists (or nurse practitioners) is not available at present. The increased responsibility that attracts many nurses to a clinical metrology post is offset by the relative lack of career prospects and long-term financial security.

Combined Care in the Outpatient Clinic— the Nurse's View

Original Role of the Clinical Metrologist

The role of clinical metrologist was originally envisaged as that of a technician whose job it was to make routine clinical assessments and measurements, normally as part of drug trials. Over recent years the role of clinical metrologist has changed, moving steadily away from that of technician towards that of nurse practitioner. With hindsight, the employment of nurses for this work made the change inevitable. The whole *raison d'être* of nursing is an active provision of patient care, whereas that of pure clinical metrology is the passive taking and recording of measurements.

It became apparent that by adhering to pure metrology an enormous potential benefit was being wasted; a move towards a nursing model could make drug trials therapeutic, whether or not the drugs were efficacious, and this could be achieved without invalidating the trial. In fact the change has been found to be positively advantageous, as the drop-out rate through non-compliance has been reduced to about 2%.

Organisation of Clinics

The rheumatology outpatient clinics at the General Infirmary at Leeds are arranged to accommodate physicians and nurses, who are all involved in patient care. Adjoining consulting rooms allow each professional easy access to the other's expertise. As a result of this ease of access patients benefit from the skills of both, working together as professional equals to give a truly integrated system of care.

Patients are initially seen by the physician, who makes his diagnosis and initiates drug treatment. He can then refer the patient to the nurse for one or more of the following reasons:

1. For inclusion in clinical drug trials
2. To monitor for efficacy and side-effects of long-term agents
3. For patient education
4. At the patient's own request

For whichever reasons the patient is referred, the nurse initiates a programme of 'total care'. Each patient is given a series of booked appointments with their nurse. The length of the consultation will vary depending upon the patient's needs, but it is never less than 15 min. For a patient with a chronic disease the opportunity to talk is often the most beneficial treatment that can be prescribed, and this time spent with the patient allows a nurse/patient relationship to develop.

The appointment system also ensures the continuity of care which both patient and staff value highly. Our experience confirms the results of studies made in the United States that the patient enjoys seeing the same person at each visit (Kubala and Clever 1974; Runyan 1975) and feels better able to discuss the more personal aspects of their disease. Continuity also allows nursing staff to plan patient care over a period of time with the certainty that they will be able to set goals and evaluate the care which they have instigated.

In order to foster this trusting/caring relationship the atmosphere during nurse-run clinics is kept as informal as possible. It has been amply demonstrated that patients value open access to the nursing team (Lewis and Resnick 1967; Bystran 1974; Linn 1976), and this we encourage. Patients often telephone whilst clinics are in progress or attend without an appointment. They may simply be seeking advice on, for example, how to take their medications or how to cope with a flare, but sometimes a patient will contact us to clarify a physician's advice. This is not because they feel the advice of the nurse is better, but rather that some patients stand in awe of their physician, or they feel that he is too busy to worry over their small problems. Nurses, on the other hand, appear to many patients as more accessible and approachable. This phenomenon is best illustrated by a phrase freqently used by our patients, 'but I can talk to you'.

Patient Care During Clinical Trials

Much of our work in the outpatient department is devoted to the conduct of clinical trials. The running of these trials is the responsibility of the metrologist, and once a physician has referred a patient for inclusion in a trial he will not see him again until the end of the trial, unless the patient suffers side-effects or specifically requests a consultation with the physician. All the biochemical assessments are initiated and evaluated by the nurse, who can seek medical advice if abnormalities occur.

The conduct of trials is laid down in the trial protocol. Metrologists are involved at an early stage in the formulation of protocols, advising about the clinical measurements, aids to compliance and the design of data collection forms.

The protocol governs the conduct of the trial and is strictly adhered to. One of the parameters that it specifies is the frequency of visits over the trial period, which can vary from 6 weeks to a number of years. These predetermined consultations form the framework around which we build our care plan for each patient, based on the principles of the nursing process. This plan is drawn up using the holistic approach of the nurse practitioner to enable us to give 'total individualised care'. The nursing assessment is not made immediately a patient enters a trial. A delay is necessary for two reasons. First, trials are often very complicated, and patients who are unfamiliar with trial procedures take a while to settle and feel at ease with the routine. Second, this initial period allows time for the nurse/patient relationship to develop and makes a well-founded assessment possible. It is necessary to find out about the physical, social and psychological needs of patients, and to achieve this we gather information about their:

1. Acceptance of the disease
2. Understanding of the disease and its progress
3. Knowledge of the drug regimen
4. Acceptance of the importance of exercise and rest
5. Knowledge of methods of joint protection
6. Social and home conditions
7. Possible sexual problems

From this information patient needs are identified, and, because we have access to the same departments and facilities as our medical colleagues, we are able to refer patients to the other paramedical workers within the multidisciplinary team as necessary. For example, patients with early rheumatoid arthritis are given an exercise pamphlet and then referred to the physiotherapy department for a detailed explanation and assessment. We try to motivate the patients to carry out their exercises daily by teaching them about their disease and its cause and explaining the long-term benefits which they will gain from daily exercise. An appointment is made with the occupational therapist for an ADL assessment and an explanation of methods of joint protection. Referrals can also be made to the medical social worker and dietician, and, if necessary, specialised footwear and aids and appliances can be provided.

Patient education plays a major part in our work. We assess the patients' understanding of the disease and teach them on an individual basis, providing them with booklets and drug sheets as written back-up to our verbal explanation. (A full account of patient education is given in Chap. 7.)

Evaluation of the care and treatment that we give is important; constant re-evaluation is essential as the status of patients suffering from a chronic and potentially crippling disease can alter so slowly that changes may go unnoticed by both patient and nurse.

At the end of a trial the data which has been collected must be analysed. If the trial has been carried out for a pharmaceutical company their own statistician usually analyses the results. When we carry out studies of scientific interest initiated by our own Unit, we are encouraged to analyse the data ourselves. This gives an added overall interest, especially when the statistical proof confirms one's own clinical judgement!

At the end of a trial a patient will sometimes request to stay in our care. Providing that both physician and nurse are in agreement, this is acceptable, but as a safeguard a combined appointment is made, which enables the physician to carry out a medical check-up. Patients can also be referred to us for monitoring when they are treated with one of the proven but more toxic long-term agents such as gold or penicillamine. Because of the slow-acting properties of these drugs patients will need more care and support during the first few months of treatment until the beneficial effects begin to be felt. Close scrutiny of their haematological and biochemical tests is also required to check for efficacy and side-effects. Patients tend to feel 'safer' when monitored by someone whom they know and have come to trust and so will persevere for longer. It is sometimes necessary to refer the patient to the physician for a re-evaluation of their medication. This is discussed with the physician, who must then take the final decision. A patient whose condition is deteriorating may need hospitalisation for intensive physiotherapy or rest, and this can also be arranged at the nurse's request via the physician.

Rheumatology Nurse Practitioner

The spectrum of problems encountered in the treatment of illness is too broad to be encompassed by a single profession. Historically two main professional groupings have evolved, namely medicine and nursing, each complementary but having a distinctly separate function. There has always been an overlap of knowledge between the two professions, and because medicine is a dynamic science the interface between the two is constantly changing. A recent manifestation of this occurred in the 1960s with the emergence in the United States of the nurse practitioner. Her role first become established as a result of the lack of medical facilities in the poorer rural areas, where she serves as a 'pseudo-physician' (MacGuire 1980; Ross 1982). Because of this her training and outlook are closely aligned with that of the medical profession and in the environment in which she works there is no doubt that she fulfils a real need to a very high professional standard. The nurse practitioner role in the United States has since diversified to include specialist nurse practitioners who have moved away from the original medical model back towards their nursing foundations. In the United Kingdom, because of the different health care system and the way in which it is funded, the economic pressures which gave rise to the original physician-type of nurse practitioner have not existed. However, one of the main areas where the nurse practitioner is able to make a major contribution in the United Kingdom is in the treatment of chronic disease. In the chronic diseases the most important elements of treatment are the provision of care, education and support, all of which are major nursing functions, and the medical profession has a smaller part to play than in the acute diseases. Indeed, there is evidence that the supportive nursing approach to chronic illness results in a better outcome for the patient than does the purely medical approach (Stoeckle et al. 1963; Lewis and Resmick 1967; Jordan and Shipp 1971). Our experience in the outpatient clinics at Leeds has demonstrated the value of spending adequate time with patients but has also taught us that, with a deeper understanding of the disease process and of the biochemical and clinical indicators, we can use this time to provide a greatly enhanced standard of patient care.

Detailed knowledge of the disease equips us to carry out some of the following functions of the rheumatology nurse practitioner:

1. Assessing and managing patients suffering from rheumatic disease using the methodology of the nursing process
2. Detecting deviations from the normal course of the disease

3. Educating patients and relatives to enable them to cope with the illness
4. Acting as a knowledgeable source of referral to other members of the multidisciplinary team
5. Interpreting laboratory data
6. Adapting and developing protocols to provide a systematic and safe basis for treatment and referral
7. Acting as professional adviser to both patients and family.

Our job has evolved from that of clinical metrologist towards that of the rheumatology nurse practitioner in response to the needs of our patients. The encouragement that we receive from them indicates that, to a large extent, we are fulfilling those needs. However, we have not yet reached the point where we can regard ourselves as true nurse practitioners because, although we carry out the functions of the nurse practitioner, we cannot practise in our own right. Within our own Unit we act as autonomous practitioners, but all dealings with other departments have to be in the name of our consultant physician. Indeed it is only because of his enlightened attitude that we have been allowed to develop our job along the path that we have.

Future Developments

We believe that the nurse practitioner could be of enormous benefit to patients suffering from a chronic disease, and experience elsewhere supports this view (Stoeckle et al. 1963; Lewis and Resmick 1967; Jordan and Shipp 1971). Nurses given appropriate support from physicians could safely provide much more of the care required by the majority of patients suffering from chronic disease. Evidence suggests that this can be achieved without any lowering of standards (Sackett et al. 1974); indeed, patients who have been cared for by both physicians and nurse practitioners tend to prefer the latter (Lewis and Resmick 1967; Day et al. 1970), are less likely to break appointments (Fink et al. 1969; Charney and Kitzman 1971; Fairweather and Kifulo 1972), and are more likely to comply with their treatment programmes (Chappell and Drogos, 1972; Fairweather and Kifulo 1972).

An essential prerequisite for the development of the role of nurse practitioner in the United Kingdom is that she be recognised as an autonomous professional, able to practise as a nurse in her own right. This would end the unsatisfactory present situation in which most nurse practitioners can function only through the 'patronage' and in the presence of a physician. Before this recognition can be achieved, however, nurse practitioners must prove their ability to practise safely, demonstrate their acceptability to patients and show that they have a unique and valuable contribution to make. In the United States and Canada a number of studies (some of which are referred to above) have shown that, given the appropriate training, a nurse practitioner can practise safely to a high professional standard. Whilst we may be encouraged by their findings, we cannot take them as proof that the nurse practitioner is acceptable in the United Kingdom. Several factors combine to make patients' attitudes to physicians and nurses in the United Kingdom different from those in North America—a different system of nurse education, different social and cultural attitudes and different systems of health care. Consequently, it will be necessary to carry out independent investigations in the United Kingdom along similar lines. This will require greater cooperation among nurses working in this field, particularly with regard to the scientific evaluation of their role and their education and training.

At present in the United Kingdom, because of the lack of a formal training course, the nurse practitioner can obtain education and training only by 'apprenticeship' to a physician and through specialist courses not specifically designed for her. If the role is to develop and be used to its full potential, it will be necessary to provide a period of recognised training, preferably leading to a formal qualification. Unfortunately, this is unlikely to happen until the concept of the nurse practitioner is widely accepted and understood.

Professional Conflicts

The multidisciplinary approach is essential when caring for patients with chronic disease. Because the nurse practitioner will use the 'holistic' approach to care, she will inevitably carry out some tasks which, historically, have been the sole province of other health professionals. Without understanding on all sides, this can lay the foundation for potential professional rivalries which can jeopardise the working of an integrated system of care.

The work of the nurse practitioner includes some management decisions and assessments which are normally regarded as the sole prerogative of the physician. This should not be taken as an attempt to usurp his position. It is only with his scientific knowledge and lengthy training that differential diagnosis and initiation of drug therapy can be safely carried out. The role of the rheumatology nurse practitioner is an extended nursing role, and to be able to manage chronic conditions safely and efficiently she needs access to information and expertise which were formerly thought of as outside the nursing sphere. It is not the undoubted difference in the depth of knowledge that distinguishes physicians from nurses, but rather the way in which each profession uses shared knowledge. For example, a raised ESR to a physician may indicate a flare or that the disease requires stronger drug therapy. The nurse will understand the necessity for the physician's actions, but her priorities will be centred around patient care: Has the patient the knowledge to take adequate rest, protect his joints, carry out passive exercises, does he know how to pace himself, when to take prescribed drugs, use heat and ice etc? It can be seen that the roles of the physician and the nurse are not in rivalry but complement each other to the benefit of the patient.

It is not only doctors that can feel threatened by nurse practitioners but the nursing profession itself. Whether nurses in general accept nurse practitioners as nurses carrying out nursing duties will depend upon their fundamental concept of the profession. A nurse who believes that her function is simply to carry out the instructions of a physician and provide physical comfort to the patient is less likely to accept the nurse practitioner than one who believes in the wider definition expressed by Virginia Henderson in her book entitled, *The Nature of Nursing* (1966)

The unique function of the nurse is to assist the individual, sick or well, in the performance of those activities, contributing to health or its recovery (or to peaceful death), that he would perform unaided had he the necessary strength, will or knowledge. And to do this in such a way as to help him gain independence as rapidly as possible.

If the role of the nurse practitioner is to become established, it has to be recognised by nurses as a nursing role and not that of a pseudo-doctor. This misconception may be perpetuated by the apprenticeship method of training that has to be followed at the moment, and the nurse practitioner herself must be aware of the pitfalls of modelling herself too closely on her medical colleagues.

References

Bird HA (1983) Divided rheumatological care; the advent of the nurse practitioner? Ann Rheum Dis 42: 354–355

Bird HA, Galloway D and Wright V (1980) Clinical metrology—A future career grade? Lancet II: 138–140

Bird HA, Leatham P and le Gallez (1981) Clinical metrology. Nurs Times 77(45): 1926–1927

Bystran SF, Knight CC, Soper MR, Collis PB, Ward Morgan T and Cello JP (1974) An evaluation of nurse practitioners in chronic care clinics. Int J Nurs Stud 11: 185–194

Chappell JA and Drogos PA (1972) Evaluation of infant health care by a nurse practitioner. Pediatrics 49(6): 871–877

Charney E and Kitzman H (1971) The child-health nurse (pediatric nurse practitioner) in private practice: A controlled trial. N Engl J Med 285: 1353–1358

Day LR, Engli R and Silver HK (1970) Acceptance of pediatric nurse practitioners: parent's opinion of combined care by a pediatrician and pediatric nurse practitioner in private practice. Am J Dis Child 119: 204–208

Fairweather JC and Kifulo A (1972) Improvement of patient care in a solo OB-GJN practice using an RN physician's assistant. Am J Public Health 62: 361–363

Fink DL, Greycloud MA, Cohen M, Malloy MJ and Martin F (1969) Improving pediatric ambulatory care. Am J Nurs 69: 316–319

Henderson V (1966) The nature of nursing. Collier-MacMillan, London

Jordan JD and Shipp JC (1971) The primary health care professional was a nurse. Am J Nurs 71(5): 922–925

Kubala S and Clever LH (1974) Acceptance of the nurse practitioner. Am J Nurs 74(3): 451–452

Lewis CE and Resmick BA (1967) Nurse clinics and progressive ambulatory care. N Engl J Med 277: 1236–1241

Linn LS (1976) Patient acceptance of the family nurse practitioner. Med Care 14(4): 357–364

MacGuire JM (1980) The expanded role of the nurse. King's Fund Project Paper. King's Fund, London

Ross F (1982) The American experience. An expanded role. Nurs Times 78: Community Outlook: 301–302

Runyan JW Jr (1975) The Memphis Chronic Disease Program: Comparisons in outcome and the nurse's extended role. JAMA 231: 264–267

Sackett DL, Spitzer WO, Gent M and Roberts RS (1974) The Burlington randomised trial of the nurse practitioners: health outcomes of patients. Ann Intern Med 80: 137–142

Stoeckle JS, Noonan B, Farrisey RM and Sweatt A (1963) Medical nursing clinic for the chronically ill. Am J Nurs 63(7): 87–89

11

Combined Care in the Community

Introduction

In the United Kingdom, out of a population of 55 million, 3 million are impaired to some degree by a rheumatic complaint; of these, 1 million are suffering some degree of handicap (Harris 1971). Of patients between the ages of 50 and 65 years on the handicap register, 25% are suffering from a rheumatic disorder, and amongst the elderly this rises to 40%. The majority of these people will never enter hospital as inpatients but will be treated either as outpatients or as patients in the community. Rheumatic disease does not alter with the patient's environment. Whether the patient is at home or in hospital, the disease process remains unchanged, requiring the same care and treatment. It is not the need for care which alters, but the person who provides it and the place where it is provided.

Ideally, patients in the community would have access to exactly the same skills as they would in hospital, including those of the occupational therapist and physiotherapist, both of whom play a major role in the treatment of rheumatic disease. In practice, the responsibility for treating the majority of patients in the community will fall upon the primary health care team, the patients themselves and their relatives, with the physiotherapist and occupational therapist acting as consultants and advisers. Because of these role interchanges, those providing care in the community have a broader and less specialised role than is customary in hospital, where each professional has a well-defined area of responsibility.

Primary Health Care Team

The concept of the primary health care team came into being in the 1970s. In 1971 a report was published by the Standing Medical Advisory Committee (1971) to help medical and nursing staff organise their multidisciplinary teams in the most effective way. The primary health care team comprises doctors, nurses, health visitors and, in some instances, social workers. Secretarial and reception staff are also invaluable team members. The most successful teams work as professional equals, the leadership of the team changing with the circumstances, personality and needs of the individual patients and families concerned. Some patients need more care from the doctor, whereas in the case of patients with a chronic disabling disease, such as rheumatoid arthritis, the nurse and the social worker will play a more predominant role.

In the care of rheumatic patients, the skills of other health professionals such as physiotherapists and occupational therapists may well be called upon by the team, but resources are limited and few local authorities can afford to employ them in sufficient numbers to visit all patients in need. In these circumstances it falls to members of the primary health care team to acquire the knowledge and skill to rehabilitate immobile and dependent patients and so improve the quality of life for disabled persons and their families.

General Practitioner

Diagnosis is the exclusive province of the physician. The general practitioner will use his medical skills to make a diagnosis and will usually refer the patient to a rheumatologist for confirmation and advice on the management of the disease. Medications are often initiated by the general practitioner before hospital referral but will need to be kept constantly under review. Patients taking the more toxic slow-acting drugs such as gold and penicillamine will need to be carefully monitored for efficacy and side-effects.

Drugs available at present for the treatment of rheumatic disease may alleviate the pain or, at best, slow down the progress of the disease. To date, medical science has failed to find either a cause or a cure. As a result the essence of treatment is the provision of care, the foundation upon which the nursing profession has been built. It is in these circumstances that the primary responsibility for treatment is entrusted to the other members of the primary health care team. This does not mean that the doctor does not have a key role to play, but rather that his role alters to that of coordinator because he, of all members of the primary health care team, has the authority to initiate treatment and has easy access to other health professionals and agencies.

District Nurse

Patient Care

The aims of caring for rheumatic patients living within the community are identical to those of caring for the same patients in hospital, namely that the patients are helped to lead as pain-free, functional and independent a life style as is possible whilst accepting the limitations which their disease imposes upon both themselves and their families.

When a patient suffering from a chronic illness is passed into the care of the district nurse the achievement of these aims can indeed seem a daunting task. Unlike a rheumatic patient in hospital, who will only be there for a limited stay, the patient suffering from a chronic disease in the community will remain a patient until death or until admission to hospital or to an institution.

For patients to maintain their maximum fitness and psychological stability, they will need constant counselling and stimulation, which will require all the nursing team's resources and ingenuity. The most satisfactory approach to caring for these patients is by using the logical problem-solving approach of the nursing process (Crow 1977; Kratz 1979). When caring for patients with chronic illness, changes in their condition can easily be missed as they can take place very slowly. Evaluation is the essential component of the nursing process; it can be the final phase and also a new beginning, either for re-assessment or adjustment of care. Patients suffering from chronic diseases should be re-assessed at frequent intervals.

The district nurse can come into contact with the patient at any stage of the disease process. Patients suffering from rheumatic diseases can be referred to the nurse for a number of reasons, such as the treatment of leg ulcers following steroid therapy or for the administration of gold injections or for help with bathing and dressing. Most of these procedures apply to patients at a later stage of the disease.

Early Stage

District nurses are less likely to have patients referred to them at an early stage in the disease, but a nurse who is knowledgeable about the disease process and its treatment will know that with careful management and teaching of the patients and their families much can be achieved, both physically and psychologically.

The patients are likely to be distressed and confused if their diagnosis has only recently been confirmed. They will have fears for the future for themselves and their families and may harbour feelings of anger and frustration regarding their disease. (These psychological aspects are discussed in Chap. 9.)

The major nursing function at this early stage is to help the patients and their families to accept the diagnosis, whilst also acting as a counsellor and giving support. If the diagnosis has been confirmed in hospital, some teaching about the disease and its treatment and an ADL assessment may have been given, but this will vary according to the attitude of the physician and the time and space available in the clinic. In the Leeds clinics much emphasis is placed on the education of patients and their families as part of their overall treatment. If patient education has been given, as shown in Chapter 7, one of the functions of the district nurse will be to reinforce this teaching. If patient education has not been given, the teaching process should begin as soon as the initial shock has passed and the patient expresses a readiness to learn. Patients and families should be taught about the disease and its treatment. This will include information about the drug regimen, exercises, joint protection, pacing and priorities, how to cope with a flare, diet and some psychology. Teaching does not have to take place formally; indeed, the informal atmosphere of the patient's home can make it an ideal place in which to pass on informtion. When taught correctly, patient education can help to keep the patient independent, aid in compliance and allay much of the fear of the disease. This early contact will also help build a relationship between the nurse and her patient which will be helpful should the disease not abate but continue on its relentless path to the chronic stage.

Later Stage

As the disease progresses and necessitates more potent but toxic therapy, patients are passed into the care of the nursing team for the administration and careful monitoring of their medications. These drugs are given in the hope of controlling the disease but are slow acting and can have severe adverse effects. The most common drugs in current use are gold and penicillamine. Penicillamine is administered orally, whereas gold is given by intramuscular injection by the nursing team. Both drugs take up to 12 weeks before there is any perceptible benefit, and patients will continue to take their NSAIDs and analgesics. Because both penicillamine and gold are slow acting and highly toxic, the nursing team will need to give constant reassurance during this initial period as to their eventual efficacy and safety or patients will lose faith and may become non-compliant.

Before each gold injection is given patients should be asked if they have experienced itching or skin rash, and urine should be tested for blood and proteinuria. Treatment should be withheld until advice has been sought from the doctor if any of these symptoms are present. Patients on penicillamine should test their urine weekly. Patients on either drug should have a venous blood sample taken every 6 weeks, as bone marrow suppression leading to thrombocytopenia or leucopenia can occur. Patients should be advised to consult their doctor if they experience influenza-like symptoms accompanied by a sore throat, as these can be the first signs of a severe blood dyscrasia.

Care of the Feet

A common reason for referral to the district nurse is for treatment of leg ulcers which have occurred as a result of steroid therapy. These ulcers are usually slow to heal and can require many visits, which provide an ideal opportunity to assess patients' needs and form a good nurse/patient relationship. When dressing a leg ulcer it is a good idea to ask patients to remove their shoes and stockings, thus giving an excellent opportunity to check their feet. The services of a chiropodist can be invaluable to rheumatic patients. They often have problems with the formation of callosities beneath the metatarsal heads, which can make walking on what are already painful and deformed feet even more difficult; in extreme cases this can cause the patient to become chairbound. Some patients are unable to reach their feet to cut their toenails because of hip or knee involvement; even if they can, scissors can be very difficult to manipulate if there is muscle weakness or deformities of the hands. When replacing the patient's shoes a check should be made that they are of sensible design and are well fitting. Shoes in a poor state of repair with loose soles or fraying laces can be very dangerous.

Personal Hygiene

The district nurse is often required to assist patients who have difficulty in carrying out their personal toilet. By this stage the patient is either walking with difficulty with the use of an aid or is bedridden. If the patient uses an aid to walk, carpets and rugs should be checked for fraying edges and curled corners as a fall could be disastrous. If the patient is still capable of using the bath, handrails should be checked, and a non-slip mat is essential. Bath-seats and planks can be of considerable help to patients who are unable to sit low down in the bath or who experience difficulty when getting out. For patients unable to get into the bath manually a special seat or hoist can be provided which can be raised and then placed into the bath. Unfortunately, not all bathrooms are large enough to accommodate this facility but it can be a great boon to some patients. Showers can be very useful, and patients can sit on a plastic chair if unable to stand. However, many older patients prefer their bath, and many houses do not have showers installed. If patients are confined to bed at any stage, bed bathing is indicated. Patients must be encouraged to help themselves as far as it is possible, and their relatives will need to be taught how to carry out this procedure. Some patients find it embarrassing to be washed by their relatives, and their feelings should be respected.

If a patient is confined to bed the importance of positioning of limbs and avoidance of contractures must be stressed. Resting splints may be necessary, and patients will need to be encouraged to use them as they can be very uncomfortable to begin with.

In the past, steroid therapy was prescribed for many rheumatic patients, and so many now have fragile skin. Pressure sores can develop very quickly but may take months to heal; this is a definite case of prevention being better than cure. Lightweight covers and the use of a bed cradle will enable patients to move about the bed more easily and so help to avoid pressure sores and prevent stiffness.

Unlike hospital beds, the patient's own bed is likely to be very low and may cause unnecessary back strain for either the nurse or relatives. Blocks can be placed under the bed to raise it to a more useful level for bending and lifting. The patient's relatives must be taught how to lift correctly and so not endanger their own health and cause discomfort to the patient. Patients suffering from rheumatoid arthritis must be encouraged to become ambulant as soon as their physical condition allows, as enforced bed rest can cause them much pain and stiffness and contractures can occur.

Family Care

The patient is usually a member of a family. The district nurse is responsible for their care as well as that of the patient, and so the family wellbeing must be taken into account when treatment is planned. Many families can cope well with short-term illness that lasts for only a few weeks, but chronic diseases may carry on for years. This can lead to stress within the family unit, as caring for loved ones for a long period is very tiring both mentally and physically, especially if the relatives responsible have their own families of small children or are in full-time employment. In these circumstances short-term admission to hospital can give useful respite to the family as well as the patient.

Nursing care is ultimately the responsibility of the nurse, but it is not possible for the district nurse to give all the care needed herself. The family and the patient will need to be taught basic skills, such as lifting and bathing, in the correct manner to avoid causing injury to themselves and discomfort to the patient. If relatives are carrying out caring tasks then it is important that they are involved at the planning and decision-making stage of care. At times this can be frustrating for the nurse, particularly if the patient is less than cooperative or has an overprotective family.

Health Visitor

The health visitor is part of the primary health care team and can play a very important role in the care of the patient and the family. Health visitors are qualified nurses who have received a specialist training in preventive health care. Traditionally their primary responsibility has been preventive care and the assessment of children aged 5 years and under. Some health visitors feel that the care of the family as a whole is a more satisfactory method of practising preventive health care, and other health visitors are beginning to specialise in the care of the elderly. A chronic disabling disease such as rheumatoid arthritis places much more stress on the family infrastructure, necessitating changes in both attitude and aspiration of all close members of the family. The health visitor is trained to perceive stressful situations within the family and to act as counsellor and adviser on family health and associated welfare problems. The patient may be a child, and if this is the case the local education authority will be notified by the health visitor, who will also put the parents in contact with the appropriate voluntary bodies. She will continue to monitor the progress of the child and the child's family by giving advice and support and helping them adjust to new situations as they arise. Some health visitors act as liaison between hospital and home or vice versa. The health visitor can follow patients from hospital to community, ensuring that a planned programme of care initiated in hospital is continued when the patient arrives home.

Social Worker

Social workers are employed by local authorities and can be based in hospitals, community health centres, social services departments or attached to general practitioners' practices, where they form part of the primary health care team. Rheumatoid arthritis, in common with many other chronic diseases, is unpredictable in its course. The uncertainty this produces, when added to the enormous mental and physical re-adjustments required for coping with the chronic disease, generates stress not only for the patient but also for the immediate family. It is the task of the social worker to help patients (or clients) to cope with their social, domestic, financial and emotional problems, all of which are experienced to a greater or lesser degree by rheumatic patients. They are experts in the field of statutory services, benefits and allowances and have a wide knowledge of the availability and location of the voluntary services. The social worker can be a valuable liaison officer and patient advocate within the social services department itself.

Physiotherapist and Occupational Therapist

Physiotherapy and occupational therapy play a large part in the integrated treatment of rheumatic diseases (see Chap. 6). When patients are lucky enough to be admitted to hospital they will be referred to the appropriate departments and will doubtless receive excellent and beneficial care. Unfortunately, the care available in the community falls far short of this hospital Utopia because of inadequate funding, difficulty of access to hospital facilities or lack of communication. Even when access is available a proportion of patients are unable to take advantage of it because of their immobility, or simply because they are too ill to withstand a long and painful journey. Another factor is that rheumatic patients, probably because of their chronic condition, are reluctant to keep asking for help.

The traditional and still the most common source of access to physio-therapy or occupational therapy is referral by a hospital physician to a hospital department. This is a slow process, with the general practitioner having to refer the patient to a hospital consultant, who in turn refers him to the appropriate department. By this time the patient may well have seized up or caused immeasurable damage to their joints. Only a small number of direct or open-access schemes are currently available, but their services can be a great boon to the primary health care team and the patient. They allow the general practitioner to refer the patient directly to the department concerned making it a much quicker access route than the two-stage traditional method. Some hospitals hold special evening clinics for patients referred directly from the community, and these are invaluable for patients in full-time employment. Many schemes accept referrals from any member of the primary health care team or even from the patients or their relatives. Physiotherapists are sometimes employed to hold clinics in local health centres in conjunction with general practitioners. They treat acute cases which are referred directly from the general practitioner's clinic. Because treatment is immediately available when this system is used, patients need less treatment than if an equivalent condition is treated in hospital.

Domiciliary Remedial Therapists

Therapists working within the community can be employed by the local authority or the NHS. Whichever authority employs them there is no doubt that they can save time and money by either helping to keep patients out of hospital or enabling earlier discharge.

Domiciliary Physiotherapist

Physiotherapists are trained in hospital departments and very little formal training is given to staff working in the relatively new domiciliary service. To be successful in the community, the physiotherapist must be an innovator and have more than her fair share of commonsense. In the community, along with all other health professionals, the physiotherapist is a guest in the patient's home and will soon come to realise that not all her recommendations, such as re-positioning of furniture or the acquisition of a firmer mattress, will be accepted with heartfelt thanks!

Many hospital physiotherapy departments are packed with fearsome-looking equipment most of which would be impossible to use in the patient's home. Items which are of use are portable heatlamps, ice packs, hot packs and ultrasound machines.

The primary aims of the physiotherapist working in the community are the same as those of a physiotherapist working within the hospital:

1. Reduction of pain
2. Restoration of maximum function
3. Correction and prevention of deformities
4. Improvement of muscular power

The community physiotherapist will need to spend a greater proportion of her time teaching and motivating the patient and relatives than does her hospital counterpart. She will define the goals to be reached and explain the part that she and they will be expected to play in achieving these goals. It is important to set realistic achievable goals, and the aims of treatment should be made clear at the outset so that when the aims are met there is a feeling of success. Unfortunately, when treating rheumatic patients a successful outcome cannot be final because of the progressive nature of the disease, and so re-assessment will inevitably be necessary.

One of the major problems facing domiciliary physiotherapists can be the professional isolation which it can impose. This can be alleviated by making herself aware of the other professional agencies which are available for her to call upon and to communicate frequently with members of the primary health care team.

Domiciliary care can prove to be a major challenge to a physiotherapist, but its rewards can be very satisfying indeed.

Domiciliary Occupational Therapist

The occupational therapist plays a major role in the care of rheumatic patients. She helps the patient with physical disability to bridge the gap which appears when environmental needs outstrip physical capabilities. She does this by providing aids and appliances where necessary, adapting existing equipment and clothing and by teaching the patient how to use personal resources more effectively. She will also advise the patient on joint protection and is skilled in the making of splints (see Chap. 6. p. 168). It may be necessary to advise about re-housing if the existing home is considered unadaptable or unsuitable for the patient's needs. The domiciliary occupational therapist is in a unique position as the ideal place to see a patient's needs is in their home environment. Often patients are given aids whilst they are in hospital which prove to be ineffectual when they try to use them at home. This is less likely to happen when a domiciliary occupational therapist is in attendence or when the hospital occupational therapist has made a home visit. As with physiotherapy, re-assessment is invaluable, as splints or aids provided today will be useless in 5 years' time.

Future Developments

A very small percentage of primary health care teams now include a physiotherapist and an occupational therapist. With a growing aged population and the increasing emphasis now being placed on care in the community, the inclusion of remedial therapists as members of the primary health care team is the next logical step in the development of community care. The number of patients will always outstrip the number of therapists available, and so the emphasis on who gives the treatment may have to be changed. Relatives can be taught to carry out simple procedures under the supervision of the therapists, and this innovation may become increasingly commonplace.

Disablement Resettlement Officer

As patients become more severely handicapped by their disease it may become necessary for them to find more suitable employment. The services of a disablement resettlement officer (DRO) can be invaluable in this situation.

DROs are employed by the Manpower Services Commission and usually work from Jobcentres. Their aim is to help disabled persons to find a job in which they can reach their maximum employment potential following illness or injury. They will give the patient guidance and advice on further training and assistance with aids necessary to help them at work.

Employers are asked to employ one registered disabled person per 20 employees, and DROs usually supervise this quota scheme. DROs can also recommend that a patient attends an employment rehabilitation centre (ERC) for further assessment or vocational guidance. There are 26 ERCs in the United Kingdom and about 13 000 people benefit from their rehabilitation courses each year.

Sexual Difficulties

Many patients suffering from rheumatic diseases experience sexual difficulties. These may be due to physical discomfort or painful joints or the inability of either partner to adjust to the loss of body image. Whatever the reason for sexual difficulty, the opportunity to talk about it can be a great help. Patients can feel too embarrassed to bring up the subject of sexual intercourse, but many arthritic patients find that their disease interferes with their sexual lives but not their sexual needs. However, it should not be assumed that sexual activity is important to all patients, and they must be allowed to express their true feelings. The important factor is to introduce the subject of sexuality and if the patient wishes they will seek further advice. It is important to be able to give advice in an uncritical manner when a patient asks a question. This is often accepted by the patient not just as information but as permission to experiment with behaviour which previously they would have thought unacceptable. There are many books and leaflets published on the subject of sexual activity and the disabled or chronically ill (see Appendix C). The ARC has produced a leaflet which can be useful. Wendy Greengross has written an excellent book called *Entitled to Love*. It is written with great sensitivity but is sensible and practical and should be read by those who are disabled and those caring for them. SPOD (Sexual Problems of the Disabled) is an advisory organisation which was established in 1973 under the auspices of the National Fund for Research into Crippling Diseases. Its officers will provide general information either by information sheets or in correspondence about specific sexual problems. Although they are unable to offer counselling help, the Disabled Living Foundation has on display a selection of aids and prostheses.

In addition, the Family Planning Association (FPA) will help with advice as well as prescribing contraceptives free of charge. It does not deal solely with contraception and will provide a reading list on request, which includes many aspects of family life. The FPA also publish a series of fact sheets, including one entitled, *Sex Education for Handicapped People*.

Rheumatoid arthritis can have a devastating effect on a marriage. In a survey carried out in Leeds and Harrogate of young married women with rheumatoid arthritis, it was found that those couples who were aware of the disease before marriage were more able to cope than those where the disease developed after marriage (Wright and Owen 1976). The aim of the National Marriage Guidance Council is to provide a confidential counselling service to couples experiencing difficulties in their marital and family relationships. They also provide a reading list related to marriage and family life.

Social Services Department

The Chronically Sick and Disabled Persons Act 1970 made it the responsibility of local authorities to keep themselves informed of the number of disabled persons living in their locality and to provide help and assistance for them. Local authorities must satisfy themselves, by their own criteria, that the help requested is necessary. In addition to the employment of social workers, the local social services department makes available a wide range of services to the community. In the rehabilitation of patients suffering from rheumatic diseases many of these services may be essential to a satisfactory outcome. Community support systems such as the provision of home helps, Meals on Wheels, hoists, aids, the installation of equipment and adaptations to existing fitments are all the responsibility of this department. Patients are asked to make a financial contribution to the cost of some of these facilities, the amount depending upon their income.

Residential and day care centres, where a physiotherapist may be in attendance, are also provided by the social services department. Day centres with this facility may well help to keep a patient mobile and able to live within the community instead of filling a hospital bed.

Mobility and Independence

Of all the losses which a rheumatic patient endures during the course of the disease the loss of independence is the one most feared, for with it comes loss of self-esteem and dignity, which to many patients is intolerable. Mobility is vital to independence, and so any re-training equipment or transport which can be supplied to maintain mobility must be regarded as essential.

The functions performed by the hands and arms are far more complex and difficult to substitute artificially than those of the legs. Therefore, when planning long-term care, it is important to preserve the functions of the upper limbs, if necessary at the expense of the lower. Unfortunately, to the majority of patients mobility means the ability to walk; many struggle to continue walking for too long, using methods which are to the long-term detriment of the upper limbs. Consequently, when selecting walking aids, it is important to consider the possible long-term effects on the joints of the upper limbs as well as the short-term improvement in walking ability.

A minority of patients become so severely disabled that the use of a wheelchair becomes necessary. Wheelchairs are supplied from the local aids and appliance centre on either short- or long-term loan. Electrically powered chairs can be made available for patients who are unable to propel themselves. The type of wheelchair needed will depend upon the individual's physical requirements and where it is to be used. However, the provision of a wheelchair will not aid mobility unless the patient is able to use it. Most houses are designed for healthy walking adults and are likely to require adaptation. These adaptations will range from the provision of simple ramps in place of steps to the widening of doorways or the complete re-designing of kitchens and bathrooms.

Loneliness, depression and financial hardship can result from being confined to the home. Public transport is very often useless to the severe arthritic who cannot walk, stand for long periods or negotiate the high step of a bus. These difficulties make working or shopping almost impossible for some patients, and personal transport then becomes an essential aid to independence. Financial help is available in the form of a Mobility Allowance (see Appendix C). To qualify, the patient must be unable or virtually unable to walk and be between the ages of 5 and 60 years. Modifications to the patient's own car may be possible. Personnel from the Artificial Limb and Appliance Centre (ALAC) undertake to make assessments for motorised transport.

Communication

Continuity of care is essential in the rehabilitation of a patient, and this cannot be achieved without effective communication by all who are involved in the programme. If a patient is discharged from hospital without effective hospital/community liaison the gains made whilst in hospital can be lost very rapidly. Hospital/community liaison is often a responsibility of a nurse/health visitor, who will inform hospital staff of the patient's environmental and social conditions on admission and then ensure that the home environment is suitable when the patient is ready for discharge. She will also enlist the help of the primary health care team and support services so that when the patient returns home rehabilitation can continue effectively.

When a patient is admitted to hospital as much information as possible should be given in the admission letter. In addition to current and past diagnoses this should include details of medication, social and family support services, and appliances and adaptations already provided. Upon discharge from hospital the discharge summary should include medical information, such as alteration in drug regimens, and an outline of the programme initiated by the remedial therapists, stating progress and future goals. A list of any aids or appliances provided or support groups contacted is also useful. The discharge summary should be sent to the general practitioner or members of the primary health care team immediately upon the patient's discharge, enabling them to visit as soon as possible. This will relieve some of the anxiety and give reassurance to the patient and the patient's family and ensure continuity of care.

Communication between members of the primary health care team is important. Combined meetings are useful to discuss individual cases and allow teams to define their roles in relation to each patient. Ineffectual communication, either written or verbal, can lead to misunderstanding. Meaningful case histories can be compiled by combining accurate well-written reports to provide an overall picture of the patient's problems. From this an integrated care plan can be formulated and the care given can then be evaluated by all members of the team.

Good communication between the patient and members of the health care team is essential, as the information gathered from the patient is the basis on which the health care plan will be formulated. If communication is poor at the outset, the care plan may bear little relationship to the patient's needs and expectations. The health professionals will need to impart a realistic view of what is achievable and of what part the patient is expected to play in treatment, so that the patient's needs and expectations can be fulfilled as far as possible.

Conclusion

There are large numbers of people living in the community who are suffering from a rheumatic disease. To care for them adequately we require an integrated and comprehensive rehabilitation service which is accessible to all those in need.

When defining rehabilitation of the disabled and chronically sick, the World Health Organisation (1969) states, 'as applied to disability this [rehabilitation] is a combined and co-ordinated use of medical, social, educational and vocational measures for training and re-training the individual to the highest possible level of functional ability'. If these high standards for our rheumatic patients in the community are to be attained, it will be necessary for the primary health care team to engage the assistance of physiotherapists, occupational therapists, DROs and social services and enlist the help of the voluntary organisations.

For rehabilitation to be successful and enduring it is essential that there is continuity of care and good communication between all concerned parties.

No matter how excellent the services available, they are useless to a patient who is unaware of their existence. It is the responsibility of health professionals to assess patient's needs and ensure that they have the benefit of all of the available resources so that they may fulfil their maximum potential and independence.

Lord Amulree coined the phrase, 'adding life to years'. If the members of the primary health care team can come even close to this definition of rehabilitation, then their aims will indeed have been achieved.

References

Crow J (1977a) The nursing process—1: theoretical background. Nurs Times 73 (16 June): 892–896

Crow J (1977b) The nursing process—2; how and why to take a nursing history. Nurs Times 73 (23 June): 950–957

Crow J (1977c) The nursing process—3: a nursing history questionnaire for two patients. Nurs Times 73 (30 June): 978–982 (see also pp 983–944 for Care Studies and centre pages for Care Plans)

Kratz C (ed) (1979) The nursing process. Baillière Tindall, London

Standing Medical Advisory Committee (1971) The organisation of group practice. A report of a subcommittee of the Standing Medical Advisory Committee. HMSO, London

World Health Organisation (1969) Expert Committee on Medical Rehabilitation. Second Report. World Health Organisation, Geneva

Wright V and Owen S (1976) The effect of RA on the social situation of housewives. Rheum Rehab 15: 156

12
Clinical Research and Trial Methodology

Introduction

This chapter introduces nurses, physiotherapists and occupational therapists to some basic research techniques in the hope that they will be encouraged to make critical evaluations of some time-honoured practices. Only a small number of projects to which research techniques might be applied can be discussed here, and the interested reader should refer elsewhere for more detail (Clark and Hockey 1979).

General Aspects of Research

The first principle in conducting research is to decide upon and define the question which is to be answered. Ideally the researcher may have started from a simple clinical observation or impression in one patient. He or she is likely to collect more such observations, and once the observation has been made on a group of three or four patients, this will form a small uncontrolled series. At this point the researcher will perhaps formulate a hypothesis as to why this unexpected observation might have occurred. Having done this, the researcher will then go on to design a prospective controlled study that will clarify beyond all doubt whether the hypothesis is correct. As a result, the hypothesis may be unproven, which constitutes a negative finding, or may be proven, which constitutes a positive finding. The latter is always more valuable and of more interest than the former. If a positive finding is confirmed, this represents a genuine advance for medical science and may have important practical applications in dictating modified forms of treatment. Alternatively, it may be a more fundamental question that has been answered that will simply be a link in a chain leading to further hypotheses and further advance of knowledge.

This attractive and logical sequence of events is rarely enacted in its entirety in clinical medicine. Every investigator knows the experience of having chanced upon an astounding clinical observation in one isolated patient only to find that the observation is not substantiated in the following two or three similar patients. Alternatively, the investigator may be thrilled to have a finding substantiated by the collection of a personal series, only to discover that the finding has already been noted in the literature some 10 or 20 years earlier. Although investigators may be familiar with the medical literature of their own country and that of other key countries such as the United States, Canada and Australia, all of them English speaking, they may be ignorant of the equally large literature that emanates from Eastern Europe and Japan. This is not always easily available (except through translations in comprehensive university libraries). Previous publication in the literature should not necessarily deter the investigator. If the purpose of the research work is to gain a diploma or to provide evidence of the ability to conduct original research for a postgraduate nursing qualification or a 1-year higher degree, an unoriginal finding may well suffice. However, the intending author should not be disappointed if his subsequent report of the research is rejected for publication by eminent medical or nursing journals, the editors of which will be well acquainted with the precise world expert who can indicate where such findings have previously been published.

As already stated, a positive finding is always of more value than a negative finding. Prospective studies (those that are planned in advance and which require a wait of a period of time before the conclusion can be reached) are always of more value than retrospective studies (which are based on a search through past literature or case notes and are thus dependent upon the ability to make observations on the part of a large number of people unconnected with the research project). Controlled trials are usually of more value than uncontrolled trials. In a controlled trial the treatment under investigation is formally tested against a placebo or apparently exactly similar treatment that lacks the active principle or crucial variable. Only in this way can it be verified that improvement is actually due to the treatment under investigation and not caused by 'placebo' effect (i.e. the patient deriving benefit through psychological factors linked to the administration of the treatment or the extra care engendered by its administration).

Planning the Study—Questions to be Asked

Biological research is more difficult than any other form. There are many variables inherent in living beings, particularly those who are diseased, and research studies to test hypotheses involve the use of more compromise than in other branches of science. In rheumatic disease in particular, the cyclical variation is disease activity that often occurs requires a background knowledge of the variables to be measured in the untreated disease.

It is very important to define the problem under investigation and make certain that the proposed study will be relevant. A literature search may be necessary to determine what is already known about the problem, and a local librarian may be of assistance. The proposed study should contribute to knowledge and understanding and not be a waste of time and energy, either because it is ill-planned or because it has been done before.

Some investigators favour the use of a pilot study before the main study, but in our experience these are unsatisfactory and, although at first sight representing economy of resources, may fail to answer questions because they are inadequate in scope and planning and thus ultimately waste resources.

A controlled study in which the treatment (e.g. drug)· that may be efficacious is compared to a placebo is always preferable. The study may be designed as single (observer) blind, single (patient) blind or double blind. In a single (observer)-blind study the observer is unaware of the treatment received by the patient until the code is broken, but the patient, possibly because the drug has distinctive appearance, cannot be kept in the dark. In a single (patient)-blind study the patient will be unaware whether they are receiving the active drug or a placebo, since both types of treatment (usually a tablet or capsule) will have identical appearance. In a double-blind study the patient will be unaware of the identity of the medication, be it active ingredient or placebo, and the observer will also be unaware whether each patient is receiving active drug or placebo until the study is completed and the code to the study is broken prior to analysis of results. This last design is by far the most satisfactory since it prevents patients deriving a strong placebo effect from any therapy, and also eliminates possible bias on the part of researchers, who may have a vested interest in trying to prove that their particular favoured treatment is efficacious. The same principles apply to the evaluation of other treatments, for example local applications for ulcers or mechanical methods of physiotherapy.

Thought must be given to the study population; this should be carefully defined with adequate exclusion criteria and inclusion criteria, both for subjects and controls. If a sample is taken it should be representative of the whole population.

Most nurses undertaking research are likely to be working by themselves, and their studies will therefore be termed 'single-centre'. However, nurses working in different hospitals may collaborate to produce a 'multicentre' study, particularly if a quick answer is required or if, as is usually the case, a single nurse working in a single hospital cannot produce enough clinical material to answer the question posed in the protocol. Although the advantages of multicentre studies include speed of execution and greater clinical material, there are many disadvantages. Normally, multicentre studies involve a large number of observers (unless a single nurse acting as observer can visit all the centres in rotation), and there may be variation in the way in which different nurses notice and record findings, thus producing a significant 'inter'-observer error. In some trials the inter-observer error may be so large as to completely engulf the modest improvement that is produced by the treatment under question. Single-centre studies are therefore preferable whenever possible, but observers should also be aware that their own observations may alter week by week, producing an 'intra'-observer error. Multicentre studies may require laboratory assessment in addition to clinical observation. Although these are more reproducible with less variation than findings recorded by observers, there may still be quite different normal ranges for even routine variables produced by different laboratories. This inter-laboratory variation needs to be determined and considered in planning the study.

Careful thought should be given to the measurements made. Frequently the measurements taken lack relevance to the study being performed. Although routine measurements of range of movement at the hip and knee are often requested in trials of NSAIDs in osteoarthrosis of the hip and knee joints, our own experiences suggests that they add little to the overall evaluation of the drugs and can often be omitted. Measurements made should be reliable, specific (i.e. they cannot be produced by factors other than those under investigation) and sensitive (i.e. they should be accurate measurements of the changes involved). Consideration should also be given to how the data will be processed and analysed. The investigator may be responsible for this, or may need to invoke the help of a professional statistician or mathematician.

If the research involves patients, particularly if it includes an invasive procedure, such as injections, approval of a local ethical committee may be required. Ethical committees protect the patients and, in so doing, protect the investigator. The majority contain members well experienced in research techniques who can draw the attention of the investigator to any deficiencies or pitfalls in the protocol or study design. Independent members of the ethics committee will consider whether the treatment to be evaluated may represent a true advance and whether its testing constitutes too great a risk to the patient. All projects, not just those involving drugs, should be referred to ethics committees. The ethics committee may want details of what will happen to patients on completion of the study—as in the following hypothetical example: A comparative study of a new drug for rheumatoid arthritis shows it to be more effective than all earlier existing therapies. Clearly those patients who were allocated by chancce to receive the drug will clamour to have the treatment continued; it may be considered unethical to withdraw supplies from them at the end of the study. Equally, the other half of the patients in the study who were unlucky enough to draw the less satisfactory treatment will want access to the new drug. Adequate supplies should be available. In addition, the ethics committee may want to know that the investigator has provided adequate safeguards to detect possible side-effects that might occur as a result of treatment and that all patients can be speedily recalled for the withdrawal of therapy in the unlikely event that this becomes necessary. Some ethics committees may insist upon the preservation of confidentiality for the medical detail of patients who fall under their jurisdiction; however, too strict attention to confidentiality sometimes makes patient recall more difficult, and patient safety may be compromised (if, for example, an investigator leaves the area).

Finally the anticipated timetable and cost of the study should be considered. There is little point in embarking on a study estimated to be of 2 years' duration if the principal investigator is likely to leave the area for a new appointment after only 1 year.

Statistical Aspects

It may be wise to take advice from a statistician before starting to write a protocol. Once a hypothesis has been established, attention must be given to ensuring that the study group size is adequate enough to provide an answer. Formulae are available for guarding against a type I error (concluding erroneously that the difference between treatments is larger than it actually is) and a type II error (concluding that a specified real difference does not exist). Fuller accounts of these are to be found elsewhere (May 1976; Bird and Wright 1982).

Attention should also be given to the statistical analysis of results of the trial. The statistical test used may depend on whether the variable measured is spread across an even distribution or non-even (skewed) distribution. The former requires a parametric statistical test (such as the Student t test) to evaluate significance between the means of two populations. If comparison requires a non-parametric test (such as the Wilcoxon Rank Sum Test) to evaluate significance between the means of two populations. If comparison between two sets of groups of data is required the Chi square test will be used. Full details of these are available elsewhere (Bradford Hill 1971; Swinscow 1976).

The Protocol

Writing the protocol provides an important first step. Many experienced investigators may be tempted to bypass this important stage. If they do so their study is more likely to contain basic errors of design and execution, and, since compilation of the final study report is a close approximation to the writing of the original protocol, it makes sense to direct time to this basic planning at the earliest possible stage.

Introduction

The ideal protocol is likely to start with a short introduction outlining the background to the study, explaining why it is important to perform it, and giving literature references to occasions on which similar studies have been performed in the past. In the case of a trial designed to evaluate a piece of physiotherapy equipment, brief details of the rationale behind the design of such a machine are likely to be included here. For a trial involving a nursing procedure (e.g. a new dressing), details of the new treatment, its manufacture and its anticipated advantages over existing methods should be stated. Any previous uses should also be cited, together with details of its anticipated problems.

The protocol should then state the basic aim of the study in clear unambiguous terms. At this stage it may be advisable to summarise how the outcome of the study is going to be determined. This may be by simple clinical assessment (see Chap. 8.) in the case of a drug, or may be by a health questionnaire, completed by the patient at the end of the study, in the case of an occupational therapy manoeuvre that may or may not improve the quality of the patient's subsequent life.

Study Design

The protocol will then give a brief summary of the study design. In parallel group design half the patients are allocated at random to one treatment and the other half to the second treatment. Patients receive their treatment for the whole duration of the study, and assessments are made at the start, possibly at serial intervals throughout the study and at the end of the treatment period. This method assumes that both groups of patients to be studied are comparable at the start of the study. The random allocation should ensure this, but the statistician will want to check that in fact both groups were comparable in terms of age, numbers of men and women, disease of similar duration and similar previous therapy. In order to avoid this risk of mismatch of the two groups, some investigators will opt for a crossover design. In this type of study all patients receive both the treatments being compared. Half the patients are allocated at random to treatment A and the other half to treatment B. After an appropriate period of time (long enough for the treatment to be judged efficacious or not) patients who receive treatment A switch to treatment B and those who receive treatment B switch to treatment A, and both groups proceed for an equal length of time to the end of the study. Assessments are made at the start of the study, just prior to the changeover of therapy and at the end of the study. Since all patients receive both treatments the patients act 'as their own controls', but a major drawback of this study is that there must be no interaction between the two treatments. In general, this is true for short-acting drugs in the rheumatic diseases, but one could never finally exclude the possibility that treatment B, for example, only works if treatment A has been given first. On this basis there may be a 'carryover effect' of the first treatment into the second treatment period thus biasing the results recorded during and at the end of the second treatment period.

A further consideration may be the length of the study. Much can be said in favour of studies that do not exceed 6 months in duration, since patient (and investigator) interest wains after this time. If the therapeutic effect of a drug, as in the case of penicillamine, is not observed for 2–3 months, the 6-month trial period may be essential, and here a parallel group study is clearly preferable. Otherwise, our own preference would be for a crossover study design, both treatment periods being accommodated within the 3 or 6 months of the study; this method also has the advantage that smaller numbers of patients are required in the final statistical analysis, and so the study may not be so large as with the parallel group design.

Randomisation

Randomisation of patients between the two treatment groups is clearly essential, and randomisation tables should be used. These are to be found in all good statistical textbooks. As already discussed, the study may be double blind (the best), single (observer) blind or single (patient) blind. Double-blind study design is complex and may create expense. For example, if a tablet is being tested, identical 'placebo' tablets which look and smell the same but do not contain the active drug are required. In the case of a study on physiotherapy equipment, a period of time with the machine connected to the patient but the machine not switched on would be required, with the patient under the impression that active treatment is being given. In the case of an assessment of a topically applied healing agent, bandages soaked in the new agent might be compared to bandages soaked in saline.

Number of Patients Required

Statistical advice on the avoidance of type I and II errors may be taken. This will have to be balanced against local factors in deciding the number of patients that any one individual working from a single centre can provide. A parallel goup design is likely to need more patients than a crossover design.

Inclusion Criteria

The inclusion criteria must be carefully set out, starting with a list of an adequate number of features to ensure that patients with only a single disease are entered into the study. For patients with rheumatoid arthritis the American Rheumatism Association (ARA) criteria may be stipulated so that only patients having either classic or definite rheumatoid arthritis are included. The ARA criteria are an amalgam of clinical and laboratory features, but a positive rheumatoid factor is not necessarily a prerequisite for entry. For a study in osteoarthrosis, radiological criteria may be selected in addition to clinical signs, and such a study may be restricted to patients with osteoarthrosis of a particular joint, for example the knee, the hip, or both the knee and the hip. The inclusion criteria will also state whether both males and females are to be studied and the age range throughout which it is proposed to study patients. The purpose of these criteria is to ensure that the population group being assessed is as homogeneous as possible. Studies using radioactive compounds or radioactive investigational procedures may be restricted to post-menopausal females and males over the age of 50 years.

Exclusion Criteria

The exclusion criteria should then be stated. Some of these may reflect the desire to ensure that all patients entering the study have a single disease. Thus in a study to evaluate a drug in osteoarthrosis, a high serum uric acid level or a previous history of gout may be an exclusion criteria, since this disease may be hard to distinguish radiologically from osteoarthrosis. In a study on rheumatoid arthritis, patients who have clinical or radiological evidence of ankylosing spondylitis may similarly be excluded. In drug studies, exclusion criteria may be applicable to the drug under test. If the drug is aspirin or a relative of aspirin, patients who have previously developed hypersensitivity to this drug or side-effects following its use may also be excluded. If the drug is potent in inducing ulcers, patients with existing duodenal ulcer or a previous history of duodenal ulcer may be excluded. If the drug is suspected of causing adverse liver or kidney effects (or if the toxicological testing of the drug has not yet been adequate to confirm whether these might occur), patients with pre-existing liver or kidney disease are likely to be excluded from the protocol. In addition, patients with neoplasm or significant other diseases may also be excluded. If the drug is suspected of being teratogenic or if adequate teratogenic studies have not been performed, pregnant females or females of childbearing age will be excluded from the study. Patients who are deaf, blind or dumb will have difficulty in completing clinical assessments and are therefore excluded. If a questionnaire is to be used, illiterate patients may also be excluded from the study, unless they can be interviewed.

Treatment Regimens

The treatment to be given must be fully described and the drug dosage, frequency or specific instructions stated. If the study is designed to evaluate a new style of bandage, a complete description of the bandaging and the period of its use should be included. The treatment time should be long enough to ensure that the desired effect could be achieved.

Clinic Visits

The number of clinic visits and the duration of the study is then stated. This depends upon the duration of action of the treatment, the time course over which it might become effective and the speed with which the improvement first occurs. A treatment that has toxic side-effects is likely to be evaluated in more frequent clinic visits than a long-standing treatment that is safe.

Assessments

The protocol should next list the assessments that are going to be performed. (These are comprehensively covered in Chap. 8.) The selection of assessments appropriate to the particular disease under study and its possible response to the drug under study will be incorporated in the protocol. The baseline assessment is clearly essential. Many studies take baseline assessment both immediately prior to starting therapy and either 1 or 2 weeks before this time so that the intrinsic variability of the assessments in a particular patient can be determined. This is of value to clinicians in interpreting the final result at the end of the study.

Side-effects

Consideration should also be given to the monitoring of side-effects. In a drug study we prefer a standard question, 'Have the tablets upset you in any way?', which can be linked directly to side-effects. The vaguer question, 'How do the tablets suit you?' could be interpreted by the patient as referring to side-effects or referring to efficacy. If a detailed side-effect profile of the drug is required, it may be safest to submit the patient to a standard questionnaire of possible side-effects prior to starting the study. This guards against the erroneous attribution to a particular drug of a side-effect that might have occurred by chance anyway. It is interesting that some patients describe all their side-effects much more readily than others prior to receiving drug therapy in a study, and that, in general, the frequency with which side-effects are reported falls throughout the course of a drug study, patients perhaps becoming less anxious about the particular drugs under test as the study advances.

Handling Withdrawals

Consideration will then be given to the way data is handled in relation to withdrawals. On the one hand, an adequate number of patients completing a study is needed to provide enough material for statistical analysis; on the other hand, the frequency with which patients refuse to take a particular treatment because of side-effects will provide much information in the overall clinical picture that needs to be built up by the clinician before he prescribes the treatment regularly. If a study is designed only to demonstrate efficacy, there is an argument in favour of replacing all patients who withdraw. This would apply both to patients who withdraw because of side-effects and to patients who withdraw for reasons unconnected with the study, for example concomitant illness, such as a stroke or heart attack, or leaving the area during the course of the study. However, we generally prefer not to replace drop-outs, on the basis that this provides a combined picture both of the treatment efficacy and of its toxicity profile. We would only replace drop-outs arising for reasons unconnected with the study. If patients drop out because of side-effects, they should still be included in the statistical analysis. Restricting analysis only to patients who complete the study may well give an overoptimistic picture for the treatment.

Ethical Aspects

The protocol should also clarify the ethical aspects of the study. The consent of a local ethics committee is likely to be sought for the majority of research projects; if this is the case, it should be clearly stated in the protocol. Other ethical considerations such as whether follow-up supplies of the treatment will be available and brief details of the risk to the patient and the way in which this risk will be minimised might usefully be included at this point. Information will also be required on the extent to which confidentiality of the patients' medical records will be observed.

Patients should also be told of their right to refuse entry to a trial and the fact that if they exercise their right it will not prejudice their treatment in the hands of the present physician or in the hands of other physicians. In general, we feel patients should be told if they are likely to receive a placebo during the course of the study; however, at the same time they should be told that it has been built into the study design that if they fail to improve during any of the treatment periods (including the placebo period) they may proceed immediately to the next active treatment period. The investigator—be it physician or clinical metrologist—is likely to have personal insurance cover for inappropriate medical practice either from a medical defence organisation or from the Royal College of Nursing respectively.

Many protocols provide a brief description of the statistical methods that will be applied to the study. This allows the ethics committee and the investigator to confirm that adequate conclusions will be reached from the data that is provided.

Conduct of a Clinical Trial or Research Project

The investigator who has given full attention to the protocol will be well equipped to perform the study, but inevitably teething problems will arise. It is surprising how research invariably takes far longer than one has ever anticipated. A safe rule is to work out an estimated time for a project and double it.

Once the trial has commenced, the investigator has a moral and ethical obligation to proceed with all speed until a conclusion is reached. It is possible that a conclusion may be reached at a stage earlier than the final end point of the trial, and the investigator may give consideration to sequential analysis, possibly analysing results on completion of every group of ten patients, certainly if one of the available treatments is likely to be life-saving. In general, however, this does not apply in rheumatic diseases.

Another major problem in the conduct of clinical trials is that of investigators overreaching themselves in protocol design. We have seen this happen on several occasions. As a general rule it is best to design a study that only answers one simple question. If an attempt is made to draw too many conclusions from a study, correspondingly large numbers of patients will be needed to give all the answers and interest will flag as the study reaches into its third or fourth year. Even if a study is restricted to a particular question, it is important to ascertain that this question can be resolved with the facilities available.

Funding of Research

It is amazing how frequently investigators with ingenuity and perseverance, can find locally administered funds available for research. One useful advantage of such funds is that they often have to be spent locally, possibly on specific research projects, and there may be very little competition for their acquisition. For example, elderly patients who wish to express their gratitude to the ward on which they receive their terminal care, may bequeath a donation that is specific to that particular ward or specific to the disease suffered by the patient. A research project may well be planned around such funds, which might otherwise remain unspent with subsequent depreciation in value over the years.

Regional health authorities or area health authorities often have locally administered research funds that have to be spent within their area. Indeed one of the provisions in the original charter of the NHS was that this service should be used to propagate research into the causes, prevention and treatment of disease. Such funds are likely to be administered on the advice of an expert and an experienced research subcommittee that is convened each year for the consideration of applications. Such funds will not be granted lightly (and quite correctly so), but in many health authorities they may be available to paramedical professionals as well as to physicians, and competition may be less intense at the local level than at a national level.

Charitable bodies such as the ARC also grant research awards from funds donated by the general public and are receptive to applications from health service professionals as well as to applications from physicians and basic scientists. Competition is high and the peer review of such applications searching and thorough. Applications for grants take several months to process, but this may be faster than the NHS-administered funds either at the local area health authority or central DHSS level, where applications are only considered once a year and for which applications have to be made several months in advance off the application date to allow clearance by the appropriate ethical committees and so on. Regrettably, a delay of almost 2 years in some cases between the conception of a research project and the granting of funds that would allow it to commence can be counterproductive in the world of scientific research.

Money may probably be obtained most quickly from private enterprise— the pharmaceutical industry. Such money may well be granted at a few weeks' notice, though it is more likely to be granted for physicians than paramedical workers applying in their own right. The problem is that this research has to be profit orientated, and a pharmaceutical company will only meet the cost of research if there is likely to be a commercial benefit at the end of the day.

Dissemination of Results

The presentation of results is every bit as important as the design of the study and the conduct of the research work. If the research is externally funded, the grant-giving body is likely to need an annual report on progress and photocopies of all publications emanating from the work they are funding. They may also require a more comprehensive final report; and in any case, if the research is being used simultaneously for the acquisition of a higher degree, there will be a lengthy period at the end of the research project that will be used for the compilation of the thesis or dissertation. The body that funds the research may also feel that they have a certain claim on the research workers' time for publicity purposes. If the research worker is therefore asked to lecture on their behalf on topics that do not involve the premature breaking of codes and publication of preliminary findings', he or she should probably oblige.

In addition to these reports to grant-giving bodies, the research worker will also wish to disseminate the results of the research to the appropriate professional colleagues. The standards of presentation required are likely to be higher than that required by grant-giving bodies, and there is likely to be a system of peer review or professional refereeing of such results. The research worker can choose between verbal presentation of results at a meeting or conference and written publication of results in a journal or book; however, these options are not necessarily mutually exclusive.

Communications to Learned Societies

At the simplest level the paramedical research worker might start by rehearsing the verbal presentation of results to a group of friends and departmental colleagues. Overhead projection facilities will be adequate for illustrating this, and the cost of preparing coloured acetate sheets is much less than the cost of preparing slides. The presentation should be kept within a strict time limit and an almost equal time allowed for questions and criticisms, as this would form an essential part of a subsequent presentation to a larger meeting. Many hospitals may have clinical meetings that could be used as a forum for the rehearsal of such results to a group of doctors as well as other health professionals. Here it may be preferable to use slides for illustration, and the help of a physician colleague may be required in gaining access to slide-preparing facilities; these should be available in all teaching hospitals and most provincial hospitals in the United Kingdom, although the wait for slides may be correspondingly longer in district general hospitals. Allowance for the cost of preparing slides should be made in applications for research grants.

Subsequently the research findings can be offered for presentation at meetings of national professional societies or at national or international conferences attended by doctors and paramedical workers.

Publication of Results

The presentation of results to a learned society may be a natural prelude to the formal writing-up of the research work. The readership of journals and the style in which articles are written for that readership vary enormously. Before writing the paper it is useful to become conversant with the style of the journal to which one proposes to submit the work. The style in which the paper is written should exactly follow the style of the particular journal, not only from the point of view of 'instructions to typist' that are normally published at 6-monthly or annual intervals by most journals, but also from the point of view of capturing the attention and interest of the particular readership. The paper is likely to be written in standard format, divided into sections as follows: (1) introduction, (2) patients and methods, (3) results and (4) discussion. There should be brief acknowledgements, a list of references, a title and, most importantly, a summary (possibly written last though often placed first). The summary may be the only part of the paper that is read by the majority of the readership and a great deal of care should go into its compilation. The author would be well advised to write the article in the style of the original protocol, drawing attention to most of the points included therein, and to write the results section as a series of paragraphs following the outline of the original protocol. The draft of the paper should be circulated to all the author's professional colleagues, particularly those who are involved in the work, and our own view is that the first author should have the final say if there are points of disagreement between the others as to the paper's content. The author should not be deterred if the first journal to which the paper is submitted turns it down, but the author may have to be prepared to re-write the paper slightly to match the style of each subsequent journal to which the paper is submitted.

Once the paper has been accepted there will be an inevitable delay before publication. When page proofs arrive they should be checked carefully, and editorial constraint may dictate that only minor and essential corrections may be made. Once the paper has appeared in print it is courteous to send copies to all co-authors and to the grant-awarding body, if applicable; in any case the paper is likely to be incorporated in the annual report to a grant-giving body.

References

Bird HA and Wright V (1982) Applied drug therapy in the rheumatic diseases. Wright, Bristol, pp 264–266

Bradford Hill A (1971) Principles of medical statistics. Lancet, London

Clark JM and Hockey L (1979) Research for nursing. HM & M, Aylesbury

May D (1976) Significance in medical statistics. Lancet I: 1025

Swinscow TDV (1976) Statistics at square one. British Medical Association, London

Appendix A

Normal Laboratory Values and Indicators of Inflammation

Normal Haematological Values

Haemoglobin
Men	13.5–18.0 g/dl
Women	11.5–16.5 g/dl
Children 1 year	11.0–13.0 g/dl
Children 10–12 years	11.5–14.8 g/dl

Packed cell volume
Men	40%–54%
Women	35%–47%

Red Cells
Men	$4.5–6.5 \times 10^{12}$/litre
Women	$3.9–5.6 \times 10^{12}$/litre.

Mean corpuscular volume (MCV)
Adults 76–96 fl

Mean corpuscular haemoglobin (MCH)
Adults 27–32 pg

Mean corpuscular haemoglobin concentration MCHC
Adults 30–35 g/dl

Reticulocytes
Adults 0.2%–2.0%

Total leucocytes
Adults	$4.0–10.0 \times 10^{9}$/litre
Infants (1 year)	$6.0–18.0 \times 10^{9}$/litre
Childhood (4–7 years)	$6.0–15.0 \times 10^{9}$/litre
Childhood (8–12 years)	$4.5–13.5 \times 13.5 \times 10^{9}$/litre

Differential leucocyte count

Adults	Neutrophils	40%–75%	or 2.5–7.5 $\times$ 10^9/litre
	Lymphocytes	20%–50%	or 1.5–3.0 $\times$ 10^9/litre
	Monocytes	2%–10%	or 0.2–0.8 $\times$ 10^9/litre
	Eosinophils	1%–6%	or 0.04–0.4 $\times$ 10^9/litre
	Basophils	1%	or 0.01–0.1 $\times$ 10^9/litre

Platelets
Adults 160–600 $\times$ 10^9/litre

Normal Biochemical Values

Sodium	135–145 mmol/litre
Potassium	3.6–5.0 mmol/litre
Chloride	98–107 mmol/litre
Bicarbonate	21–28 mmol/litre

Anion-gap   13–18 mmol/litre
(sodium + potassium)—(chloride + bicarbonate)

Urea   2.5–7.1 mmol/litre
Creatinine 50–140 mmol/litre

Total bilirubin	3–15 μmol/litre
Total protein	67–82 g/litre
Albumin	37–49 g/litre
Globulins	24–37 g/litre
Glutamyl oxalate transaminase (GOT)	11–35 IU/litre
Alkaline phosphatase	4–13 King Armstrong units

Calcium   2.25–2.60 mmol/l
Standard calcium 2.13–2.43 mmol/l
standard calcium = measured calcium − [(albumin − 40) $\times$ 0.0225]
Phosphorous 0.8–1.3 mmol/l

Uric acid Males   0.20–0.45 mmol/l
          Females 0.14–0.38 mmol/l

Indicators of Inflammation (Normal Range)

ESR
Males   4–20 mm/h
Females 10–25 mm/h

CRP 0.0 mg/100 ml
Plasma viscosity 1.50–1.72 centipoise

Haptoglobin 0.3–2.0 g/litre
Serum sulphydryl 450–600 μmol/litre
Serum histidine 1.5–1.8 mg/100 ml
Fibrinogen 2.0–4.0 g/litre
Gamma glutamyl transpeptidase
  Males   6–28 units/1
  Females 4–18 units/1
IgG   128–199 IU/ml
IgA   97–181 IU/ml
IgM   60–129 IU/ml
C$_3$ 80–140 mg%

Typical Abnormal Values for Indicators of Inflammation in Rheumatoid Arthritis (with acknowledgements to Dr. J.S. Dixon)

Test	Mean value in patients with active disease
ESR	53 mm/h
Haemoglobin	11.7 g/dl
Platelets	418×10^9/litre
CRP	5.74 mg/100 ml
IgM	318 IU/ml
Serum sulphydryl	313 μmol/litre
Serum histidine	1.23 mg/100 ml
Fibrinogen	3.4 g/litre

Appendix B

Appointment of Clinical Metrologist – Clinical Pharmacology Unit (Rheumatism Research), University of Leeds

The Clinical Pharmacology Unit is part of the Rheumatism Research Unit of the Department of Medicine, University of Leeds. Its function is the evaluation of new drugs in the treatment of the rheumatic diseases and also to conduct basic research into the possible cause of these complaints. The Unit is situated in the grounds of the Royal Bath Hospital, Cornwall Road, Harrogate, which, with 125 beds, is the largest hospital devoted entirely to the treatment of the rheumatic diseases in the country. Studies are performed here on inpatients and also on outpatients. The outpatient clinics are at the Leeds General Infirmary, Great George Street, Leeds.

The Unit is under the direction of the Professor of Rheumatology. It is headed by a consultant physician, who supervises the activities of the two metrologists employed, one of whom we have to replace. There is a large laboratory supervised by a biochemist, who heads a team of three technical officers. The staff is completed by a unit secretary, a part-time typist, a part-time pharmacist and a part-time phlebotomist.

The successful appointee, who will receive full training, will be personally responsible for conducting an outpatient clinic at Leeds General Infirmary on Monday mornings and Friday afternoons. This is run on an appointment basis under the supervision of the physicians with the other metrologist, in post. All patients referred to this clinic will be undergoing clinical trials and the appointee will be responsible for checking the entry criteria of patients against a protocol, monitoring their subsequent progress by using a series of clinical and biochemical tests, prescribing further medication and supervising the collection of specimens, including blood samples. The remaining time is spent at the Clinical Pharmacology Unit, Harrogate, where similar studies are done on inpatients and where most of the paperwork is completed. Additional duties at Harrogate, after appropriate training, will include the collection of blood samples and the use of intravenous cannulae. Experience in other techniques, e.g. radioisotope studies, infrared thermography, arthrography etc. may be available. The appointee will be encouraged to join the Association for Clinical Research in the Pharmaceutical Industry, the national representative body for the expanding profession of metrology. In addition, the appointee will be encouraged to attend relevant conferences at home and abroad at which scientific communications may be given and for which financial support will be available.

The successful candidate is likely to be a state registered nurse with at least 2 years, wide post-registration experience. They are likely to value patient contact and, when trained, will enjoy taking a high degree of responsibility for the supervision of patients' treatment. They will be meticulous in their keeping of patient records and will be equipped to act as ambassadors for the Unit in their contacts with physicians and scientists employed by the pharmaceutical industry. Independent transport would be an advantage, particularly if the appointee lived in Leeds.

The post to be filled is likely to be for a total of 24 hours per week (6 half-day sessions). Two of these sessions are in Leeds (Monday morning and Friday afternoon), the remaining four in Harrogate (probably Tuesdays and Wednesdays). This commitment could be modified slightly according to the wishes of the appointee, though attendance at the Monday morning and Friday afternoon clinics in Leeds is essential. The salary, dependent upon the experience of the applicant, is likely to be on the Whitley scales. A 24-hour week would give 64% of the annual salary. Annual paid holiday leave appropriate to this salary scale will be allowed. The job, which is funded mainly from non-University sources, will be for a fixed term of 3 years but is likely to be renewable.

The post falls vacant on 1 September 1981, and it is hoped that the appointee would be able to start on or as soon as possible after this date. Interested candidates should apply in writing to Dr. H.A. Bird, Clinical Pharmacology Unit, Royal Bath Hospital, Cornwall Road, Harrogate HG1 2PS, before 10 July 1981. Applications should give full details of training, qualifications and experience in whatever field, as well as naming two referees. Prospective candidates are invited to visit the Harrogate Unit and/or Leeds General Infirmary to meet existing members of staff, in particular our two current metrologists. Appointments for this can be made by telephoning Harrogate 57526. It is hoped to interview short-listed candidates in Leeds on Wednesday 22 July.

Appendix C
Advisory Services and Sources of Information

DHSS Benefits

Attendance Allowance—leaflet NI. 205. Attendance allowance is payable to severely disabled persons over 2 years of age needing much care and attention for at least 6 months.

Invalid Care Allowance—leaflet NI. 212. This benefit is payable to persons under retirement age who are prevented from working because they are caring full-time for a severely disabled person (not necessarily a relative). The disabled person being cared for must be receiving attendance allowance or constant attendance allowance. (Invalid care allowance is not payable to a woman living with a man as his wife, whether she is married to him or not.)

Invalidity Benefit—leaflet NI. 16A. This benefit is dependent on the patient's national insurance contributions record and is composed of (1) invalidity pension and (2) invalidity allowance. Invalidity pension replaces sickness benefit after a period of 28 weeks. If the patient has dependants, greater benefits may be payable and in these circumstances may exceed the allowances of sickness benefit.

Invalidity allowance is an additional benefit payable to patients who become chronically sick and unable to work before the age of retirement.

Mobility Allowance—leaflet NI. 211. This benefit is payable to people who are unable or are virtually unable to walk as a result of their disability. They do not have to be drivers.

Non-Contributory Invalidity Pension—leaflet NI. 210. This benefit is payable to people of working age who do not qualify for sickness or invalidity benefit because of insufficient national insurance contributions. They must have been incapable of work for at least 28 consecutive weeks.

This benefit is only payable to married women (leaflet NI. 214) who are also unable to carry out their normal household duties.

Sickness Benefit—leaflet NI. 16.   This is a short-term benefit paid for a maximum of 28 weeks after which the patient becomes eligible for invalidity benefit.

The DHSS publishes a guide to family benefits and pensions—leaflet FB. 1. Further advice can be obtained from a local social security officer or social worker.

Useful Addresses

Arthritis and Rheumatism Council for Research, 41 Eagle Street, London WC1R 4 AR.
The Council supports many research teams at universities and hospitals throughout the United Kingdom. It also publishes many useful leaflets for sufferers and their families.

British Council for the Rehabilitation of the Disabled, Tavistock House (South), Tavistock Square, London WC1H 9LB.
The Council provides a free information and advisory service and further education courses for hospitalised and housebound persons. It also publishes a quarterly journal.

British Rheumatism and Arthritis Association, 6–7 Grosvenor Crescent, London SW1X 7ER.
The Association caters for the social and welfare needs of arthritis sufferers.

British School of Motoring Disability Training Centre, 269 Kensington High Street, London W8.

British Sports Association for the Disabled, Stoke Mandeville Stadium, Harvey Road, Aylesbury, Bucks.

Disabled Drivers' Association, Ashwellthorpe Hall, Ashwellthorpe, Norwich NR16 1EX.

Disabled Living Foundation, 346 Kensington High Street, London W14 8NS.
The Disabled Living Foundation maintains a permanent exhibition of aids of all kinds and provides a comprehensive information service covering all aspects of coping with disability.

Family Planning Association, 27–35 Mortimer Street, London W1N 8BQ.

National Marriage Guidance Council, Herbert Gray College, Little Church Street, Rugby CV21 3AP.

Royal Association for Disability and Rehabilitation, 23–25 Mortimer Street, London W1N 8AB.

SPOD Committee on Sexual and Personal Relationships of the Disabled, Brook House, 2–16 Torrington Place, London WC1E 7HN.

Books and Publications

Darnbrough A and Kinrade D (1979) The directory for the disabled. Woodhead-Faulkner, Cambridge
Greengross W (1983) Entitled to love: sexual and emotional needs of the handicapped. National Marriage Guidance Council, Rugby
Joseph M (1976) One step at a time. Heinemann, London
Holidays for the physically handicapped. (1977) Available from the Central Council for the Disabled, 34 Eccleston Square, London SW1V 1PE
The easy path to gardening. (1972) The Readers Digest Association, London

Subject Index